Dedication

*To my mother, now 87 and post
femoral fracture, who with her canes
and walker continues regular, leisure
time physical activity including house
and yard work. I wish her much content as she anticipates her ninth
decade.*

EXERCISE IN THE PRACTICE OF MEDICINE

Second Revised Edition

edited by
Gerald F. Fletcher, M.D.

Professor and Chairman
Department of Rehabilitation Medicine
Professor of Medicine (Cardiology)
Emory University School of Medicine
Atlanta, Georgia

Futura Publishing Company, Inc.
Mount Kisco, New York
1988

Library of Congress Cataloging-in-Publication Data

Exercise in the practice of medicine.

Revised ed. of: Exercise in the practice of medicine/
Gerald F. Fletcher. 1982.
Includes bibliographies and index.
1. Exercise therapy. I. Fletcher, Gerald F.,
1935– . [DNLM: 1. Exercise Therapy. 2. Exertion.
WE 103 E961]
RM725.E93 1987   615.8′2   87-19669
IBSN 0-87993-310-0

Copyright 1988
Futura Publishing Company, Inc.

Published by:
Futura Publishing Company, Inc.
295 Main Street
Mount Kisco, New York 10549

L.C. #: 87993-3100
ISBN #: 0-87993-310-0

Printed in the United States of America.

Contributors

J. Brand Brickman, M.D.
Department of Psychiatry
University of California at San Diego
School of Medicine
LaJolla, California

Edwin Dale, Ph.D.
Associate Professor of Gynecology and Obstetrics
Emory University School of Medicine
Atlanta, Georgia

Barbara Johnston Fletcher, R.N., M.N.
Nurse Coordinator
Emory Health Enhancement Program
Clinical Associate
Nell Hodgson Woodruff School of Nursing
Emory University
Atlanta, Georgia

Gerald F. Fletcher, M.D.
Professor and Chairman
Department of Rehabilitation Medicine
Professor of Medicine (Cardiology)
Emory University School of Medicine
Atlanta, Georgia

Robert T. Hyde, M.A.
Epidemiologist
Department of Family, Community and Preventive Medicine
Stanford University
Palo Alto, California

J. Ronald Mikolich, M.D.
Assistant Professor of Internal Medicine (Cardiology)
Northeastern Ohio Universities College of Medicine
Youngstown, Ohio

Ralph S. Paffenbarger, Jr., M.D.
Professor of Epidemiology
Department of Family, Community and Preventive Medicine
School of Medicine
Stanford University
Palo Alto, California

Thomas A. Rodgers, M.D.
Department of Psychiatry
University of California at San Diego
School of Medicine
La Jolla, California

Robert C. Schlant, M.D.
Professor of Medicine (Cardiology)
Emory University School of Medicine
Atlanta, Georgia

L. Thomas Sheffield, M.D.
Professor of Medicine (Cardiovascular)
Director, Electrocardiogram Laboratory
Allison Laboratory of Exercise Electrophysiology
University of Alabama School of Medicine
Birmingham, Alabama

Harvey B. Simon, M.D.
Assistant Professor of Medicine
Harvard University School of Medicine
Massachusetts General Hospital
Boston, Massachusetts

Jonne B. Walter, M.D.
Medical Director
Pulmonary Function Laboratories
Georgia Baptist Medical Center
Associate Clinical Professor of Medicine
Emory University School of Medicine
Atlanta, Georgia

Preface

Gerald Fletcher's book on exercise is a classic. He combines his own extensive knowledge of the subject with a number of authoritative experts in the field, including such notables as Robert Schlant, Ralph Paffenbarger, Thomas Sheffield, and a number of others. The guest author's chapters are written so as not to overlap with the material in the other parts of the book which is a departure from the usual multi-authored work.

The book provides not only in-depth discussions of the usual subjects, such as exercise physiology, exercise testing, and exercise prescriptions, but excellent reviews of subjects not ordinarily covered, such as the effects of exercise on immunology, hemotology, psychiatry, and pregnancy.

Dr. Fletcher provides a treasure trove of details from the important papers published on exercise over the last 20 years. The work is heavily referenced and many of the chapters have 100 or more references, many of which are very current. The figures are appropriate and well done and clearly explained by the legends. He not only provides data in support of his primary thesis, that exercise is, on the whole, beneficial for both normal subjects and those with illness, but amply documents research work that both supports and contradicts this thesis in special cases. Indeed, there is a whole chapter dealing with the dangers of unwise exercise.

I found the chapters dealing with immunology, obstetrics, endocrinology, psychiatry, and hypertension especially interesting and well written. These are areas where a great deal of new knowledge is now becoming available, and the thorough presentation of the latest research in exercise in these areas is especially well done.

This book is a must for the serious student of exercise physiology and cardiac rehabilitation whether they be physicians, physiologists, or rehabilitation personnel. Over the years Dr. Fletcher has established himself as one of the recognized experts in the field of exercise, and his second edition is the best and most comprehensive book available in a crowded field of competitors.

Myrvin H. Ellestad, M.D.
Medical Director, Memorial Heart Institute
Memorial Medical Center of Long Beach
and
Clinical Professor of Medicine
University of California, Irvine

Introduction

As the late 1980s evolve, physical activity and exercise are assuming an increasingly important role in the day-to-day lifestyle of the American public. Exercise enthusiasm prevails in both the allegedly healthy and unhealthy populations. Numerous programs for organized and medically supervised physical activity in cardiac patients (post infarction, post myocardial revascularization, and post angioplasty) exist throughout the country. These programs offer a multifactoral approach including efforts to modify dietary habits and body weight, control blood pressure, eliminate smoking, and modify certain behavioral characteristics.

The history of physical activity relating to health and medicine is to some degree becoming cyclic or repetitive. Before the era of machines and conveniences of life, our population, by necessity, was more involved in physical activity and physical labor. Then with the industrial revolution and the evolution of our "mechanized society," people became less physically active and the sedentary way of life became more "the rule than the exception." Of late (within the last 15 years) as the public has become more "health conscious," there has been a resurgence of exercise and physical activity.

An historically important phase of exercise evolved in 1818 when William Cubitt, a British civil engineer, designed an elongated "stepping wheel" on which dozens of prisoners could work side by side. In accord with this, "treading the wheel" for punishment became prevalent throughout English prisons.[1] In 1846, however, because reformers considered treading the wheel a cruel, inhumane, and unhealthy practice, Edward Smith began to investigate physical performance by utilizing new physiologic techniques during treadmill exercise.[2] These studies were the first systematic inquiry into the respiratory and metabolic responses of the human to muscular exercise, and provided the groundwork for extensive studies that have followed in the evaluation of exercise performance in patients with coronary heart disease. Smith's early studies included measurements of inspired air, respiratory rate, stroke volume, pulse rate, and oxygen production. By 1857, measurements were made for other types of exercise including swimming, rowing, and horseback riding.[3]

With the acquisition of exercise habits early in history and the insight into methods of evaluation of exercise performance, observations[4] in some instances began to reveal a higher mortality rate in people with sedentary occupations compared to those who were physically active. These observations were to be the forerunners of more studies relating physical inactivity to morbidity from coronary heart disease.

Later in the 1900s, Dr. Paul Dudley White became part of history but his influence continues in both professional and lay circles. He was a strong advocate of exercise and believed that exercise was of value, both physiologically and psychologically. He advocated that people who walk a great deal have less early arteriosclerosis. He felt that people today have a life that is much too easy—using elevators instead of stairs and having lunch brought in rather than going out. He believed that "work alone never killed a man unless he was already sick."

Dr. White advised walking as probably the best exercise and was averse to activities with weight-lifting. His own personal exercise included climbing stairs, walking to lunch, gardening, cutting trees, splitting logs, shoveling snow, and "working in the soil." He believed that "one feels so much better with exercise" and his formula for long life was to "work hard mentally, physically, and spiritually." He referred to our easy way of living as a "real pity" and felt that our ancestors were in better physical health because of their active lives spent in clearing the forests and plowing the land. He believed that exercise was the "best tranquilizer there is." In farewell comments to friends and acquaintances, he was never known to say "take it easy" but rather "take it hard."[5]

With continued interest in exercise, physicans are repeatedly confronted with the problem of the proper prescription for the individual patient. In all subsets of medical practice, physicans have increasing need to be familiar with the application of exercise testing and the exercise prescription within the safe limits for the individual's need and the residual disease involved.

The second edition of this book is highlighted by four chapters from new contributors and significant revisions and update of other chapters. Dr. Edwin Dale of Emory University has provided a new and in-depth coverage of Exercise in Obstetrics and Gynecology. Dr. Harvey Simon of Harvard addresses many current perspectives in his chapter on Exercise, Immunology, and Infectious Diseases. Dr. Ralph Paffenbarger and Robert Hyde of Stanford summarize many of their important contributions in a new chapter on Exercise in Occupational Medicine. Drs. Brand Brickman and Tom Rodgers (University of California at San Diego) present a very intuitive, clinical insight into Exercise and Psychiatry.

With these new chapters and extensive revisions in the topics of exercise in primary and secondary prevention of coronary disease, exercise testing (Sheffield), physiology (Schlant), prescription (Mikolich), endocrinology, hematology, high blood pressure, pulmonology, environmental factors, and dangers, we feel exercise in medical practice has been well addressed and updated.

As this book is finalized, new information continues to evolve. The major specialties of medicine and the subspecialties of internal medicine recognize the role of exercise with regard to both preventive and therapeutic measures. It is our hope that this book will be informative and of benefit to all health professionals who are involved in health enhancement for the public and who care for patients with both congenital and acquired disease.

GERALD F. FLETCHER, M.D.
Emory University
Atlanta, Georgia

REFERENCES

1. Fletcher GF, Cantwell JD: Historical aspects of exercise and coronary heart disease. In: *Exercise and Coronary Heart Disease*. 2nd ed. Springfield, Illinois, Charles C. Thomas, 1979; 7.
2. Chapman CB, Smith E (1818–1864): Physiologist, human ecologist reformer. *J Hist Med* 1967; 22:1–26.
3. Smith E: Inquiries into the quantity of air inspired throughout the day and night and under the influence of exercise, food, medicine and temperature. *Proc Roy Soc Med* 1857; 8:451–456.
4. Smith E: Report on the sanitary circumstances of tailors in London. In: 6th Edition Rep Med Officer Primary Council with Appendix, 1862. London, H.M. Stationary Office, 1864; 416–430.
5. White PD: Personal communication, 1969.

Contents

Physiology of Exercise

Robert C. Schlant, M.D.

*Exercise ferments the humors, casts them into their proper chan-
nels, throws off redundancies, and helps nature in those secret
distributions, without which the body cannot subsist in its vigor,
nor the soul act with cheerfulness.*

Joseph Addison 1711

INTRODUCTION

Exercise is one of the most common activities, and some form
of exercise is performed by all normal individuals. On the other
hand, the neural, metabolic, and physiological adjustments and
control systems that must be integrated during ordinary exercise
are extraordinarily complex. The purpose of this chapter is to
review briefly the physiology of exercise, more detailed reviews of
which are available.[1-7]

TYPES OF EXERCISE

Exercise is usually divided into the following two types: (1)
Rhythmic or dynamic (isotonic) exercise is the usual, repetitive,

From: Fletcher GF: *Exercise in the Practice of Medicine*, 2nd Revised Edition. Mount
Kisco, NY, Futura Publishing Co., Inc., ©1988.

rhythmic contraction of muscle groups associated with nearly continuous motion of part of the body. Examples include walking, running, and swimming. (2) Static or isometric exercise consists of sustained muscle contractions that produce no or relatively little motion of the involved body part. Examples include squeezing a hand dynamometer, carrying a heavy suitcase, and water skiing. Obviously, many forms of exercise involve both dynamic and static exercise. The following discussion will refer to dynamic exercise except when specifically stated otherwise.

PHASES OF EXERCISE

The cardiovascular responses to continued dynamic exercise can be divided into the following four phases:[5] (1) the anticipatory or expectant phase, (2) the on-transient or initiation phase, (3) the adjustment or fine-tuning phase, and (4) the "drift" period.

Anticipatory Phase

This phase occurs immediately prior to the onset of exercise. The effects are produced by the autonomic nervous system and are under conscious and subconscious cerebral influences probably initiated from the cerebral cortex and diencephalon. It is associ-

---

Figure 1: Cardiac output ($\dot{Q}$) in L/min and estimates of its regional distribution in relation to the oxygen uptake ($\dot{V}O_2$) at rest and during submaximal and maximal leg exercise (bicycling) and arm exercise (arm cranking). At any $\dot{V}O_2$, values apply to the situation after 5–7 minutes of exercise when $\dot{V}O_2$ and Q have reached a steady state. In the diagrams, corresponding values are shown for heart rate (HR) in beats/min, for stroke volume (SV) in ml, and for aortic pressures (BP): systolic, mean, and diastolic in mmHg. Based on data from Clausen et al.,[25] Rowell,[74] Kitamura et al.,[331] and Wade and Bishop.[15] It should be noted that during maximal exercise as well as at any relative $\dot{V}O_2$, the perfusion of nonworking tissues and the heart can be assumed to be the same during arm exercise as during leg exercise and at any absolute $\dot{V}O_2$, Q is the same for the two types of exercise. MBF = muscle blood flow; cor = coronary blood flow; skin = skin blood flow; viscera = visceral blood flow; CBF = cerebral blood flow; HR = heart rate; SV = stroke volume; and BP = blood pressure. (From Clausen JP: Circulatory adjustments to dynamic exercise and effect of physical training in normal subjects and in patients with coronary artery disease. *Prog Cardiovasc Dis* 1976; 18:459, by permission)

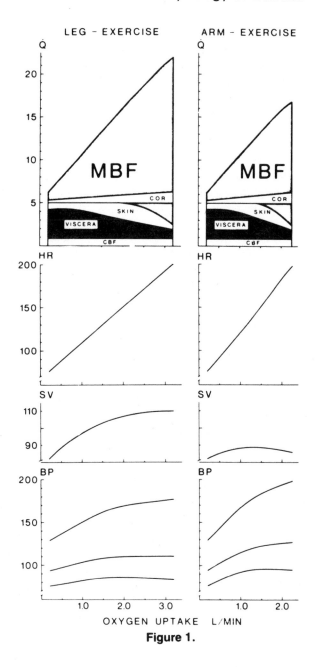

Figure 1.

ated with increases in heart rate (HR), blood pressure, and cardiac output (Q) in association with a decrease in venous compliance and an increase in venous return to the heart. Vasodilatation of the arterioles in the skeletal muscles may be produced by sympathetic cholinergic impulses.[6-8]

Initiation Phase

An intense increase in autonomic nervous system activity occurs almost immediately with the onset of exercise and produces further increases in heart rate, blood pressure, and cardiac output (Fig. 1).[9]

The heart rate increases rapidly, within seconds. The initial increase in heart rate is due to vagal withdrawal, whereas after 8-10 seconds, there is a large sympathetic accelerator component.[10-12] At times, the heart rate overshoots and then comes back down to a steady rate.[13] The increase in heart rate is a function of the relative intensity of the work.[14] The heart rate may increase 2½ to 4 times normal during very severe exercise;[15-18] in some highly trained individuals, the heart rate may increase from 50 to 220.[9,16,19,20] The increase in heart rate may also be partly due to the large increase in venous return activating the Bainbridge reflex and producing cardiac acceleration.[9,10,21] In addition, it appears likely that afferent impulses originating from the exercising muscles also contribute to the increased sympathetic stimulation of the heart and to the tachycardia during steady-state exercise.[22] In general, the heart rate is faster during arm cranking than during bicycling,[23-25] faster during bicycling than running,[26,27] and faster during running than walking with ski sticks ("ski-walking").[27]

The usual increase in cuff arterial blood pressure during exercise is due both to the increased cardiac output and to the sympathetic vasoconstriction of nonexercising muscles, viscera, and skin.[12,18,28,29] It appears that the arterial baroreceptor reflex is markedly inhibited during severe exercise.[30] It is important to note that studies have demonstrated that systolic blood pressure in the aorta during exercise increases much less than radial systolic blood pressure but that the increases in mean pressures were nearly identical.[31-34] Of interest, the same amount of upper arm exercise produces a greater increase in blood pressure than the same amount of work by the legs, apparently due to more intense vasoconstriction in nonexercising tissues during arm exercise (Fig. 1).[24,25]

The increase in cardiac output, which may reach a plateau in less than a minute,[35] goes mainly to the exercising muscles and to the myocardium (Fig. 1).[36,37] In general, the increase in cardiac output is nearly proportional to the increase in total oxygen consumption, which can increase from 250 ml/min (or 3.5 to 4.5 ml O_2/Kg/min) to 6.0 liters per minute (or 75 to 80 ml O_2/Kg/min) in physically trained men (Fig. 2).[4,38,39] The increase in cardiac output is the combined result of an increased venous return produced by mechanical compression ("milking") of the veins in the exercising muscles, compression of the intra-abdominal veins by the abdominal wall and the action of the thoracic "respiratory pump;"[40−43] an increase in heart rate; an increase in myocardial contractility (and the rate of relaxation) from the positive inotropic sympathetic impulses to the heart and from the increase in heart rate (Treppe effect); and, especially, an acute decrease in afterload from the marked decrease in the peripheral resistance of the exercising muscles.[1,4,18,35,43−49] In some highly trained athletes, the cardiac output may increase 5 to 6 times the normal value, or from 5.0 liters per minute to 35−42 liters per minute. In general, the cardiac output at a given oxygen uptake during submaximal exercise in the upright position is 1−2 liters less than during exercise in the supine position.[15,50,51]

Changes in stroke volume during exercise depend upon whether the exercise is performed in the supine position or in the upright position.[26,52−56] In the supine position, the stroke volume and end-diastolic volume are at a near-maximum level at rest and thus do not increase or only increase relatively little, perhaps 10 to 20 percent, during supine exercise.[57] When one stands upright, however, stroke volume may decrease by 40% in association with a shift of 300−800 ml blood to the legs (Fig. 3).[58−60] During mild upright exercise, the increase in heart rate may be sufficient to produce all of the required increase in cardiac output.[61,62] Soon after the onset of vigorous upright exercise, however, stroke volume begins to increase, and during severe exercise, it may increase up to twice the resting value (Fig. 3).[12,17,25,26,29,54,56,60,63−65] Cardiovascular endurance training increases the increase in stroke volume during exercise;[16] this increase in stroke volume during exercise is one of the better indicators of physical

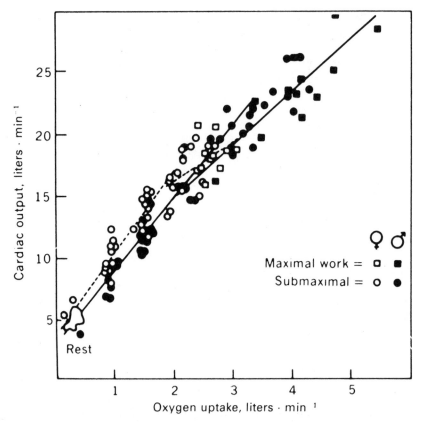

Figure 2: Individual values on cardiac output in relation to oxygen uptake at rest, during submaximal, and during maximal exercise on 23 subjects sitting on a bicycle ergometer. Regression lines (broken lines for women) were calculated for experiments where the oxygen uptake was (1) below 70 percent and (2) above 70 percent of the individual's maximum. (From Astrand P-O, Rodahl K: *Textbook of Work Physiology*, 2nd Edition. New York, McGraw-Hill Book Company, Inc, 1977. Used with the permission of McGraw-Hill Book Company.)

training. As an example, a highly trained athlete may increase his stroke volume from 85 ml to 170 ml. In general, stroke volume is greater during leg exercise than during arm exercise at all absolute and relative work levels.[12,24,25]

During moderately severe upright exercise, the left ventricular end-diastolic volume normally does not increase,[9,60,66-68] and any increase in stroke volume is produced by a decrease in

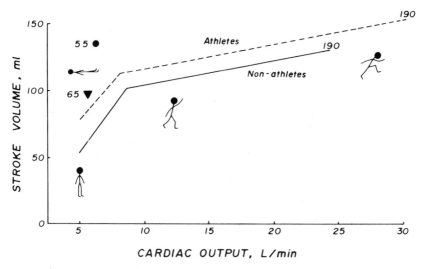

Figure 3: Cardiac output and stroke volume in athletes (●) and nonathletes (Δ), during resting supine, quiet standing, and graded upright exercise. Figures represent the heart rate (beats/minute). The pattern in both groups is the same, except the athletes have a larger stroke volume and a slower heart rate when resting. On standing, the stroke volume decreases because of pooling of blood in the lower limbs. Even with mild exercise the muscle pump restores the pooled blood to the heart and lungs, and the stroke volume approaches the supine value. As exercise increases in severity, the stroke volume continues to increase slightly, so that as maximal exercise is approached it exceeds by about 10 percent the values obtained in the supine position at rest. Oxygen consumption in both groups at rest is about 300 ml/min, and at maximal effort, it is about 3,000 ml/min in the nonathletes and about 5,000 ml/min in the athletes. (From Shepherd JT, Vanhoutte PM: *The Human Cardiovascular System*, 1979, reprinted by permission of Raven Press, New York.)

end-systolic volume secondary to the combined effects of the increased contractility from beta-adrenergic stimulation and the decrease in afterload, rather than by an increase in end-diastolic volume or preload. Thus, in human beings at least, the Frank-Starling mechanism appears to play only a slight role in the normal ventricular response to exercise.[9] With extreme exercise, however, healthy dogs have been shown to have both a decrease in ventricular end-systolic volume and an increase in end-diastolic volume.[17,19] With most forms of exercise, the right atrial pressure decreases slightly, although it may increase slightly with very severe exercise.[18]

The vascular resistance of working muscles decreases within 0.5 seconds after the onset of exercise, almost instantaneously with muscle contraction.[1,18,35,44-47,49,69] When many muscles are used, therefore, the total systemic (peripheral) resistance and cardiac afterload decrease markedly. The large decrease in vascular resistance of exercising muscles appears to be largely of local metabolic origin, perhaps mediated by ATP or adenosine.[45,47,48,70] Blood flow to the exercising muscles is also significantly aided by the rhythmic pumping effect of the muscles upon the arteries and veins, which increase local perfusion pressures and increase muscle oxygenation.[42,49] The intense sympathetic adrenergic outflow to the splanchnic area and to nonexercising muscles produces both arterial vasoconstriction, which decreases blood flow to the nonexercising muscles, skin, kidney, spleen, liver, and intestines, and venoconstriction, which increases venous return from the splanchnic capacitance vessels.[12,15,18,25,49,71-74] Reduction in splanchine-hepatic-renal blood flow produced by sympathetic vasoconstriction is a function of the relative work load and is similar to the increase in heart rate.[25,74] In contrast to most studies in human beings, however, studies in exercising dogs have indicated that visceral flow is relatively well maintained so long as all other compensatory mechanisms remain intact, indicating that the normal dog uses his sympathetic system less than man under stress.[9,36,37,74-81] Cerebral blood flow (CBF) in man probably stays the same or increases slightly during exercise,[82] while coronary blood flow normally increases markedly during sustained exercise.[12,83-87]

Exercising muscles may extract 20 times more oxygen than usual, producing a widened arteriovenous oxygen difference together with increased K^+ in the venous blood and increased tissue osmolality.[88-91] The arteriovenous oxygen difference of the body can increase approximately 2.5 to 3.0 times its resting value, or from 5 to 15 ml oxygen per 100 ml blood. In addition, during heavy exercise, exercising skeletal muscles utilize some "anaerobic" metabolism and release lactate. In general, it would appear that the limiting factor in whole body exercise is the capacity of the heart, not the skeletal muscles, to deliver oxygen.[92]

Working muscles may develop a temperature above 40°C and a pH lower than 7.0 from the formation of CO_2 and lactic acid.[90,91,93] The increase in body temperature and lower pH may produce a "Bohr effect" on the oxygen-hemoglobin dissociation curve, helping to deliver more oxygen to the working muscles. On the other hand, arterial saturation may decrease slightly during strenuous exertion due to the same Bohr effect in the pulmonary capillaries.[4]

At low levels of exercise and low levels of force development, skeletal muscles appear to use predominately "red" slow twitch (ST) or Type 1 muscle fibers, which are rich in mitochondria and intramitochondrial enzymes necessary for the citric acid cycle, the fatty acid cycle, and the electron transport chain.[94] Such Type 1 fibers can sustain rhythmic contraction for long periods of time. When greater force is necessary, however, the muscle units appear to recruit "white" fast twitch (FTb) or Type IIb muscle fibers, which have fewer mitochondria but have a high content of enzymes for anaerobic glycosis. Some of the progressive release of lactate during heavy work loads is probably explained by the recruitment of Type IIb muscle fibers rather than by hypoxia.[12,95]

Untrained individuals may develop pain or a "stitch" in the side during this or a later phase, presumably from hypoxia of the diaphragm resulting from increased respiratory work prior to the redistribution of blood flow. Alternative explanations include tension of the hepatic capsule and splenic contraction.

Adjustment Phase

During this phase, there is a complex integration of central and peripheral mechanisms to maintain cardiac output, venous return, and adequate distribution of the cardiac output to the working muscles. The shift in blood flow away from the liver, kidneys, and intestines is associated with a shift of blood volume and flow away from these areas and to the active muscles.

The plasma volume decreases for the first 10 to 15 minutes of moderately strenuous exercise, due to a functional increase in systemic capillary pressure in the working muscles.[18,96−101] Eventually, the interstitial fluid pressure in the working muscles increases and opposes the increased capillary pressure. On the other hand, there is a decrease in mean capillary pressure in the nonworking muscles and tissues, as a result of which some interstitial fluid re-enters the circulation and partially compensates for the fluid loss into the active muscles.[18,98] During prolonged exercise, there is hemoconcentration of blood due to these changes as well as the loss of fluid from the skin and lungs.[96−98,100,101]

Cardiovascular Drift Phase

A true steady state cannot exist for long if the level of exercise is above the "endurance level" or a level that can be tolerated continuously for 8 hours. In most subjects exercising above this level, the heart rate gradually increases up to a maximum during the "cardiovascular drift" phase due to a gradual increase in the intensity of sympathetic activation (Fig. 4).[74,101–105] Associated changes which occur during this phase include a gradual decrease in venous pressure, stroke volume, and arterial pressure while heart rate increases and cardiac output is maintained relatively constant.[106] An important factor during this phase is the competition between the need for blood flow to working muscles and the need for blood flow to the skin to eliminate the increased heat load produced by the muscular work. In most individuals if the cardiac output and the work level are not near maximal, heat can be eliminated in this phase by an increased sympathetic vasoconstriction of the viscera in association with reflex sympathetic vasodilatation of skin vessels.[74,107,108] This vasodilatation is the direct opposite of the sympathetic vasoconstriction of skin vessels that occurs during the initiation of exercise. This increase in skin blood flow to eliminate heat is associated with a constant or gradually decreasing blood volume, decrease in central venous pressure, and, later, decrease in arterial pressure.[18] At very high $\dot{V}O_2$, skin blood flow may again decrease, and at maximal $\dot{V}O_2$, vasoconstriction of the skin may occur even in a hot environment.[74,109]

EFFECTS OF ENDURANCE EXERCISE TRAINING

In general, it appears that many of the circulatory effects of endurance exercise training are predominantly upon the peripheral muscles and blood vessels rather than primarily upon the heart.[110]

Hypertrophy

For many years it has been recognized that endurance training produces eccentric cardiac hypertrophy.[111] In marked instances, this has been referred to as the "athletic heart syndrome."[112–116]

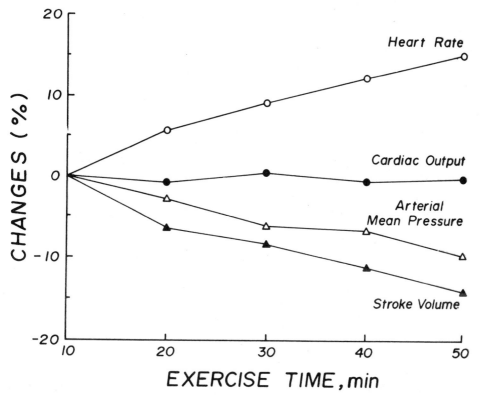

Figure 4: Response to prolonged exercise. The mean arterial pressure and stroke volume decrease slightly, and the cardiac output is maintained by a further increase in heart rate. These changes are due to the increasing dilatation of the cutaneous veins to meet the need for body temperature regulation. With the consequent reduction in the volume of blood in the heart and lungs, the filling pressure decreases and stroke volume falls. (From Shepherd JT, Vanhoutte PM: *The Human Cardiovascular System*, 1979, reprinted by permission of Raven Press, New York.) (Data from Ekelund and Holmgren.[103])

There is no evidence that this is harmful in any way. In pigs, exercise-induced cardiac hypertrophy is associated with the production of new arterioles but not capillaries.[117]

Hemodynamics at Rest

The primary consistent hemodynamic finding of training athletes at rest is a slower heart rate,[16,25,118–120] apparently due to parasympathetic dominance and perhaps also due to changes in the intrinsic rate of the sinus node or to an increase in blood volume.[3,121-123] The cardiac output at rest usually shows no consistent change although it may occasionally decrease slightly.[25,124-127]

Adjustments to Exercise

One of the hallmarks of endurance training is an increase in the maximal oxygen consumption ($\dot{V}O_2$max or maximal aerobic power) (Fig. 5). In young and middle-aged persons, this may increase about 10-30% during moderate training, while the maximal heart rate at $\dot{V}O_2$max is either unchanged or reduced.[3,17,25, 61,74,127-134] An additional benefit of training is the ability to use a greater percentage of maximal oxygen uptake during the prolonged work (Fig. 6). In general, the increase in $\dot{V}O_2$max results about equally from an increase in cardiac output due to tachycardia and an increased stroke volume and from an increased arteriovenous oxygen difference due to increased oxygen extraction.[16,74,93,130,131,135,136] The usual criteria for determining $\dot{V}O_2$max are that no further increase in O_2 uptake occurs despite a further increase in work load and that the blood lactate is above 70-80 mg or 8-9 mM per 100 ml.[27,74]

The ratio of cardiac output to oxygen consumption ($Q/\dot{V}O_2$) during submaximal exercise with trained arm or leg muscles or untrained leg muscles is not changed significantly by training.[16, 25,137,138] During heavy exercise with untrained arms after leg training, however, there is a greater increase in both cardiac output and arterial blood pressure for the same oxygen consumption.[25]

The maximal cardiac output (Qmax) after training is largely the result of an increase in stroke volume produced by an increase in venous return, a reduction in total peripheral resistance due to vasodilatation in the exercising muscles, cardiac hypertrophy, tachycardia, increase in blood volume, and, perhaps, by a possible increase in myocardial contractility.[3,139,140] The increase in maximal stroke volume is another hallmark of endurance cardiovascular training. Cardiac output values up to 42 L/min have been reported in highly trained athletes.[4] Well-trained athletes have a relatively small maximal arteriovenous oxygen difference ($AVDO_2$max) and do not appear to increase total systemic $AVDO_2$max with

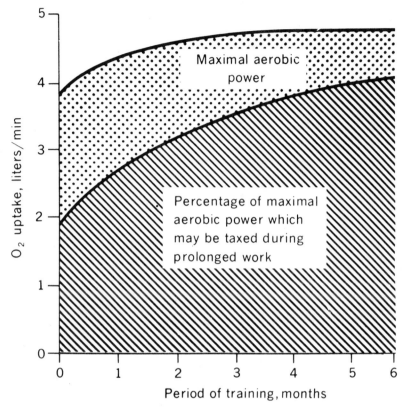

Figure 5: Training causes an increase in maximal oxygen uptake. With training, a subject is also able to tax a greater percentage of his maximal oxygen uptake during prolonged work. (From Astrand P-O, Rodahl K: *Textbook of Work Physiology*, New York, McGraw-Hill Book Company, Inc, 1970. Used with the permission of McGraw-Hill Book Company.)

training.[141] Although several studies have suggested that athletes tend to have an increase in blood volume[142-146] but slightly lower hemoglobin concentrations at rest,[12,142] these findings have not been uniformly confirmed.[38,147-149] If true, a lower hematocrit might lower blood viscosity and assist them to achieve a very high cardiac output and very high muscle blood flow.[12]

Training results in a decreased heart rate response during submaximal exercise, in association with the increase in stroke

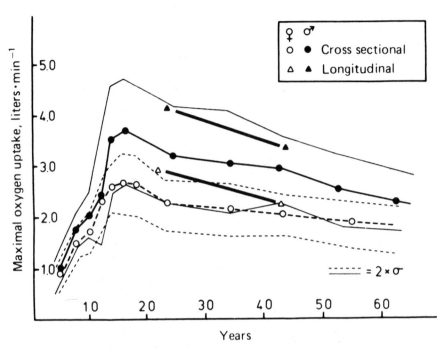

Figure 6: Mean values for maximal oxygen uptake (maximal aerobic power) measured during exercise on treadmill or bicycle ergometer in 350 female and male subjects 4 to 65 years of age. Included are values from a group of 86 trained students in physical education (from Astrand P-O, Christensen EH, 1964),[332] and measured maximal oxygen uptakes in a longitudinal study (21 years) of 35 female and 31 male subjects of the former students (Astrand I, et al., 1973).[231] (From Astrand P-O, Rodahl K: *Textbook of Work Physiology*, 2nd Edition. New York, McGraw-Hill Book Company, Inc, 1977. Used with the permission of McGraw-Hill Book Company.)

volume.[3,12,16,25,129,130,135] The decrease in heart rate increase may be due to the increased stroke volume. Most studies have shown that the maximal heart rate (HRmax) can be decreased by training.[3,17,135,150–153] Although the exact mechanism of the decrease in maximal heart rate response produced by training is unknown, it has been suggested that training reduces the sympathetic drive to the heart during exercise.[3] It may also be related to down-regulation of beta-receptors due to the prolonged exposure to high levels of catecholamines that occur during exercise training.[154] In general, the decrease in heart rate response during exercise with trained muscles is more marked with higher work loads, while the decrease in heart rate response with nontrained muscles is more marked during light exercise. Of interest, the decrease in heart rate that results from training with arm exercises does not carry over to leg exercise.[3,12,25,155,156] This suggests an involvement of the central nervous system (Table 1).

Table 1
Systemic Effects of Training and Effects that are Confined to Exercise with Trained Muscles*

Systemic Effects	Effects Confined to Exercise with Trained Muscles
Reduction in HR at rest and during submaximal exercise with nontrained muscles	Reduction of ΔHR during submaximal exercise
Increase in $\dot{Q}$ and BP. Only seen heavy submaximal exercise with nontrained arms after leg training	Reduction of sympathetic vasoconstriction in nonexercising tissues during submaximal exercise
Decrease in blood hemoglobin concentration	Reduction in MBF during submaximal exercise and concomitant increase of regional and/or systemic $AVDo_2$
Displacement to the right of O_2 hemoglobin dissociation curve	Reduction in $\dot{Q}/\dot{V}o_2$ during submaximal exercise. Most often seen in patients with CAD
Increase in $\dot{V}o_2$max attended by an increase in MBPmax	Reduction in BP during submaximal exercise
	Decrease in $\Delta\dot{V}E/\Delta\dot{V}o_2$ during submaximal exercise
	Increase in mechanical efficiency
	Decrease in blood lactate content and lactate release from exercising extremity during submaximal exercise
	Decrease in RQ during submaximal exercise
	Increase in pH and decrease of pCO_2 in venous blood from exercising extremity
	Decrease in acute postexercise expansion of upper arm volume
	Increase in $\dot{V}o_2$max caused by increased O_2 extraction or decrease in TPR

*From Clausen[12] based on data from Clausen et al.,[25] Rasmussen et al.,[167] and Klausen et al.[169]

Training has no consistent effect upon resting arterial blood pressure [146] though several studies have suggested modest reductions in hypertensive subjects.[157-159] In normal subjects, there is also little effect of training upon the mean blood pressure response to submaximal exercise.[126,150] Training does seem to lower the blood pressure response to exercise in older,[143] less fit, or hypertensive subjects.[3,143,158,160,161]

Blood flow per gram of working muscle is actually lower in trained individuals than in untrained individuals at the same levels of work.[12,25,137,159,162-165] On the other hand, trained muscles extract more oxygen per 100 ml blood flow than do untrained muscles. Thus, for the same amount of external work, the trained individual requires less muscle blood flow, and exercise is associated with a widened arteriovenous oxygen difference for the working, trained extremity.[16,124,127,130,166] The decrease in exercise-induced vasodilatation in the exercising muscles of trained individuals allows relatively more blood flow to nonexercising muscles and splanchnic-renal areas[25] during exercise than in untrained individuals.

Noncirculatory parameters are also altered by training. Thus, the ventilatory equivalent ($\dot{V}E/\dot{V}O_2$) is reduced during exercise with trained muscles.[167] This is more marked after arm training than after leg training. In addition, there is a reduced respiratory quotient (RQ), an increased mechanical efficiency, and a decrease in the lactate released from the exercising extremity and in the blood lactate concentration.[168] Training increases red cell 2,3-diphosphoglycerate[93,169,170] and increases the size of the heart including the end-diastolic volume, wall thickness, and heart weight.[171-176] On the other hand, despite many studies, it is still uncertain whether or not training produces any change in intrinsic myocardial contractility.[173-187] The enlargement of the heart that occurs with endurance training may persist for many years after the disappearance of other training effects.[132,188-190]

The optimal length, frequency, and intensity of training sessions, as well as the exercise pattern, have not been satisfactorily studied.[168] A training frequency less than twice a week does not appear to be sufficient,[191] and sessions of 30-60 minutes three to five times a week are frequently used. The intensity of exercise may be relatively more important than the duration or amount of exercise,[191,192] but it is uncertain whether continuous or intermittent exercise produces greater training effect.

Training also decreases both the release of catecholamines from the heart[193] and the plasma levels of norepinephrine and epinephrine during exercise.[194,195] Training also increases the number of beta-adrenergic binding cells on polymorphonuclear leukocytes, perhaps reflecting an increased sensitivity to catecholamines.[196]

Mitochondrial Oxidative Enzymes in Skeletal Muscles

Training skeletal muscles produces a significant increase in the capillaries[197] and in the number and size of mitochondria in the muscles[3,134,198-205] as well as an increase in the activity and concentration of many enzymes involved in aerobic metabolism and an increased capacity to generate ATP by oxidative phosphorylation.[134] These enzymes include those involved in fatty acid oxidation, the enzymes of the citrate cycle, and the components of the respiratory chain that link the oxidation of succinate and NADH to oxygen and coupling factor 1.[134,163,166,200,206-211] As a consequence, trained muscles are better able to metabolize fat, carbohydrates, and ketones. This increase in respiratory capacity occurs in all three types of skeletal muscle, slow twitch (ST) or Type I, fast twitch FTa or Type IIa, and fast twitch FTb or Type IIb. Since fast twitch (FT) muscle fibers appear to be less involved in endurance exercise, it is not surprising that they change their enzyme patterns less than slow twitch (ST), Type I, or red muscle fibers.[94,134] In general, the changes in skeletal muscle enzymes in response to training tend to make the skeletal muscles more like cardiac muscle in their enzyme patterns and activity. Exercise also increases the hexokinase activity of the trained skeletal muscle but produces only small changes in the activity of the other enzymes concerned with glycolysis.[134,212] Interestingly, endurance training does not produce adaptive increases in respiratory enzymes in heart muscle although myosin ATPase activity is increased.[213] Trained muscles are also better able to function at a lower PO_2 because of increased skeletal muscle myoglobin,[134,166,214] which facilitates oxygen diffusion to the mitochondria,[215,216] and a shift to the right of the oxygen-hemoglobin dissociation curve.[91,149,167]

Trained individuals have more glycogen and glycogen synthetase in their active muscles, and they deplete their skeletal muscle glycogen more slowly than when they are untrained.[138,200,217,218] In part, this may be due to the fact that they obtain relatively more energy from the oxidation of fatty acids.[128,138,217,219,220] The increase in fatty acid oxidation tends to decrease glucose uptake and glycogen depletion in the exercising muscles, thereby tending to protect against hypoglycemia and exhaustion during prolonged exercise. Trained individuals also have lower blood and muscle lactate levels than untrained individuals at the same work level.[127,138,217,218,221,222] On the other hand, training increases the level of maximal work, and the trained individual is usually able to achieve a higher concentration of lactate in the blood and a lower pH at maximal work than an untrained individual. Endurance training often decreases blood levels of triglycerides and of free fatty acids at rest,[166,223-226] while producing a greater release of fatty acids from adipose tissue during exercise.[227,228]

ADJUSTMENTS TO EXERCISE IN PATIENTS WITH ATHEROSCLEROTIC CORONARY HEART DISEASE

There is a wide spectrum of circulatory adjustments to exercise in patients with atherosclerotic coronary heart disease (CHD). Some patients can hardly be distinguished from normal, whereas others are in continual severe congestive heart failure, even at rest. In general, however, patients with CHD have a diminished maximal oxygen consumption, diminished maximal cardiac output, decreased maximal heart rate, and decreased maximal stroke volume.[150,229-233] The blood pressure response may be normal, but in some patients with severe CHD, exercise may result in a decrease in stroke volume and cardiac output and a fall in arterial blood pressure. In most individuals with CHD, the increase in cardiac output relative to the increase in oxygen consumption ($\dot{Q}/\dot{V}O_2$) is usually the same as in other individuals of the same age, although it may decline in patients with very severe CHD.[150,229,232,233] Often the heart rate response to exercise is greater than normal while the stroke volume response is less than normal. With work loads above 60–70 percent of maximal, the stroke volume frequently decreases or fails to increase in patients with CHD.[160,230,232,234] Associated with the above, the left ventricular end-diastolic pressure frequently becomes elevated during exercise; in general, the increase in end-diastolic pressure correlates with the severity of the coronary disease.[235-238] When the end-diastolic pressure and stroke volume are normal at rest and become abnormal during exercise, it suggests that the changes are due to reversible myocardial ischemia. In general, patients with CHD can perform higher levels of exercise in the upright position than in the supine position.

In patients who develop agina pectoris during upright leg exercise, the product of heart rate and systolic pressure at which angina pectoris occurs is relatively constant for different types and levels of exercise. During supine exercise, angina pectoris often occurs at a lower pressure−rate product, perhaps because supine exercise frequently occurs at a larger diastolic volume.[26,239] The latter increases ventricular myocardial consumption by increasing mean ventricular diameter which increases wall tension by the LaPlace relationship. Similarly, arm exercise, which is associated with smaller increases in stroke volume, may permit the achievement of a higher pressure-rate product before the onset of angina pectoris.[240] Patients with CHD tend to have higher levels of total peripheral resistance at all levels of work than normal young subjects.[25] In general, however, patients with CHD and exercise-induced angina pectoris do not differ significantly from normal in respect to their circulatory regulation during exercise, which is limited primarily by myocardial ischemia.

EFFECTS OF TRAINING ON CIRCULATORY ADJUSTMENTS TO EXERCISE IN PATIENTS WITH ATHEROSCLEROTIC CORONARY HEART DISEASE (CHD)

Resting Hemodynamics

The decrease in heart rate at rest tends to be less than in normal individuals,[156,160,240−243] while the cardiac output at rest may decrease,[16,25,244] or show no significant change.[129,137,150,160,241,242]

Submaximal Exercise

Training increases the maximal oxygen consumption ($\dot{V}O_2$ max) from 16 percent to 56 percent in those patients who are able to undergo training.[150,161,214,230,245-250] Some patients with CHD who undergo training increase their $\dot{V}O_2$max primarily by increasing their maximal arteriovenous oxygen difference ($AVDO_2$ max), rather than increasing their maximum cardiac output.[74,230,234] The heart rate response to submaximal exercise may be reduced even without an increase in stroke volume in patients with CHD.[243,251,252] The maximal heart rate (HRmax) is unchanged or reduced by training, as in normal subjects. Training also decreases the maximal norepinephrine and epinephrine responses to exercise.[253]

In patients with CHD, as in normal subjects, training results in less blood flow to the exercising trained muscles, with relatively more going to nonexercising muscles and splanchnic organs.[142,163,164,165] As in normal subjects, training results in an improved aerobic metabolic capacity of the trained muscles.

After a period of training, the same work load usually results in a lower heart rate and frequently a lower systolic blood pressure.[158,178,243] The tension-time index or triple product (heart rate × systolic blood pressure × duration of left ventricular ejection) at a given work load are often reduced 8–18 percent by training.[252] Clinically, this results in increased exercise tolerance in many patients with angina pectoris. In patients with angina pectoris, training may increase the lowest work load needed to produce angina pectoris, increase the time to onset of pain at a given work load, and increase the highest work load a patient can sustain during a given period of time. These efforts are due primarily to a reduced myocardial oxygen need for the same oxygen consumption by the body.

Most of the effects of training are due to changes in the trained muscles rather than the heart itself, although the fact that some patients are able to tolerate a 13–22 percent higher triple product before the onset of angina pectoris suggests that there may be additional effects of training upon the heart. On the other hand, the slope of the relation between triple product and ST segment depression does not appear to be changed by training.[248]

AGE CHANGES IN THE PHYSIOLOGIC RESPONSE TO EXERCISE

In the resting state, the heart of the aged has a prolongation of mechanical systole in the pre-ejection phase and during isovolumic diastole, together with a slower rate of ventricular relaxation.[254–256] The resting heart rate does not appear to vary with age,[257] if one excludes subjects with primary conduction system disorders. There is, however, a gradual decrease in stroke volume that is responsible for the decrease in cardiac output with age.[249, 258–261]

The decreased responsiveness of the aged heart to stress has been termed "presbycardia" by Dock, in analogy with the loss of visual accommodation to near vision referred to as presbyopia.[262] The general decrease in cardiovascular responsiveness can be appropriately measured by the maximal oxygen consumption ($\dot{V}O_2max$). In one study, this decreased from a mean of 3.53L/min for men at mean age of 24.5 years to 1.71 L/min at a mean age of 75 years.[263] This age-related decrease in $\dot{V}O_2max$ occurs in both men and women and in both physically active and inactive individuals.[69,231,249,264]

In addition to a lower maximal oxygen uptake (aerobic capacity), older individuals have a lower maximal heart rate, maximal stroke volume, maximal AV oxygen difference, and maximal cardiac output.[229,260,261,264–267] In contrast, recent studies by Rodeheffer et al. indicated that healthy individuals of advanced age maintained their exercise cardiac output by increased stroke volume, possibly related to an age-related diminution in the cardiovascular response to beta-adrenergic stimulation.[268] At any given $\dot{V}O_2$, the stroke volume and cardiac output in older subjects tend to be lower while the arterial pressure tends to be higher.[249, 259–261] The systemic (peripheral) vascular resistance does not decrease during exercise to the same degree in the elderly.[259,269] In addition, the pulmonary capillary pressure, pulmonary artery, and the right ventricular end-diastolic pressures tend to become elevated in aged individuals during recumbent exercise.[246,259] It is not known whether these changes are due to decreases in ventricular systolic function or to decreased ventricular compliance and diastolic relaxation. The age-associated increase in diastolic stiffness[270] and decreased relaxing ability may be due to physical–chemical changes in either the myocardial connective tissue[271,272] or the high molecular weight proteins of heart muscle.[256] Other factors that may contribute include possible changes in pericardial stiffness[256,273] or decreased cardiac responsiveness to catecholamines.[256] In addition, the aging aorta loses much of its elasticity and Windkessel effect.[274–276] At age 85, the aorta is almost a rigid tube.[276,277] As a result, aging is associated with an almost inevitable increase in the instantaneous impedance to left ventricular ejection. Furthermore, arterial rigidity or stiffness may also increase with age due to a loss of elastin and an increase in collagen.[278]

In animal studies of aging, there is evidence of an age-associated decrease in the maximal velocity of contractile element shortening (Vmax) together with a decrease in myofibrillar ATPase.[279,280] There is also a decreased responsiveness to catecholamines[256] and a decrease in the density of myocardial capillaries and in the capillary–fiber ratio.[272,281] Interestingly, when aged rats perform exercise, there is a decrease in heart weight suggesting that exercise might actually produce a dropout of myocardial fibers.[282]

The trainability of the cardiovascular system persists but decreases with age (Fig. 7).[129,144,283] There is some evidence that training in the 20's and 30's may influence certain circulatory dimensions such as heart volume and blood volume, whereas training at older ages may utilize other previously improved parameters.[139] Benestad[284] noted no significant effect of a training program in 70- to 80-year old men, and other studies[285] have shown diminished effects of training women above 50 years of age. In general, however, older individuals are generally capable of developing cardiovascular training effects, although less than in young individuals.

METABOLIC FUELS DURING EXERCISE

Normally, the body stores most of its fuel energy in the form of fat. A 70 kg man has approximately 140,000 kcal of fat, while stored carbohydrate totals less than 2,000 kcal: 350 gm of muscle glycogen, 90 gm of liver glycogen, and 20 gm of glucose in extracellular water.[286,287] Muscle glycogen can be used only for the energy requirements of the muscle fibers but cannot be transformed back to blood glucose. Protein forms the remaining 15–20 percent of body fuel reserves; however, its metabolism necessarily consumes either muscle or parenchymal tissue.

At rest, skeletal muscles use fatty acids for over 90 percent of their energy.[288] During acute maximal exertion, such as running, which can be sustained only for a few seconds, the exercising muscles utilize adenosine triphosphate (ATP) and creatine phosphate (CP).[286] After a few seconds of exercise, the aerobic metabolism of glycogen is rapidly accelerated; during the first 5 to 10

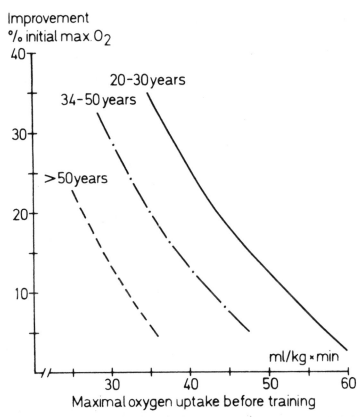

Figure 7: Improvement in maximal oxygen uptake with 2 to 6 months' physical conditioning calculated in young individuals from the studies by Rowell,[130] Ekblom,[131] and Saltin[133] in 34- to 50-year-old subjects and in men over 50 years old from the studies by Kihlbom[283] and Saltin[144] in relation to the initial level of their maximal oxygen uptake. (From Grimby,[168] with permission.)

minutes of heavy exercise, the rate of glycogenolysis is most rapid, [287,289] following which the utilization of blood-borne glucose and fatty acids becomes more important. Although this glycogenolysis is primarily aerobic, some lactate is also produced during this period.[286,290] After 10–40 minutes of prolonged moderately heavy exercise, glucose uptake and utilization by exercising skeletal muscles may increase 7 to 20 times the basal level and may account for 30 to 40 percent of the muscle oxygen consumption, while fatty acids also provide about 40 percent of energy (Fig. 8).[291–293]

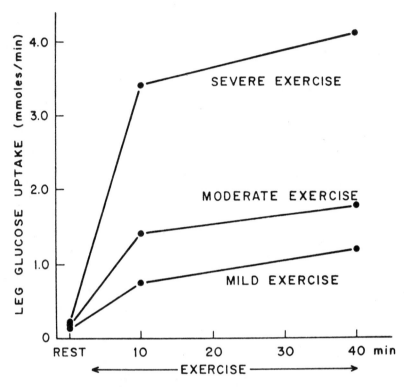

Figure 8: Glucose uptake by the legs during bicycle ergometer exercise. (From Felig and Wahren,[287] with permission.) (Reprinted by permission of the *New England Journal of Medicine* 1975; 293:1078.)

After 40 minutes of sustained exercise, muscle glycogen is significantly depleted, and blood glucose hepatic glycogenolysis and gluconeogenesis provides 75 to 90 percent of the glucose utilized. [217,287,289,292,294,295] When the exercise is continued beyond 40 minutes, glucose utilization by exercising muscles continues to increase until it peaks at 90 to 180 minutes, following which it decreases slightly (Fig. 9).[292,295,296]

The utilization of fatty acids continues to increase during prolonged exercise until, at 4 hours of exercise, fatty acids contribute 62 percent of total oxygen usage, while glucose accounts for only 30 percent (Fig. 10).[295] Intramuscular triglyceride stores provide important amounts of fatty acids during exercise.[286]

During exercise, the arterial concentration of alanine increases, reflecting the increased glucose utilization by exercising muscles,

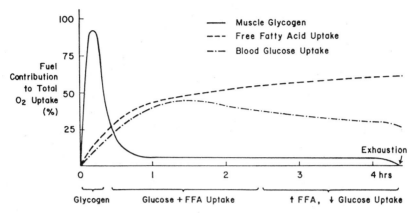

Figure 9: Triphasic response of body fuels to acute exercise. During the first few minutes of exercise breakdown of muscle glycogen is the major source of ATP for contracting muscle. As exercise extends beyond 10 minutes, blood-borne fuels in the form of glucose and free fatty acids become increasingly important. As exercise extends beyond 90–120 min (e.g., in marathon runners), there is an increasing dependence on fat and lesser uptake of glucose. Muscle glycogen contributes a small proportion of the fuel requirements even in prolonged exercise, and its depletion is associated with exhaustion. Not shown is the small contribution of body protein breakdown to total fuel utilization in prolonged exercise (generally < 5–10% of total caloric utilization). (From Felig, [296] in Bove AA, Lowenthal DT (eds). *Exercise Medicine: Physiologic Principles and Clinical Applications.* New York, Academic Press, 1983. Used with permission of Academic Press.)

the synthesis of alanine in exercising muscles by transamination of pyruvate with the utilization of free ammonia from purine nucleotides, and, perhaps, the increased utilization of leucine, isoleucine, and valine for energy.[287,297–302] Alanine returning to the liver is reconverted to glucose.[286,303]

Blood glucose concentrations do not change significantly during mild to moderate exercise of short duration. During more severe exercise, however, blood glucose concentration may increase 20 to 30 mg/dl.[304] On the other hand, when exercise continues for 90 minutes or longer, blood glucose concentration may decrease 10–40 mg/dl in association with a gradual decrease in insulin concentration and a gradual increase in glucagon concentration.[295,305,306] Blood glucose levels below 40 mg/dl are rare, but have been observed in marathon runners [307] or subjects on low carbohydrate diets.[308] Of interest, the capacity to perform prolonged, heavy exercise appears to be related to the amount of

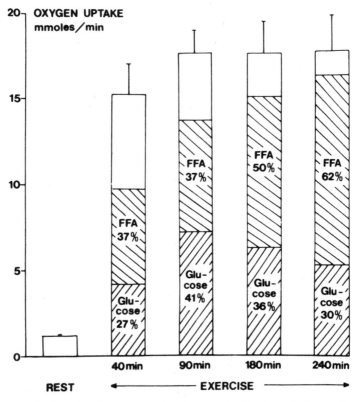

Figure 10: Uptake of oxygen and substrates by the legs during prolonged exercise. Hatched areas represent the proportion of total oxygen uptake contributed by oxidation of free fatty acids (FFA) and blood glucose. Open portions indicate oxidation of nonblood-borne fuels (muscle glycogen and intramuscular lipids), and I bars indicate 1 SEM. (From Ahlborg, Felig, Hagenfeldt, Hendler, and Wahren[295] with permission.)

glycogen stored in the muscles,[309–311] and exhaustion is associated with the depletion of muscle glycogen even though there are adequate blood concentrations of glucose and fatty acids.[310,312, 313] During light exercise and the ordinary activities of daily living, the skeletal muscles receive adequate oxygen for their needs. At the onset of exercise of moderate intensity, some anaerobic metabolism is used and some lactate is produced by skeletal muscles, but the blood lactate level gradually decreases as the exercise is continued.[292,314] During very strenuous exercise, however, the increase in blood lactate is greater and the level remains elevated throughout the work period.[12] In general, trained individuals can work at about 60 to 70 percent of maximal $\dot{V}O_2$ without a marked elevation of blood lactate,[315] whereas untrained individuals begin to elevate blood lactate significantly at about 50 percent of their maximal $\dot{V}O_2$.

After the cessation of exercise, glycogen stores in both liver and muscle are rapidly repleted in association with increased hepatic uptake of lactate, pyruvate, and alanine. Most of the lactate formed during exercise is resynthesized to glycogen and the rest is metabolized to CO_2 and H_2O. Extra oxygen is required for these processes, and this so-called *lactacid* oxygen debt is about twice as high as the oxygen deficit.

During exercise of more than mild intensity, the oxygen uptake during the first few minutes of exercise does not equal the oxygen actually consumed. This "oxygen debt," which is repaid at the end of the exercise, has classically been said to be used to restore oxygen stores in blood and myoglobin, to restore ATP and phosphocreatine stores, to provide for increased cardiac and respiratory activities during this recovery phase, and to repay a slower lactacid oxygen debt and resynthesize glycogen (Fig. 11). It is likely that the original concept of the lactic acid explanation of the oxygen debt was too simplistic, and it has been recommended that

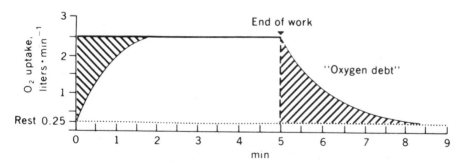

Figure 11: During the first minutes of exercise the oxygen uptake increases, then levels off as the oxygen uptake reaches a level adequate to meet the demand of the tissues. At the cessation of exercise, there is a gradual decrease in the oxygen uptake, as the "oxygen debt" is being paid off. (From Astrand P-O, Rodahl K: *Textbook of Work Physiology*, 2nd Edition. New York, McGraw-Hill Book Company, Inc, 1977. Used with the permission of McGraw-Hill Book Company.)

the term "oxygen debt" be used to explain a complex set of phenomena during recovery from exercise.[316]

After the onset of mild or moderate exercise, the arterial free fatty acid (FFA) concentration increases. When the exercise involves large leg muscles, however, the arterial FFA concentration may abruptly fall at the onset of heavy exercise and then increase above resting values after 20–30 minutes of exercise.[297,317,318] When the exercise is of long duration, the arterial levels of FFA continue to increase slowly for 10–12 hours, reaching concentrations 4 to 5 times resting.[319] Eighteen hours after prolonged exercise, the clearance rate of plasma triglyceride is augmented, postheparin lipase activity is increased, and the high density lipoprotein (HDL) level is increased.[320] Training is associated with a greater release of fatty acids from adipose tissue and higher plasma levels of FFA during exercise.

ISOMETRIC EXERCISE

When sustained isometric (static) exercise is performed, there is a marked increase in systemic arterial pressure that progressively increases over 5–45 seconds in association with lesser increases in heart rate, cardiac output, and ventilation.[321–329] The progressive increase in blood pressure tends to rise more proportionately to the relative intensity of the sustained contraction rather than to the mass of muscle involved. The increase in arterial blood pressure tends to oppose the external pressure on the blood vessels produced by the contracting muscle cells and thereby helps to maintain muscle blood flow. When the force of the sustained contraction is above 50 to 75 percent of the muscle's maximal voluntary force, however, muscle blood flow is significantly impeded, and the muscles must utilize anaerobic metabolism with the rapid development of fatigue. Repeated training using only isometric exercise increases the mass and strength of the involved muscles, but does not produce the training effects on the skeletal muscles or the cardiovascular system produced by rhythmic, dynamic exercise training. When simultaneous dynamic and isometric exercise is performed, the hemodynamic responses are additive.[330] Of interest, the hearts of athletes performing extensive isometric exercise, such as weight lifting, tend to have evidence of concentric hypertrophy.[6,333]

REFERENCES

1. Bevegard BS, Shepherd JT: Regulation of the circulation during exercise in man, *Physiol Rev* 1967; 47:178–232.
2. Ekelund L-G: Circulatory and respiratory adaptation during prolonged exercise. *Acta Physiol Scand* 1967; 70 (Suppl. 292).
3. Scheuer J, Tipton CM: Cardiovascular adaptations to physical training. *Ann Rev Physiol* 1977; 39:221–251.
4. Astrand P-O, Rodahl K: *Textbook of Work Physiology: Physiological Bases of Exercise.* 2nd ed., New York, McGraw-Hill, 1977.
5. Dowell RT: Cardiovascular physiology of exercise. In *Exercise Medicine: Physiological Principles and Clinical Applications.* Bove AA, Lowenthal DT (eds.). Orlando, Academic Press, 1983, pp. 19–27.
6. Schaible TF, Scheuer J: Cardiac adaptations to chronic exercise. *Prog Cardiovas Dis* 1985; 27:297–324.
7. Rost R: *Athletics and The Heart.* Chicago, Year Book, 1987.
8. Uvnas B: Cholinergic vasodilator innervation to skeletal muscles. *Circ Res* 1967; 20:83–90.
9. Vatner SF, Pagani M: Cardiovascular adjustments to exercise: Hemodynamics and mechanisms. *Prog Cardiovasc Dis* 1976; 19:91.
10. Horwitz LD, Bishop VS: Effect of acute volume loading on heart rate in the conscious dog. *Circ Res* 1972; 30:316.
11. Vatner SF, Boettcher DH, Heyndrickx GR, McRitchie RJ: Reduced baroreflex sensitivity with volume loading in conscious dogs. *Circ Res* 1975; 37:236.
12. Clausen JP: Circulatory adjustments to dynamic exercise and effect of physical training in normal subjects and in patients with coronary artery disease. *Prog Cardiovasc Dis* 1976; 18:459.
13. Fujihara Y, Hildebrandt J, Hildebrandt JR: Cardiorespiratory transients in exercising man. II. Linear models. *J Appl Physiol* 1973; 35: 68–76.
14. Simonson E: Evaluation of cardiac performance in exercise. *Am J Cardiol* 1972; 30:722–726.
15. Wade OL, Bishop JM: *Cardiac Output and Regional Blood Flow.* Oxford, Blackwell, 1962.
16. Saltin B, Blomqvist G, Mitchell JH, Johnson RL, Wildenthal K, Chapman CB, in collaboration with Frenkel E, Norton W, Siderstein M, Suki W: Response to exercise after bed rest and after training: A longitudinal study of adaptive changes in oxygen transport and body composition. *Circulation* 1968; 38 (Suppl. 7):1.
17. Vatner SF, Franklin D, Higgins CB, Patrick T, and Braunwald E: Left ventricular response to severe exertion in untethered dogs. *J Clin Invest* 1972; 51:3052.
18. Smith EE, Guyton AC, Manning RD, White RJ: Integrated mechanisms of cardiovascular response and control during exercise in the normal human.*Prog Cardiovasc Dis* 1976; 18:421.
19. Saltin B, Astrand P: Maximal oxygen uptake in athletes. *J Appl Physiol* 1967; 23:353.

20. McArdle WD, Foglia GF, Patti AV: Telemetered cardiac response to selected running events. *J Appl Physiol* 1967; 23:566.
21. Bainbridge FA: The influence of venous filling upon the rate of the heart. *J Physiol* 1915; 50:65.
22. Stegemann J, Kenner TH: A theory on heart rate control by muscular metabolic receptors. *Arch Kreislaufforschg* 1971; 64:185.
23. Asmussen E, Hemmingsen I: Determination of maximum working capacity at different ages in work with the legs or with the arms. *Scand J Clin Lab Invest* 1958; 10:67.
24. Astrand P-O and Saltin B: Maximal oxygen uptake and heart rate in various types of muscular activity. *J Appl Physiol* 1961; 16:977.
25. Clausen JP, Klausen K, Rasmussen B, Trap-Jensen J: Central and peripheral circulatory changes after training of the arms or legs. *Am J Physiol* 1973; 225:675.
26. Epstein SE, Beiser GD, Stampfer M, and Braunwald E. Exercise in patients with heart disease: Effects of body position and type and intensity of exercise. *Am J Cardiol* 1969; 23:572.
27. Hermansen L: Oxygen transport during exercise in human subjects. *Acta Physiol Scand* 1973; (Suppl. II):396−403.
28. Blair DA, Glover WE, Roddie IC: Vasomotor responses in the human arm during leg exercise. *Circ Res* 1961; 9:264.
29. Ekelund LG and Holmgren A. Central hemodynamics during exercise. *Circ Res* 1967; 20 (Suppl. 1):33.
30. McRitchie RJ, Vatner SF, Boettcher D, Heyndrickx GR, Patrick TA, Braunwald E: Role of arterial baroreceptors in mediating cardiovascular response to exercise. *Am J Physiol* 1976; 230:85−89.
31. Kreeker EJ, Wood EH: Comparison of simultaneously recorded central and peripheral arterial pressure pulses during rest, exercise, and tilted position in man. *Circ Res* 1955; 3:623.
32. Holmgren A: Circulatory changes during muscular work in man. *Scand J Clin Lab Invest* 1956; 14 (Suppl. 24):5.
33. Marx HJ, Rowell LB, Conn RD, Bruce RA, Kusumi F: Maintenance of aortic pressure and total peripheral resistance during exercise in heat. *J Appl Physiol* 1967; 22:519.
34. Rowell LB, Brengelmann GL, Blackmon JR, Bruce RA, Murray JA: Disparities between aortic and peripheral pulse pressures induced by upright exercise and vasomotor changes in man. *Circulation* 1968; 37:954−964.
35. Ceretelli P: Kinetics of adaptation of cardiac output in exercise. *Proc Int Symp Phys Activ* 1966; 64−73.
36. Van Citters RL, Franklin DL: Cardiovascular performance of Alaska sled dogs during exercise. *Circ Res* 1969; 24:33.
37. Vatner SF, Higgins CB, White S, Patrick T: The peripheral vascular response to severe exercise in untethered dogs before and after complete heart block. *J Clin Invest* 1971; 50:1950.
38. Astrand P-O, Rodahl K: *Textbook of Work Physiology*. New York, McGraw-Hill, 1970.
39. Gibbons LW, Cooper KH, Martin RP, Pollock ML: Medical examination and electro-cardiographic analysis of elite distance runners. *Ann NY Acad Sci* 1977; 301:283.

40. Guyton AC, Douglas BH, Langston JB, Richardson TQ: Instantaneous increase in mean circulatory pressure and cardiac output at onset of muscular activity. *Circ Res* 1962; 11:431–441.

41. Lind AR, McNicol GW, Donald KW: Circulatory adjustments to sustained (statis) muscular activity. *Proc Int Symp Physical Activity in Health and Disease.* Evang K, Anderson K (eds.). Norway, Universitetsforlaget, 1966.

42. Folkow G, Gaskell P, Wealer BA: Blood flow through limb muscles during heavy rhythmic exercise. *Acta Physiol Scand* 1970; 80:61–72.

43. Folkow B, Haglund U, Jodal M, Lundgren O: Blood flow in the calf muscle of man during heavy rhythmic exercise. *Acta Physiol Scand* 1971; 81:157–163.

44. Gaskell WH: On the changes of the blood stream in muscles through stimulation of the nerves. *J Anat* 1877; 11:360–502.

45. Grant RT: Observations on the blood circulation in voluntary muscle in man. *Clin Sci* 1938; 3:157–173.

46. Donald DE, Shepherd JT: Response to exercise in dogs with cardiac denervation. *Am J Physiol* 1963; 205:393–400.

47. Corcondilas A, Koroxenidis GT, Shepherd JT: Effect of a brief contraction of forearm muscles on forearm blood flow. *J Appl Physiol* 1964; 19:142–146.

48. Johnson PC: The microcirulation and local and humoral control of the circulation. In *MTP International Review of Science, Cardiovascular Physiology.* Guyton AC, Jones CE (eds.). Baltimore, University Park Press, 1974, p. 163.

49. Clement DL, Shepherd JT. Regulation of peripheral circulation during muscular exercise. *Prog Cardiovasc Dis* 1976; 19:23–31.

50. Reeves JT, Grover RF, Blount SG Jr, Filley GF: Cardiac output response to standing and treadmill walking. *J Appl Physiol* 1961; 16:283.

51. Bevegard S: Studies on the regulation of the circulation in man. *Acta Physiol Scand* 1962; 57 (Suppl. 200):5.

52. Chapman CB, Baker O, Mitchell JH: Left ventricular function at rest and during exercise. *J Clin Invest* 1959; 38:1202.

53. Chapman CB, Fisher JN, Sproule BJ: Behavior of stroke volume at rest and during exercise in human beings. *J Clin Invest* 1960; 39:1208.

54. Bevegard S, Holmgren A, Jonsson B: Effect of body position on the circulation at rest and during exercise, with special reference to the influence of the stroke volume. *Acta Physiol Scand* 1960; 49:279.

55. Robinson BF, Epstein SE, Kahler RL, Braunwald E: Circulatory effects of acute expansion of blood volume: studies during maximal exercise and at rest. *Circ Res* 1966; 19:26.

56. Ross J Jr, Gault JH, Mason DT, Linhart JW, Braunwald E: Left ventricular performance during muscular exercise in patients with and without cardiac dysfunction. *Circulation* 1966; 34:597–608.

57. Stein RA, Michelli D, Fox EL, Krasnow N: Continuous ventricular dimensions in man during supine exercise and recovery: An echocardiographic study. *Am J Cardiol* 1978; 41:655.

58. Sjostrand T: The regulation of blood distribution in man. *Acta Physiol Scand* 1952; 26:312–327.

59. Wang Y, Marshall RJ, Taylor HL, Shepherd JT: Cardiovascular response to exercise in sedentary man and athletes. *Physiologist* 1960; 3:173.
60. Braunwald E, Sonnenblick EH, Ross J Jr, Glick G, Epstein SE: An analysis of the cardiac response to exercise. *Circ Res* 1967; 20 (Suppl. I):44–58.
61. Rushmer RA: Constancy of stroke volume in ventricular response to exertion. *Am J Physiol* 1959; 196:745–750.
62. Rushmer RF, Smith O, Franklin D: Mechanisms of cardiac control in exercise. *Circ Res* 1959; 7:602–627.
63. Mitchell JH, Sproule BJ, Chapman CB: The physiological meaning of the maximal oxygen intake test. *J Clin Invest* 1958; 37:538–547.
64. Wang Y, Marshall RJ, Shepherd JT: The effect of changes in posture and of graded exercise on stroke volume in man. *J Clin Invest* 1960; 39:1051–1061.
65. Horwitz LD, Atkins JM, Leshin SJ: Role of the Frank-Starling mechanism in exercise. *Circ Res* 1972; 31:868.
66. Braunwald E, Goldblatt A, Harrison DC, Mason DT: Studies on cardiac dimensions in intact, unanesthetized man. III. Effects of muscular exercise. *Circ Res* 1963; 13:460.
67. Sonnenblick EH, Braunwald E, Williams JF Jr, Glick G: Effects of exercise on myocardial force-velocity relations in intact unanesthetized man: Relative roles of changes in heart rate, sympathetic activity, and ventricular dimensions. *J Clin Invest* 1965; 44:2051.
68. Gorlin R, Cohen LS, Elliott WC, Klein MD, Lane FJ: Effect of supine exercise on left ventricular volume and oxygen consumption in man. *Circulation* 1965; 32:361.
69. Folkow B: Range of control of the cardiovascular system by the central nervous system. *Physiol Rev* 1960; 40 (Suppl. 4):93–101.
70. Forrester T: An estimate of adenosine triphosphate release into the venous effluent from exercising human forearm muscle. *J Physiol* (London) 1972; 244:611–628.
71. Zelis R, Mason DT, Braunwald E: Partition of blood flow to the cutaneous and muscular beds of the forearm at rest and during exercise in normal subjects and in patients with heart failure. *Circ Res* 1969; 24:799.
72. Rowell LB: Regulation of splanchnic blood flow in man. *Pysiologist* 1973; 16:127–142.
73. Clausen JP and Trap-Jensen J: Arteriohepatic venous oxygen difference and heart rate during initial phases of exercise. *J Appl Physiol* 1974; 37:716–719.
74. Rowell LB: Human cardiovascular adjustments to exercise and thermal stress. *Physiol Rev* 1974; 54:54–75.
75. Rushmer RF, Franklin DL, Van Citters RL, Smith OA: Changes in peripheral blood flow distribution in healthy dogs. *Circ Res* 1961; 9:675.
76. LaCroix E, Leusen I: Splanchnic hemodynamics during induced muscular exercise in the anesthetized dog. *Arch Int Physiol Biochem* 1966; 74:235–250.

77. Scher AM, Ohm WW, Bumgarner K, Boynton R, Young AC: Sympathetic and parasympathetic control of heart rate in the dog, baboon, and man. *Fed Proc* 1972; 31:1219–1225.
78. Higgins CB, Vatner SF, Franklin D, Braunwald E: Effects of experimentally produced heart failure on the peripheral vascular response to severe exercise in conscious dogs. *Circ Res* 1972; 31:186.
79. Vatner SF, Higgins CB, Franklin D: Regional circulatory adjustments to moderate and severe chronic anemia in conscious dogs at rest and during exercise. *Circ Res* 1972; 30:731.
80. Millard RW, Higgins CB, Franklin D, Vatner SF: Regulation of the renal circulation during severe exercise in normal dogs and dogs with experimental heart failure. *Circ Res* 1972; 31:881.
81. Fixler DE, Atkins JM, Mitchell JE, Horowitz LD: Blood flow to respiratory, cardiac and limb muscles in dogs during graded exercise. *Am J Physiol* 1976; 231:1515.
82. Zobl EG, Talmers FN, Christensen RC, Baer LJ: Effect of exercise on the cerebral circulation and metabolism. *J Appl Physiol* 1965; 20:1289.
83. Khouri EM, Gregg DE, Rayford CR: Effect of exercise on cardiac output, left coronary flow and myocardial metabolism in the unanesthetized dog. *Circ Res* 1965; 17:427.
84. Sonnenblick EH, Ross J, Braunwald E: Oxygen consumption of the heart: Newer concepts of its multifactoral determination. *Am J Cardiol* 1968; 22:328.
85. Holmberg S, Serzysko W, Varnauskas E: Coronary circulation during heavy exercise in control subjects and patients with coronary heart disease. *Acta Med Scand* 1971; 190:465.
86. Vatner SF, Higgins CB, Franklin D, Braunwald E: Role of tachycardia in mediating the coronary hemodynamic response to severe exercise. *J Appl Physiol* 1972; 32:380.
87. Jorgensen CR, Gobel FL, Taylor HL, Wang Y: Myocardial blood flow and oxygen consumption during exercise. *Ann NY Acad Sci* 1977; 301:213.
88. Kjellmer I: The potassium ion as a vasodilator during muscular exercise. *Acta Physiol Scand* 1965; 63:460.
89. Mellander S, Lundvall J: Role of tissue hyperosmolarity in exercise hyperemia. *Circ Res* 1971; 28 (Suppl. 1):39.
90. Keul J, Doll E: Intermittent exercise: metabolites PO_2, and acid-base equilibrium in the blood. *J Appl Physiol* 1973; 34:220.
91. Thomson JM, Dempsey JA, Chosy LW, Shadihi NT, Reddan WG: Oxygen transport and oxyhemoglobin dissociation during prolonged muscular work. *J Appl Physiol* 1974; 37:658.
92. Saltin B: Hemodynamic adaptations to exercise. *Am J Cardiol* 1985; 55:42D.
93. Shappell SD, Murray JA, Bellingham AJ, Woodson RD, Detter JC, Lenfant C: Adaptation to exercise: role of hemoglobin affinity for oxygen and 2,3-diphosphoglycerate. *J Appl Physiol* 1971; 30:827–832.
94. Saltin B, Henriksson J, Nygaard E, Andersen P: Fiber types and

metabolic potentials of skeletal muscles in sedentary man and endurance runners. *Ann NY Acad Sci* 1977; 301:3.

95. Hennemann E, Olson CB: Relations between structure and function in the design of skeletal muscle. *J Neurophysiol* 1965; 28:581.

96. Astrand P-O, Saltin B: Plasma and red cell volume after prolonged severe exercise. *J Appl Physiol* 1964; 19:829–832.

97. Cade JR, Free HJ, De Quesada AN, Shires DL, Roby L: Changes in body fluid composition and volume during vigorous exercise by athletes. *J Sports Med Phys Fitness* 1971; 11:172–178.

98. Lundvall J, Mellander S, Westling H, White T: Fluid transfer between blood and tissues during exercise. *Acta Physiol Scand* 1972; 85:258–269.

99. Costill DL, Sparks KE: Rapid fluid replacement following thermal dehydration. *J Appl Physiol* 1973; 34:299–303.

100. Gill DB, Costil DL: Calculation of percentage changes in volumes of blood and red cells in dehydration. *J Appl Physiol* 1973; 37:247–248.

101. Costill DL, Finks WJ: Plasma volume changes following exercise and thermal dehydration. *J Appl Physiol* 1974; 37:521–525.

102. Astrand P-O, Cuddy TE, Saltin B, Stenberg J: Cardiac output during submaximal and maximal work. *J Appl Physiol* 1964; 19:268–274.

103. Ekelund LG, Holmgren A: Circulatory and respiratory adaptation during long-term, non-steady state exercise in the sitting position. *Acta Physiol Scand* 1964; 62:240–255.

104. Detry JM, Gerin MG, Charlier AA, Brasseur LA: Hemodynamic and thermal apsects of prolonged intermittent exercise. *Int Z Angew Physiol* 1972; 30:171–185.

105. Hartley LH: Central circulatory function during prolonged exercise. *Ann NY Acad Sci* 1977; 301:189.

106. Mole PA: Exercise metabolism. In *Exercise Medicine: Physiological Principles and Clinical Applications*. Bove AA, Lowenthal DT (eds.). Orlando, Academic Press, 1983, pp. 43–88.

107. Astrand P-O: Aerobic work capacity during maximal performance under various conditions. *Circ Res* 1967; 20:202–210.

108. Zitnik RZ, Ambrosioni E, Shepherd JT: Effect of temperature on cutaneous venomotor reflexes in man. *J Appl Physiol* 1971; 31:507–512.

109. Johnson JM: Regulation of skin circulation during prolonged exercise. *Ann NY Acad Sci* 1977; 301:195.

110. Clausen JP, Klausen K, Rasussen B, Trap-Jensen J: Effect of strenuous arm and leg training on pulmonary ventilation, metabolism and blood pH during submaximal exercise. *Acta Physiol Scand* 1971; 82:8A.

111. Henschen S: Skilanglauf und skiwettlauf. Eine medizinische Sportstudie. *Mitt Med Klin*, Upsala (Jena), 1899.

112. Rost R, Hollmann W: Athlete's heart: A review of its historical assessment and new aspects. *Int J Sport Med* 1983; 4:147.

113. Jokl E: *Sudden Death of Athletes*. Springfield, Charles C. Thomas, 1985.

114. Huston TP, Puffer JC, Rodney WM: The athletic heart syndrome. *N Eng J Med* 1985; 313:24.

115. Bekaert I: The athlete's heart: An overview. In *Sports Cardiology:*

Exercise in Health and Cardiovascular Disease. Fagard RH, Bekaert IE (eds.). Dordrecht, Martinus Nijhoff, 1986, p. 3.

116. Rost R: The athlete's heart. In *Athletics and The Heart.* Rost R. Chicago, Year Book Medical Publishers, 1987, p. 26.

117. Breisch EA, White FC, Nimmo LE, McKirnan MD, Bloor CM: Exercise-induced cardiac hypertrophy: A correlation of blood flow and microvasculature. *J Appl Physiol* 1986; 60:1259–1267.

118. Branwell C, Ellis R: Clinical observations on Olympic athletes. *Arbeitsphysiologie* 1929; 2:51–60.

119. Grande F. Taylor HL: Adaptive changes in the heart, vessels and patterns of control under chronically high loads. In *Handbook of Physiology.* Hamilton WF, Dow P (eds.). Circ Proc Am Physiol Soc. Washington, 1965, Vol. 3, p. 2615.

120. Ekblom B, Kilbom A, Soltysiak J: Physical training, bradycardia and autonomic nervous system. *Scand J Clin Lab Invest* 1973; 32:251.

121. Holmgren A, Mossfeldt F, Sjostrand T, Strom G: Effect of training on work capacity, total hemoglobin, blood volume, heart volume, and pulse rate in recumbent and upright positions. *Acta Physiol Scand* 1960; 50:72.

122. Badeer HS: Resting bradycardia of exercise training: A concept based on currently available data. In *Recent Advances in Studies on Cardiac Structure and Metabolism.* Roy PE, Rona G. (eds.). Baltimore, University Park Press, 1975, Vol. 20, p. 553.

123. Barnard RJ, Corre K, Cho H: Effect of training on the resting heart rate of rats. *Eur J Appl Physiol* 1976; 35:285.

124. Musshoff K, Reindell H, Klepzig H: Stroke volume, arteriovenous difference, cardiac output and physical working capacity, and their relationship to heart volume. *Acta Cardiol* 1959; 14:427–452.

125. Frick MH, Konttinen A, Sarajas HSS: Effects of physical training on circulation at rest and during exercise. *Am J Cardiol* 1963; 12: 142–147.

126. Tabakin BS, Hanson JS, Levy AM: Effects of physical training on the cardiovascular and respiratory response to graded upright exercise in distance runners. *Br Heart J* 1965; 27:205–210.

127. Ekblom B, Astrand P-O, Saltin B, Stenberg J, Wallstrom B: Effect of training on circulatory response to exercise. *J Appl Physiol* 1968; 24:518–528.

128. Christensen EH, Hansen O: Arbeitsfahigkeit und Ehrnahrung. *Scand Arch Physiol* 1939; 81:160.

129. Kilbom A, Astrand I: Physical training with submaximal intensities in women. II. Effect on cardiac output. *Scand J Clin Lab Invest* 1971; 28:163.

130. Rowell LB: Factors affecting the prediction of the maximal oxygen intake from measurements made during submaximal work with observations related to factors which may limit maximal oxygen intake. Thesis. Minneapolis, 1962.

131. Ekblom B: Effect on physical training on oxygen transport system in man. *Acta Physiol Scand* 1969; 77 (Suppl. 328):1–45.

132. Kihlbom A: Physical training in women. *Scand J Clin Lab Invest* 1971; 28 (Suppl. 119):345.

133. Gollnick PD, Armstrong RB, Saubertin CW, Piehl K, Saltin B:

Enzyme activity and fiber composition in skeletal muscle of untrained and trained men. *J Appl Physiol* 1972; 33:312.

134. Holloszy JO: Adaptations of muscular tissue to training. *Prog Cardiovasc Dis* 1976; 18:445–458.
135. Anderson KL: The cardiovascular system in exercise. In *Exercise Physiology*. Falls HB (ed.). New York, Academic Press, 1968, pp. 79–128.
136. Rowell LB: Cardiovascular limitations to work capacity. In *Physiology of Work Capacity and Fatigue*. Simonson E (ed.). Springfield, Thomas, 1971, pp. 132–169.
137. Clausen JP, Larsen OA, Trap-Jensen J: Physical training in the management of coronary artery disease. *Circulation* 1969; 40:143–154.
138. Saltin B, Karlsson J: Muscle glycogen utilization during work of different intensities. In *Muscle Metabolism during Exercise*. Pernow B, Saltin B (eds.). New York, Plenum, 1971, pp. 289–299.
139. Grimby G, Saltin B: Physiological effects of physical training. *Scand J Rehab Med* 1971; 3:6.
140. Higginbotham MB, Morris KG, Williams RS, McHale PA, Coleman RD, Cobb FR: Regulation of stroke volume during submaximal and maximal upright exercise in normal man. *Circ Res* 1986; 58:281–291.
141. Ekblom B, Hermansen L: Cardiac outputs in athletes. *J Appl Physiol* 1968; 25:619.
142. Oscai LB, Williams BT, Hertig BA: Effect of exercise on blood volume. *J Appl Physiol* 1968; 26:622–624.
143. Saltin B, Grimby G: Physiological analysis of middle-aged and old former athletes. Comparison with still active athletes of the same ages. *Circulation* 1968; 38:1104–1115.
144. Saltin B, Hartley LH, Kilbom A, Astrand I: Physical training in sedentary middle-aged and older men. II. Oxygen uptake, heart rate, and blood lactate concentration at submaximal and maximal exercise. *Scand J Clin Lab Invest* 1969; 24:323–334.
145. Cook DR, Gualtier WS, Galla SJ: Body fluid volumes of college athletes and non-athletes. *Med Sci Sports* 1970; 1:217–220.
146. Montage HJ, Metzner HL, Keller JB, Johnson BC, Epstein FH: Habitual physical activity and blood pressure. *Med Sci Sports* 1972; 4:175–181.
147. Bass DE, Buskirk ER, Iampietro PF, Mager M: Comparison of blood volume during physical conditioning heat acclimatization and sedentary living. *J Appl Physiol* 1958; 12:186–188.
148. Herrlick HC, Raab W, Gigee W: Influence of muscular training and of catecholamines on cardiac acetylcholine and cholinesterase. *Arch Int Pharmacodyn Ther* 1960; 129:201–215.
149. Reuschlein PS, Reddan WG, Burpee J, Gee JBL, Rankin J: Effect of physical training on the pulmonary diffusing capacity during submaximal work. *J Appl Physiol* 1968; 24:152–158.
150. Hartley LH, Grimby G, Kilbom A, Nilsson NJ, Astrand I, Bjure J, Ekblom B, Saltin B: Physical training in sedentary middle-aged and older men. *Scan J Clin Lab Invest* 1969; 24:335–344.
151. Pollock ML: The quantification of endurance training programs. In: Wilmore JH (ed.). *Exercise and Sport Sciences Reviews*. New York, Academic Press, 1973, Vol. 1, pp. 155–188.

152. Pechar GS, McArdle WD, Katch FI, Magel JR, Deluca J: Specificity of cardio-respiratory adaptation to bicycle and treadmill training. *J Appl Physiol* 1974; 36:753−756.

153. Magel JR, Foglin F, McArdle WD, Gutin B, Pechar S, Katch FI: Specificity of swim training on maximum oxygen uptake. *J Appl Physiol* 1974; 38:151−155.

154. Ohman M, Kelly J: Beta-adrenoreceptor changes in exercise and physical training. In *Sports Cardiology: Exercise in Health and Disease*. Fagard RH, Bekaert RH (eds.). Dordrecht, Martinus Nijhoff, 1986, p. 136.

155. Muller EA: Die Pulszahl als Kennzeichen fur Stoffaustausch und Ermudbarkeit des arbeitenden Muskels. *Arbeitsphysiol* 1943; 12:92.

156. Clausen JP, Trap-Jensen J, Lassen NA: The effects of training on the heart rate during arm and leg exercise. *Scand J Clin Lab Invest* 1970; 26:295.

157. Hanson JS, Nedde WH: Preliminary observations on physical training for hypertensive males. *Circ Res* 1970; 26, 27 (Suppl. 1):49−53.

158. Boyer JL, Kasch FW: Exercise therapy in hypertensive men. *JAMA* 1970; 211:1668−1771.

159. Choquette G, Ferguson RJ: Blood pressure reduction in "borderline" hypertensives following physical training. *Can Med Assoc J* 1973; 108:699−703.

160. Clausen JP, Trap-Jensen T: Effects of training on the distribution of cardiac output in patients with coronary artery disease. *Circulation* 1970; 42:611−624.

161. Redwood DR, Rosing DR, Epstein SE: Circulatory and symptomatic effects of physical training in patients with coronary artery disease and angina pectoris. *N Engl J Med* 1972; 286:459.

162. Grimby G, Haggendal E, Saltin B: Local xenon-133 clearance from the quadriceps muscle during exercise. *J Appl Physiol* 1967; 22: 305−310.

163. Varnauskas E, Bjorntorp P, Fahlen M, Prerovsky I, Stenberg J: Effects of physical training on exercise blood flow and enzymatic activity in skeletal muscle. *Cardiovasc Res* 1970; 4:418

164. Stenberg J: Muscle blood flow during exercise. Effects of training. In *Coronary Heart Disease and Physical Fitness*. Larsen OA, Malmborg RO (eds.). Copenhagen, Munksgaard, 1971, p. 80.

165. Bergman H, Bjorntorp P, Conradson T-P, Fahlen M, Stenberg J, Varnauskas E: Enzymatic and circulatory adjustments to physical training in middle-aged men. *Eur J Clin Invest* 1973; 3:414.

166. Holloszy JO, Booth FW: Biochemical adaptations to endurance exercise in muscle. *Ann Rev Physiol* 1976; 38:273−291.

167. Rasmussen B, Klausen K, Clausen JP, Trap-Jensen J: Pulmonary ventilation, blood gases and blood pH after training of the arms or the legs. *J Appl Physiol* 1975; 38:250.

168. Grimby G: The physiological background to physical training in cardiac patients. In *Progress in Cardiology*, Vol 2. Yu PN, Goodwin JF (eds.). Philadelphia, Lea and Febiger, 1973; pp. 281−290.

169. Klausen K, Rasmussen B, Clausen JP, Trap-Jensen J: Blood lactate from exercising extremities before and after arm or leg training. *Am J Physiol* 1974; 227:67.

170. Ricci G, Castaldi G, Masotti M, Lupi G, Bonetti D: 2, 3-diphospho-glycerate and P_{50} after exercise. *Acta Haematol* 1984; 7:410.
171. Carew TE, Birkett IM, Joseph MG, Covell JW: Myocardial fiber angle distribution in chronic exercise hypertrophy and chronic cardiac dilatation in the dog. (Abstr.#1185) *Fed Proc* 1973; 32:433.
172. Morganroth J, Maron BJ, Henry W, Epstein SE: Comparative left ventricular dimensions in trained athletes. *Ann Intern Med* 1975; 82:521–524.
173. Roeske WR, O'Rourke RA, Klein A, Leopold G, Karliner JS: Non-invasive evaluation of ventricular hypertrophy in professional athletes. *Circulation* 1976; 53:286–291.
174. Gilbert CA, Nutter DO, Felner JM, Perkins JV, Heymsfield SB, Schlant RC: Echocardiographic study of cardiac dimensions and function in the endurance-trained athlete. *Am J Cardiol* 1977; 40: 528–533.
175. Underwood RH, Schwade JL: Noninvasive analysis of cardiac function of elite distance runners: Echocardiography, vectorcardiography and cardiac intervals. *Ann NY Acad Sci* 1977; 301:297.
176. Ehsani AA, Hagberg JM, Hickson RC: Rapid changes in left ventricular dimensions and mass in response to physical conditioning and deconditioning. *Am J Cardiol* 1978; 42:52.
177. Crews J, Aldinger EE: Effect of chronic exercise on myocardial function. *Am Heart J* 1967; 74:536.
178. McCullagh WH, Covell JW, Ross J Jr: Left ventricular dilatation and diastolic compliance changes during chronic volume overloading. *Circulation* 1972; 45:943–951.
179. Ross J Jr, McCullagh WH: The nature of enhanced performance of the dilated left ventricle during chronic volume overloading. *Circ Res* 1972; 30:549–556.
180. Scheuer J, Penpargkul S, Bhan AK: Experimental observations on the effects of physical training upon intrinsic cardiac physiology and biochemistry. *Am J Cardiol* 1974; 33:744.
181. Bhan AK, Scheuer J: Effects of physical training on cardiac myosin ATPase activity. *Am J Physiol* 1975; 228:1178–1182.
182. Williams JF, Potter RD: Effect of exercise conditioning on the intrinsic contractile state of cat myocardium. *Circ Res* 1976; 39:425–428.
183. Bersohn MM, Scheuer J: Effects of physical training on end-diastolic volume and myocardial performance of isolated rat hearts. *Circ Res* 1977; 40:510.
184. Segal LD: Myocardial adaptations to physical conditioning. In *Exercise in Health and Disease*. Amsterdam EA, Wilmore JH, DeMaria AN (eds.). New York, Yorke Medical Books, 1977, p. 95.
185. Dowell RT, Stone HL, Sordahl L, Asimakis GS: Contractile function and myofibrillar ATPase activity in the exercise-trained dog heart. *J Appl Physiol* 1977; 43:977.
186. Carew TE, Covell JW: Left ventricular function in exercise-induced hypertrophy in dogs. *Am J Cardiol* 1978; 42:82–87.
187. DeMaria AN, Neumann A, Lee G, Fowler W, Mason DT: Alterations in ventricular mass and performance induced by exercise training in man evaluated by echocardiography. *Circulation* 1978; 57:237.

188. Holmgren A, Standell T: The relationship between heart volume, total hemoglobin and physical working capacity in former athletes. *Acta Med Scand* 1959; 163:149–160.
189. Roskamm VH, Weidenbach J, Reindell H: Nachuntersuchungen von 18 sportlern, die vor wenigsten 10 Jahren einen unvollstandigen bzw, einen physiologischen Rechtsschenkel block in EKG gehabt hatten. *Z Kreislaufforsch* 1966; 55:783–794.
190. Pyorala K, Karvonen MJ, Taskinen P, Takkunen J, Kyronseppa H, Peltokallio P: Cardiovascular studies on former endurance athletes. *Am J Cardiol* 1967; 20:191–205.
191. Saltin B: Guidelines for physical training. *Scan J Rehab Med* 1971; 3:39.
192. Roskamm H: Optimum patterns of exercise for healthy adults. *Can Med Assoc J* 1967; 96:895.
193. Cousineau D, Ferguson RJ, de Champlian J, Cauthier C, Cote P, Bourassa M: Catecholamines in coronary sinus during exercise in man before and after training. *J Appl Physiol* 1977; 43:801.
194. Lehman M, Dickhuth HH, Schmid Porzig H, Keul J: Plasma catecholamines, β-adrenergic receptors, and isoproterenol sensitivity in endurance trained and non-endurance trained volunteers. *Eur J Appl Physiol* 1984; 52:362.
195. Lehman M, Keul J: Die konjugierten Plasmakatecholamine sind bei Kraft sportlern in Ruhe und wahrend Korper arbeit niedriger als bei Untrainierten. *Klin Wochenschr* 1985; 63:37.
196. Lehman M, Schmid P, Bergdolt E: Bestimmung von β-Rezeptoren an polymorphkernigen intakten Leukocyten im autologen Plasma. *J Clin Chem Clin Biochem* 1983; 21:805.
197. Hermansen L, Wachtlova M: Capillary density of skeletal muscle in well trained and untrained men. *J Appl Physiol* 1971; 30:860–863.
198. Arcos JC, Sohol RS, Sun S-C, Argus MF, Burch GE: Changes in ultrastructure and respiratory control mitochondria of rat heart hypertrophied by exercise. *Exp Mol Pathol* 1968; 8:49–65.
199. Gollnick PD, King DW: Effect of exercise and training on mitochondria of rat skeletal muscle. *Am J Physiol* 1969; 216:1502–1509.
200. Morgan TE, Cobb LA, Short FA, Ross R, Gunn DR: Effect of long-term exercise on human muscle mitochondria. In *Muscle Metabolism during Exercise*. Pernow B, Saltin B (eds.). New York, Plenum Press, 1971, pp. 87–95.
201. Kiessling K-H, Piehl K, Lundquist C-G: Effect of physical training on ultrastructural features in human skeletal muscle. In *Muscle Metabolism during Exercise*. Pernow B, Saltin B (eds.). New York, Plenum Press, 1971, p. 505.
202. Edington DW, Cosmas AC: Effect of maturation and training on mitochondrial size distributions in rat hearts. *J Appl Physiol* 1972; 33:715–718.
203. Hoppler H, Luthi P, Claassen H, Wiebel ER, Howald H: The ultrastructure of normal human skeletal muscle: A morphometric analysis of untrained men, women, and well-trained orienteers. *Pfluegers Arch* 1973; 344:217–232.
204. Holloszy JO: Biochemical adaptations to exercise: Aerobic metabo-

lism. In: *Reviews in Exercise and Sports Sciences*. Willmore JH (eds). New York Academic Press, 1973; p. 45.

205. Brodal P, Ingjer F, Hermansen L: Capillary supply of skeletal muscle fibers in untrained and endurance trained men. *Am J Physiol* 1977; 232:705.

206. Holloszy JO, Oscai LB, Don IJ, Mole PA: Mitochondrial citric acid cycle and related enzymes: Adaptive response to exercise. *Biochem Biophys Res Commun* 1970; 40:1368–1373.

207. Mole PA, Oscai LB, Holloszy JO: Adaptation of muscle to exercise. Increase in levels of palmityl CoA synthetase, earnitine palmityltransferase and palmityl CoA dehydrogenase and in the capacity to oxidize fatty acids. *J Clin Invest* 1971; 50:2323–2330.

208. Dohm GL, Huston RL, Askew EW, Fleshnood HL: Effects of exercise, training, and diet on muscle citric acid cycle enzyme activity. *Can J Biochem* 1973; 51:849–854.

209. Holloszy JO, Mole PA, Baldwin KM, Terjung RL: Exercise induced enzymatic adaptations in muscle. In *Limiting Factors of Physical Performance*. Keul J (ed.). Stuttgart, Georg Thieme, 1973, pp. 66–80.

210. Gollnick PD, Sembrowich WL: Adaptations in human skeletal muscle as a result of training. In *Exercise in Health and Disease*. Amsterdam EA, Wilmore JH, DeMaria AN (eds.). New York, Yorke Medical Books, 1977, p. 70.

211. Holloszy JO: Biochemical adaptations in muscle: Effects of exercise on mitochondrial oxygen uptake and respiratory enzyme activity in skeletal muscle. *J Biol Chem* 1967; 242:2278.

212. Holloszy JO, Oscai LB, Mole PA, Don IJ: Biochemical adaptations to endurance exercise in skeletal muscle. In *Muscle Metabolism during Exercise*. Pernow B and Saltin B (eds.). New York, Plenum Press, 1971, p. 51.

213. Resink TJ, Gevers W, Noakes TD, Opie LH: Increased cardiac myosin ATPase activity as a biochemical adaptation to running training: Enhanced response to catecholamines and a role for myosin phosphorylation. *J Molec Cell Cardiol* 1981; 13:679–694.

214. Pattengale PK, Holloszy JO: Augmentation of skeletal muscle myoglobin by a program of treadmill running. *Am J Physiol* 1967; 213:783–785.

215. Scholander PF: Oxygen transport through hemoglobin solutions. *Science* 1960; 131:585–590.

216. Hemmingsen EA: Enhancement of oxygen transport by myoglobin. *Comp Biochem Physiol* 1963; 10:239–244.

217. Hermansen L, Hultman E, Saltin B: Muscle glycogen during prolonged severe exercise. *Acta Physiol Scand* 1967; 71:129–139.

218. Saltin B, Karlsson J: Muscle ATP, CP and lactate during exercise after physical conditioning. In *Muscle Metabolism during Exercise*. Pernow B and Saltin B (eds.). New York, Plenum, 1971, pp. 395–399.

219. Christensen EH, Hansen O: Respiratorischen Quotient und O_2-Aufnahme. *Scand Arch Physiol* 1939; 81:180–189.

220. Issekutz B, Miller HI, Rodahl K: Lipid and carbohydrate metabolism during exercise. *Fed Proc* 1966; 25:1415–1420.

221. Robinson S, Harmon PM: The lactic acid mechanism and certain properties of the blood in relation to training. *Am J Physiol* 1941; 132:757–769.
222. Cobb LA, Johnson WP: Hemodynamic relationships of anaerobic metabolism and plasma free fatty acids during prolonged strenuous exercise in trained and untrained subjects. *J Clin Invest* 1963; 42: 800–810.
223. Holloszy JO, Skinner JS, Toro G, Cureton TK: Effect of a six month program of endurance exercise on the serum lipids of middle-aged men. *Am J Cardiol* 1964; 14:753.
224. Siegel W, Blomqvist G, Mitchell JH: Effects of a quantitative physical training program on middle-aged sedentary men. *Circulation* 1970; 41:19.
225. Froberg SO: Effects of training and of acute exercise in trained rats. *Metabolism* 1971; 20:1044–51.
226. Lopez-Santolina A, Vial R, Balart L, Arrogave G: Effect of exercise and physical fitness on serum lipids and lipoproteins. *Atherosclerosis* 1974; 20:1–9.
227. Havel RJ, Carlson LA, Ekelund L-G, Holmgren A: Turnover rate and oxidation of different free fatty acids in man during exercise. *J Appl Physiol* 1964; 19:613.
228. Issekutz B Jr, Miller HI, Paul P, Rodahl K: Aerobic work capacity and plasma FFA turnover. *J Appl Physiol* 1965; 20:293.
229. Julius S, Amery A, Whitlock LS, Conway J: Influence of age on the hemodynamic response to exercise. *Circulation* 1967; 36:222.
230. Detry J-M, Rousseau M, Vandenbroucke G, Kusumi F, Brasseur LA, Bruce RA: Increased arteriovenous oxygen difference after physical training in coronary heart disease. *Circulation* 1971; 44:109.
231. Astrand I, Astrand P-O, Hollback J, Kilbom A: Reduction in maximal oxygen uptake with age. *J Appl Physiol* 1973; 35:649.
232. Bruce RA, Kusumi F, Niederberger M, Petersen JL: Cardiovascular mechanisms of functional aerobic impairment in patients with coronary heart disease. *Circulation* 1974; 49:696.
233. Adams WC, McHenry MM, Bernauer EM: Long-term physiologic adaptations to exercise with special reference to performance and cardiorespiratory function in health and disease. *Am J Cardiol* 1974; 33:765.
234. Rousseau MF, Brasseur LA, Detry J-MR: Hemodynamic determinants of maximal oxygen intake in patients with healed myocardial infarction: Influence of physical training. *Circulation* 1973; 48:943.
235. Muller O, Rorvik K: Hemodynamic consequences of coronary heart disease with observations during anginal pain and on the effect of nitroglycerine. *Br Heart J* 1958; 20:302.
236. Malmborg RO: A clinical and hemodynamic analysis of factors limiting the cardiac performance in patients with coronary heart disease. *Acta Med Scand* 1964; 177 (Suppl. 426):1–94.
237. McCallister B, Yipinstoi T, Hallerman F: Left ventricular performance during mild supine leg exercise in coronary artery disease. *Circulation* 1968; 37:922.

238. Parker JO, West RO, DiGeorgi S: The effect of nitroglycerine on coronary blood flow and the hemodynamic response to exercise in coronary artery disease. *Am J Cardiol* 1971; 27:59.

239. Bygdemon S, Wahren J: Influence of body position on the anginal threshold during leg-exercise. *Eur J Clin Invest* 1974; 4:201.

240. Clausen JP, Trap-Jensen J: Heart rate and arterial blood pressure during exercise in patients with angina pectoris: Effect of training and of nitroglycerin. *Circulation* 1976; 53:436—442.

241. Bjernulf A: Hemodynamic effects of physical training after myocardial infarction. *Acta Med Scand* 1973; 194:(Suppl. 548).

242. Frick MH, Katila M: Hemodynamic consequences of physical training after myocardial infarction. *Circulation* 1968; 37:192.

243. Varnauskas E, Bergman H, Houk P, Bjorntorp P: Hemodynamic effects of physical training in coronary patients. *Lancet* 1966; 2:8.

244. Bergman H, Varnauskas E: The hemodynamic effects of physical training in coronary patients. In *Physical Activity and Aging: Medicine and Sport*, Vol. 4. Brunner D and Jokl E (eds.). Basel, Karger, 1970, p. 138.

245. Kasch FW, Boyer JL: Changes in maximum work capacity resulting from six months training in patients with ischemic heart disease. *Med Sci Sports* 1969; 1:156.

246. Sanne H, Grimby G, Wilhelmsen L: Physical training during convalescence after myocardial infarction. In *Coronary Heart Disease and Physical Fitness*. Laren OA, Malmborg RO (eds.). Copenhagen, Munksgaard, 1971, pp. 183—188.

247. Benestad AM: *Treningsterapi vid koronare hjertesjukdomar.* Oslo, Universitets-forlaget, 1971.

248. Detry J-M, Bruce RA: Effects of physical training on exertional S-T segment depression in coronary heart disease. *Circulation* 1971; 44:390.

249. Degre S, Messin R, Vandermoten P, DeMaret B, Haissly JC, Salhadin J, Denoglin H: Aspects physio-pathologiques de l'entrainement musculaire chez des patients atteints d'infarctus du myocarde. *Acta Cardiol* (Brux) 1972; 27:445.

250. Sanne H: Exercise tolerance and physical training of non-selected patients after myocardial infarction. *Acta Med Scand* 1973; (Suppl. 551):194.

251. Frick MH, Katila M, Sjogren AL: Cardiac function and physical training after myocardial infarction. In *Coronary Heart Disease and Physical Fitness*. Laren OA, Malmborg RO (eds.). Copenhagen, Munksgaard, 1971, pp. 43—47.

252. Trap-Jensen J, Clausen JP: Effect of training on the relation of heart rate and blood pressure to the outset of pain in effort angina pectoris. In *Coronary Heart Disease and Physical Fitness*. Laren OA, Malmborg RO (eds.). Copenhagen, Munksgaard, 1971, p. 111—114.

253. Lehman M, Berg A, Keul J: Anderung der sympathischen Aktivitat bei 18 Postinfarktpatienten nach 1 Jahr Bewegungstherapie. *Z Kardiol* 1984; 73:756.

254. Harrison TR, Dixon K, Russell RO Jr, Bidwai DS, Coleman HN: The

relation of age to the duration of contraction, ejection, and relaxation of the normal human heart. *Am Heart J* 1964; 67:189–199.

255. Strandell T: Mechanical systole at rest, during and after exercise in supine and sitting position in young and old men. *Acta Physiol Scand* 1964; 60:197–216.

256. Gerstenblith G, Lakatta EG, Weisfeldt ML: Age changes in myocardial function and exercise response. *Prog Cardiovasc Dis* 1976; 19: 1–21.

257. Strandell T: Heart rate, arterial lactate concentration and oxygen uptake during exercise in old men compared with young men. *Acta Physiol Scand* 1964; 60:197–216.

258. Brandfonbrener M, Landowne M, Shock NW: Changes in cardiac output with age. *Circulation* 1955; 12:557–566.

259. Granath A, Jonsson B, Strandell T: Circulation in healthy old men studied by right heart catheterization at rest and during exercise in supine and sitting position. *Acta Med Scand* 1964; 176:425–446.

260. Strandell T: Circulatory studies on healthy old men. *Acta Med Scand* 1964; (Suppl. 414) 175:1–44.

261. Conway J, Wheeler R, Sannerstedt R: Sympathetic nervous activity during exercise in relation to age. *Cardiovasc Res* 1971; 5:577–581.

262. Dock W: Cardiomyopathies of the senescent and senile. *Cardiovasc Clin* 1972; 4:362–373.

263. Robinson S: Experimental studies of physical fitness in relation to age. *Arbeitsphysiol* 1938; 10:251–323.

264. Astrand I: Aerobic work capacity in men and women with special reference to age. *Acta Physiol Scand* 1960; (Suppl. 169) 49:1–92.

265. Astrand P-O, Rodahl K: Physical work capacity. In *Textbook of Work Physiology*, 2nd ed. Astrand P-O, Rodahl K (eds.). New York, McGraw-Hill, 1977, p. 289.

266. Tsuchiya M, Kawasoki S, Masuya K, Matsui S, Ishise S, Hara S, Funatsu T, Takeuchi N, Maeda M, Onoe T, Kin T, Takekoshi N, Murokami E, Mifune J, Murakami M: The effect of age on hemodynamics. *Jap J Geriatr* 1962; 9:364–369.

267. Kuikka JT, Lansimies E: Effect of age on cardiac index, stroke index and left ventricular ejection fraction at rest and during exercise as studied by radiocardiography. *Acta Physiol Scand* 1982; 114:339.

268. Rodeheffer RJ, Gerstenblith G, Becker LC, Fleg JL, Weisfeldt ML, Lakatta EG: Exercise cardiac output is maintained with advancing age in healthy human subjects: Cardiac dilatation and increased stroke volume compensate for a diminished heart rate. *Circulation* 1984; 69:203.

269. Tartulier M, Bourret M, Deyrieux F: Pulmonary arterial pressures in normal subjects, effects of age and exercise. *Bull Physiopathol Resp* 1972; 8:1295–1321.

270. Weisfeldt ML, Lowen WA, Shock NW: Resting and active mechanical properties of trabeculae carneae from aged male rats. *Am J Physiol* 1971; 220:1921–1927.

271. Verzar F: The stages and consequences of aging of collagen. *Gerontologia* 1969; 15:233–239.

272. Tomanek RJ, Taunton CA, Liskop KS: Relationship between age, chronic exercise, and connective tissue of the heart. *J Gerontol* 1972; 27:33–38.

273. Berglund E, Sarnoff SJ, Isaacs JP: Ventricular function. Role of the pericardium in regulation of cardiovascular hemodynamics. *Circ Res* 1955; 3:133–139.

274. Roy CS: The elastic properties of the arterial wall. *J Physiol* (London) 1880–1882; 3:125–159.

275. Learoyd BM, Taylor MG: Alterations with age in the viscollastic properties of human arterial walls. *Circ Res* 1966; 18:278–292.

276. Gonzna ER, Marble AE, Shaw A, Holland JG: Age-related changes in the mechanics of the aorta and pulmonary artery of man. *J Appl Physiol* 1974; 36:407–411.

277. Bader H: Dependence of wall stress in the human thoracic aorta on age and pressure. *Circ Res* 1967; 20:354–361.

278. Roach MR, Burton AC: The effect of age on the elasticity of human iliac arteries. *Can J Biochem* 1959; 37:557–570.

279. Alpert NR, Gale HH, Taylor N: The effect of age on contractile protein ATPase activity and the velocity of shortening. In *Factors Influencing Myocardial Contractility*. Kavaler K, Tranz RD, Roberts J (eds.). New York, Academic Press, 1967, pp. 127–133.

280. Alpert NR, Hamrell BB, Halpern W: Mechanical and biochemical correlates of cardiac hypertrophy. *Circ Res* 1974; 34–35 (Suppl. II):71–82.

281. Rakusan K, Poupa O: Capillaries and muscle fibers in the heart of the old rats. *Gerontologia* 1964; 9:107–112.

282. Bloor CM, Pasyk S, Leon AS: Interaction of age and exercise on organ and cellular development. *Am J Pathol* 1970; 58:185–199.

283. Kihlbom A, Hartley LH, Saltin B, Bjure J, Grimby G, Astrand I: Physical training in sedentary middle-aged and older men. I. Medical evaluation. *Scand J Clin Lab Invest* 1969; 24:315.

284. Benestad AM: Trainability of old men. *Acta Med Scand* 1965; 178:321.

285. Edstrom L, Nystrom B: Histochemical types and sizes of fibres in normal human muscles. *Acta Neurol Scand* 1969; 45:257.

286. Wahren J: Substrate utilization by exercising muscle in man. In *Progress in Cardiology*, Vol. 2. Yu PN, Goodwin JF (eds.). Philadelphia, Lea and Febiger, 1973, pp. 255–279.

287. Felig P, Wahren J: Fuel homeostasis in exercise. *N Engl J Med* 1975; 293:1078–1084.

288. Andres R, Cader G, Zierles KL: The quantitatively minor role of carbohydrates in oxidative metabolism by skeletal muscle in intact man in the basal state: Measurements of oxygen and glucose uptake and carbon dioxide and lactate production in the forearm. *J Clin Invest* 1956; 35:671–682.

289. Hultman E: Studies on muscle metabolism of glycogen and active phosphate in man with special reference to exercise and diet. *Scand J Clin Lab Invest* 1967; 19 (Suppl. 94):1–63.

290. Pernow B, Wahren J: Lactate and pyruvate formation and oxygen utilization in the human forearm muscles during work of high intensity and varying duration. *Acta Physiol Scand* 1962; 56:267.

291. Klassen GA, Andrew GM, Becklake MR: Effect of training on total and regional blood flow and metabolism in paddlers. *J Appl Physiol* 1970; 28:397.
292. Wahren J, Felig P, Ahlborg G, Jorfedlt L: Glucose metabolism during leg exercise in man. *J Clin Invest* 1971; 50:2715–2725.
293. Wahren J, Felig P, Hendler R, Ahlborg G: Glucose and amino acid metabolism during recovery after exercise. *J Appl Physiol* 1973; 34:838–845.
294. Jorfeldt L, Wahren J: Human forearm muscle metabolism during exercise. V. Quantitative aspects of glucose uptake and lactate production during prolonged exercise. *Scand J Clin Lab Invest* 1970; 26:73.
295. Ahlborg G, Felig P, Hagenfeldt L, Hendler R, Wahren J: Substrate turnover during prolonged exercise in man: Splanchnic and leg metabolism of glucose, free fatty acids, and amino acids. *J Clin Invest* 1974; 53:1080–1090.
296. Felig P: Metabolic and endocrine disorders and exercise. In *Exercise Medicine: Physiological Principles and Clinical Applications.* Bove AA, Lowenthal DT (eds.). Orlando, Academic Press, 1983, pp. 305–320.
297. Carlsten A, Hallgren B, Jorgenburg R, Svanborg A, Werko L: Arterial concentrations of fatty acids and free amino acids in healthy human individuals at rest and at different work loads. *Scand J Clin Lab Invest* 1962; 14:185.
298. Pozefsky T, Felig P, Tobin JD, Soeldner JS: Amino acid balance across tissues of the forearm in postabsorptive man: Effects of insulin at two dose levels. *J Clin Invest* 1969; 48:2273.
299. Felig P, Pozefsky T, Marliss E, Cahill GF Jr: Alanine: Key role in gluconeogenesis. *Science* 1970; 167:1003–1004.
300. Felig P, Wahren J. Amino acid metabolism in exercising man. *J Clin Invest* 1971; 50:2703.
301. Lowenstein JM: Ammonia production in muscle and other tissues: The purine nucleotide cycle. *Physiol Rev* 1972; 52:382–414.
302. Felig P: The glucose-alanine cycle. *Metabolism* 1973; 22:179–207.
303. Ross BD, Hems R, Krebs HA: The rate of gluconeogenesis from various precursors in the perfused rat liver. *Biochem J* 1967; 102:942.
304. Wahren J, Felig P, Havel RJ, Jorfedlt L, Pernow B, Saltin B: Amino acid metabolism in McArdle's syndrome. *N Engl J Med* 1973; 288: 774–777.
305. Young DR, Pelligra R, Shapira J, Adachi RR, Skrettingland K: Glucose oxidation and replacement during prolonged exercise in man. *J Appl Physiol* 1967; 23:734–741.
306. Felig P, Wahren J, Hendler R: Plasma glucagon levels in exercising man. *N Engl J Med* 1972; 287:184.
307. Levine SA, Godon B, Derick CL: Some changes in the chemical constituents of the blood following a marathon race. *JAMA* 1924; 82:1778–1779.
308. Hultman E, Nilsson LH: Liver glycogen in man: effect of different diets and muscular exercise. In *Muscle Metabolism during Exercise.* Pernow B, Saltin B (eds.). Proceedings of a Karolinska Institutet

Symposium Held in Stockholm, Sweden, Sept. 6–9, 1970. New York, Plenum Press, 1971, pp. 143–151.

309. Ahlborg B, Bergstrom J, Brohult J, Ekelund L-G, Hultman E, Maschio G: Human muscle glycogen content and capacity for prolonged exercise after different diets. *Forsvarsmedium* 1967; 3:85.

310. Bargstrom J, Hermansen L, Hultman E, Saltin B: Diet, muscle glycogen, and physical performance. *Acta Physiol Scand* 1967; 71:140.

311. Karlsson J, Saltin B: Diet, muscle glycogen, and endurance performance. *J Appl Physiol* 1971; 31:203.

312. Ahlborg B, Bergstrom J, Ekelund LG, Hultman E: Muscle glycogen and muscle electrolytes during prolonged physical exercise. *Acta Physiol Scand* 1967; 70:129–142.

313. Pernow B, Saltin B: Availability of substrates and capacity for prolonged heavy exercise in man. *J Appl Physiol* 1971; 31:416.

314. Galbo H, Host JJ, Christensen NJ: Glucagon and plasma catecholamine responses to graded and prolonged exercise in man. *J Appl Physiol* 1975; 38:70–76.

315. Rennie MJ, Jennet S, Johnson RH: The metabolic effects of strenuous exercise: A comparison between untrained subjects and racing cyclists. *Q J Exp Physiol* 1974; 59:201–212.

316. Gaesser GA, Brooks GA: Metabolic bases of excess post-exercise oxygen consumption: A review. *Med Sci Sports Exerc* 1984; 16:29.

317. Carlson LA, Pernow B: Studies on blood lipids during exercise. I. Arterial and venous plasma concentrations of unesterified fatty acids. *J Lab Clin Med* 1959; 53:833.

318. Rodahl K, Miller HJ, Issekutz B Jr: Plasma free fatty acids in exercise. *J Appl Physiol* 1964; 19:489.

319. Young DR, Shapira J, Forrest R, Adachi RR, Lim R, Pelligra R: Model for evaluation of fatty acid metabolism for man during prolonged exercise. *J Appl Physiol* 1967; 23:716.

320. Sady SP, Thompson PD, Cullinane EM, Kantor MA, Domagala E, Herbert PN: Prolonged exercise augments plasma triglyceride clearance. *JAMA* 1986; 256:2552–2555.

321. Lind AR, Taylor SH, Humphreys PW, Kennely BM, Donald KM: Circulatory effects of sustained voluntary muscle contraction. *Clin Sci* 1964; 27:229.

322. Donald KW, Lind AR, McNicol GW, Humphreys PW, Taylor SH, Staunton HP: Cardiovascular responses to sustained (static) contractins. *Circ Res* 1967; 20 (Suppl. 1):15.

323. Nutter DO, Schlant RC, Hurst JW: Isometric exercise and the cardiovascular system. *Mod Concepts Cardiovasc Dis* 1972; 41:11.

324. Fisher ML, Nutter DO, Jacobs W, Schlant RC: Haemodynamic responses to isometric exercise (handgrip) in patients with heart disease. *Br Heart J* 1973; 35:422–432.

325. Grossman W, McLaurin LP, Salty SB, Paraskos JA, Dalen JE, Dexter L: Changes in the inotropic state of the left ventricle during isometric exercise. *Br Heart J* 1973; 35:697.

326. Stefadouros MA, Grossman W, El Shahawy M, Witham AC: The effect of isometric exercise on the left ventricular volume in normal man. *Circulation* 1974; 49:1185.

327. Haissly J-C, Messin R, Degre S, Vandermoten P, DeMaret B, De-Nolin H: Comparative response to isometric (static) and dynamic exercise tests in coronary disease. *Am J Cardiol* 1974; 33:791−795.
328. Flessas AP, Connelly GP, Handa S, Tilney CR, Kloster CK, Rimmer RH Jr, Keefe JF, Klein MD, Ryan TJ: Effects of isometric exercise on the end-diastolic pressure, volumes, and function of the left ventricle in man. *Circulation* 1976; 53:839.
329. Ludbrook P, Karliner JS, O'Rourke RA: Effects of submaximal isometric handgrip of left ventricular size and wall motion. *Am J Cardiol* 1974; 33:30.
330. Lind AR, McNicol GW: Circulatory responses to sustained handgrip contractions performed during other exercise, both rhythmic and static. *J Physiol* 1967; 192:595.
331. Kitamura K, Jorgensen CR, Gobel FL, Taylor HL, Wang Y: Hemodynamic correlates of myocardial oxygen consumption during upright exercise. *J Appl Physiol* 1972; 32:516.
332. Astrand P-O, Christensen EH: Aerobic work capacity. In *Oxygen in the Animal Organism*. Dickens F, Neil E, Widdos WF (eds.): New York, Pergamon Press, 1964, p. 295.
333. Graettinger WF: The cardiovascular response to chronic physical exertion and exercise training: An echocardiographic review. *Am Heart J* 1984; 108:1014−1018.

2

Exercise Stress Testing

L. Thomas Sheffield, M.D.

INTRODUCTION

The Nature of Exercise Stress Testing

Stress testing aims to show how the body reacts to calibrated increases in exercise stress. The time course of increases in heart rate, blood pressure, respiration, and perceived level of exertion provide data which permit quantitative estimation of cardiovascular fitness. To a limited extent, these data also correlate with more general aspects of fitness such as flexibility and musculoskeletal strength.

In addition to numerical data, stress tests provide an opportunity for a health professional to observe a person, a human physiologic system, in the process of performing in the range of peak power. The sports trainer can learn much from the way the subjects stride, their arm motions, breathing, and facial expression. The physician can recognize anxiety and hyperventilation episodes, classic angina pectoris, and nonanginal chest wall pain. By continually observing the electrocardiogram, he or she can detect ischemic-type ST segment depression and can detect and classify disturbance in cardiac rhythm and conduction brought on or aggravated by exercise.

From: Fletcher GF: *Exercise in the Practice of Medicine*, 2nd Revised Edition. Mount Kisco, NY, Futura Publishing Co., Inc., © 1988.

Thus the exercise stress test, when employed at best advantage, is actually a multifactoral study of the subject's reaction to exercise, a detector of cardiovascular disease, and a measure of its severity.

Physiological Bases of Exercise Testing

The arterial blood supply to the myocardium, and indeed, to all muscles and organs, is normally sufficient for the maximal perfusion requirement of which the organ is capable. If obstructive disease takes place within the coronary artery, only minimal reduction in maximal blood flow will take place until the degree of arterial obstruction becomes quite advanced.[1] If the subject engages only in sedentary behavior, avoiding any activity which requires maximal or near maximal coronary blood flow, it is possible for an advanced degree of atherosclerotic coronary arterial obstruction to develop without underperfusion of the myocardium ever taking place. Individuals who experience myocardial infarction due to coronary atherosclerosis without ever having had angina pectoris represent probable instances of this. It is tempting to think that if a myocardial infarction victim had been subjected to vigorous exercise prior to his infarction, the high level of coronary blood flow required for this exertion could not have taken place through the diseased arteries, and some evidence of disparity between coronary blood flow requirement and actual delivery would have been manifested. The predictive importance of such exertional myocardial hypoxia (or "ischemia" as it is usually termed) is thought to be related to the intensity of cardiac activity at which the disparity became apparent.[2] For example, if there was no evidence of ischemia at 75 percent of maximum exercise, but there was ischemia at 90–100 percent of maximal exercise, this would represent a much less severe degree of coronary obstruction than if the ischemia had been detectable at only 25–50 percent of normal maximal exercise.

This reasoning was so simple and persuasive that near-maximal and maximal exercise testing became widely adopted. The inevitable comparisons between exercise test results and coronary angiography were made, and it was found that many patients who did not show evidence of ischemia on exercise testing had "significant" coronary obstructive lesions.[3,4] On the other hand, some patients who did show exertional ST segment depression did not have significantly abnormal coronary angiograms. Although it was repeatedly pointed out that the exercise test is a measure of physiology, not anatomy, and that it was reasonable to expect only a rough correlation between anatomical obstructive coronary disease and physiological evidence of disturbed peak myocardial blood flow, there nonetheless developed among many an attitude of skepticism regarding the diagnostic utility of exercise stress testing. It was only with the publication of large follow-up studies that it came to be realized that, when properly interpreted, exercise test results do indeed predict the subsequent course of coronary atherosclerotic disease with remarkable accuracy.[5]

Since there is strong evidence that the level of exercise required to produce ischemia is the most important part of the exercise test result, the question arises of how the exercise test work load shall be selected. There is overwhelming agreement on use of a progressively increasing exercise protocol beginning with a stage low enough to be tolerable by the weakest candidate for testing, with the highest stage being sufficiently difficult to challenge the fittest candidate. Each stage should be long enough in duration for the body to reach or closely approach steady state, and the work increments from one stage to the next should be small enough to permit the desired degree of precision in estimating work capacity.* The Bruce treadmill protocol is widely used (Table 1). Typical work output requirements for each stage in terms of oxygen consumption have been calculated, and the range of stages is adequate both for sedentary individuals and athletes.[6] To increase its applicability, two easier stages have been added below Stage 1 in order to accommodate virtually all ambulatory individuals.[7] In order for any measurements of treadmill performance, exercise time, rate-pressure response, and others, to be dependably applicable to the actual cardiac work involved, the subject must have reached or closely approached "steady state." This implies that if the subject continued to exercise at this same intensity,

---

*An interesting and physiologically sound variation of this approach involves the use of brief exercise stages consisting of tiny work increments, giving the overall effect of a slow, continuous increase in work output rather than abrupt changes as are found in protocols with three or more minute stages.[8] Although this type of protocol is not widely employed compared with the others, the results in terms of seconds of exercise performed are equally valid.

Table 1
Schedule of Treadmill Exercise for the GXT

Stage Number	Time Per Stage (Min)	Elapsed Time at End of Stage	Speed		Treadmill Slope	
			Km/H	(MPH)	Grade %	Elevation 0(degrees)
Zero*	3	3+	2.7	1.7	0 (Level)	0 (Level)
One-half*	3	3+	2.7	1.7	5	2.8
First	3	3	2.7	1.7	10	5.7
Second	3	6	4.0	2.5	12	6.8
Third	3	9	5.5	3.4	14	8.0
Fourth	3	12	6.8	4.2	16	9.0
Fifth	3	15	8.0	5.0	18	10.0
Sixth	3	18	8.9	5.5	20	11.0
Seventh	3	21	9.6	6.0	22	12.4

(Adapted from Bruce Multistage Exercise Test)
* Begin with stage zero or stage one-half if appearance and demeanor of subject suggest that walking capacity is severely limited.
+ Exercise time in these preliminary stages is not counted when tabulating functional capacity.
GXT = graded exercise test.

cardiac output, heart rate, and other parameters would stay essentially the same until fatigue set in. Steady state attainment requires at least 3 minutes, and more likely 4 or more minutes of exercise on the treadmill. Exercise times shorter than this will not yield a reliable reflection of cardiovascular capacity. A subject beginning a test at Stage 1 and stopping near the end of Stage 1 cannot be accurately evaluated for functional aerobic capacity. But if the same person begins at Stage 1/2 and is exhausted after 2 minutes in Stage 1, that 2 minute endurance time (begin timing with Stage 1) is a reproducible measure of functional capacity. Therefore, it is a challenge to those conducting treadmill tests to recognize the subjects unlikely to complete Stage 1 or 2 and start them lower on the protocol so that aerobic steady state is achieved before exhaustion and useful test data are generated (Table 1).

Rather than assign a certain stage of exercise protocol for an individual to attempt, whether based on age, history of exercise participation, or apparent fitness, it is preferable to require the test subject to exercise progressively through the protocol until it becomes excessively uncomfortable or impossible to continue. As will be seen, there are numerous means of gauging whether the subject does indeed make a good effort so that the exercise time is a

Table 2
Predicted Exercise Heart Rate: Men/Women

Age		30	35	40	45	50	55	60	65
Maximal predicted	(M)	193	191	189	187	184	182	180	178
heart rate	(W)	190	185	181	177	172	168	163	159
80% of maximal predicted heart rate	(M)	154	153	151	150	147	146	144	142
(HRi = .80)	(W)	152	148	145	142	138	134	130	127

true representation of his physical capacity, or whether the effort was only desultory and unrepresentative. The most obvious criterion is heart rate. Maximum exercise heart rate declines with age and to a lesser extent with athletic training, and can be predicted with about 90 percent accuracy.[9,10] Failure to attain an exercise tachycardia reasonably close to a predicted maximum (in the absence of propranolol or other therapy which influences heart rate) is reason to question the degree of effort put forth in an otherwise normal test response (Table 2). There are other guides to the intensity of effort put forth, as will be seen in the section on Stress Test Methodology.

Assuming that a subject has coronary atherosclerosis and in the course of exercise testing has worked sufficiently hard to develop myocardial ischemia, how may this be detected? Ischemia is usually manifested first by depression of the ST segment of the electrocardiogram.[11] Ischemia may also produce chest discomfort, a typical episode of angina pectoris.[12] Finally, ischemia may cause deterioration of the heart's mechanical performance as a pump, resulting blood pressure drop, general weakness, and inability to continue exercise.[13] Even before these gross abnormalities are apparent, peak ejection velocity into the aortic root can be seen to diminish, when this is monitored by Doppler ultrasound via the suprasternal notch.[13] If the perfusion abnormality is localized or inhomogeneous as it usually is, thallium perfusion images directly after exercise will show reduced activity in the zones of the left ventricle underperfused by the diseased arteries.[14] Wall motion studies made during exercise using either technetium pyrophosphate labeling of the blood or two-dimensional echocardiography will show one or more regions of the ventricle to be poorly contracting or actually bulging as a result of the insufficient perfusion. Cardiokymographic recording directly after exercise shows abnormality of left ventricular contraction produced by ischemia, especially if it is the anterior wall which is involved.[15] Details of ischemia detection will be presented in the section on Stress Test Methodology.

How accurate is the exercise stress test? This question is more complicated than it appears, because while the exercise test seems to indicate the presence and severity of exertional ischemia, the question we pose is whether our patient has coronary artery disease which is likely to cause clinical illness, and if so, how soon?[16] Unless we are careful we are liable to be sidetracked into the question: does this patient have advanced anatomical coronary obstructive disease? Yet many persons with coronary atherosclerosis never develop clinical heart disease.[17,18] It is the prediction of overt clinical coronary heart disease that is important in the diagnosis and management of patients. Were it possible, we would prefer to have bypass surgery performed on those patients with coronary atherosclerosis who have a poor nonsurgical prognosis, but not on those patients who have an excellent nonsurgical prognosis. This issue will be addressed further in the section on Interpretation and Prognosis. At this point, let us simply agree that about 65 percent of patients with significant coronary obstructions will be identified by exercise testing, whereas between 5 and 10 percent of patients who show some sign of ischemia on exercise testing will not have significant obstructive lesions on angiography.[2,19]

STRESS TESTING IN HEALTH AND DISEASE

Sports Training

Both treadmill and cycle ergometer exercise stress testing were employed in sports training, in physical education departments of high schools and colleges, and in academic physiology laboratories well before exercise stress testing was adopted by clinical medicine for disease diagnosis.

1. Testing is used to provide a baseline fitness measure-

ment for later comparison in order to evaluate the rate of progress being achieved by training.

2. Exercise testing also provides possible clues to the existence of musculoskeletal problems to be encountered in sports training.

3. Previously unknown disease conditions, such as congenital cardiovascular malformations, pulmonary disorders, or skeletal diseases, may be brought to light by exercise testing.

In this context, the symptom-limited maximal exercise test is most likely the procedure of choice.

Primary Disease Prevention

It is widely appreciated that individuals who engage in strenuous exercise regularly have a much lower incidence of cardiovascular disease and in general enjoy better health than those who do not.[20] Whether exercise testing is called for when exercise training is used for primary prevention depends on the individual's activity history.[21]

1. Asymptomatic habitual exercisers do not require exercise testing in order to continue their exercise. Life-long asymptomatic exercisers may be assumed to be as healthy as they look. One cannot overemphasize here the key word *asymptomatic*. Some regular exercisers with undiagnosed coronary artery disease push themselves in spite of symptoms and think their exercise regimen is all right as long as they can continue it with impunity. Unfortunately, these are the persons likely to be found collapsed beside a jogging trail.

2. Persons who took up regular strenuous exercise 1 to 5 years ago either had appropriate screening at the outset or subjected themselves to an imponderable risk which has gradually resolved.

3. The prospective adult exerciser should certainly be screened and exercise tested[22] in order to:
   a. exclude unsuspected and asymptomatic disease;
   b. establish a baseline functional capacity measurement for future comparison;

    c. provide the data needed for an appropriate exercise prescription;

    d. As progress is made in the course of exercise training, repeated exercise tests may be appropriate in order to revise the exercise prescription, especially in middle-aged and older subjects or those with known chronic diseases.[23]

Diagnosis

Exercise stress testing has been employed more and more frequently since the pioneering work of Dr. Arthur Master dating from 1940 with his development and popularization of the two-step test.[24] Since then, cycle ergometer and treadmill tests have supplanted the step test; and high performance tests, either close to or at maximal exercise capacity, have replaced the relatively mild stress of earlier tests.

1. Coronary artery disease is the principal disorder for which the exercise test is used.[25] As a diagnostic aid, it provides a greater benefit/cost ratio than any other technical procedure. In addition to aiding in detection of coronary disease, it provides valuable prognostic information which helps to choose appropriate therapy for the condition. The exercise test results provide substantial assistance in determining that a given patient has very mild disease with a good prognosis, provided cardiovascular risk factors are controlled. In others, it indicates that there is a relatively good prognosis but both risk factor modification and a medical regimen should be employed with frequent follow-up. Finally, exercise testing helps to recognize a group of patients with severe disease who most likely should be considered for early coronary bypass operation.[4]

2. Treatment evaluation is another important use of exercise testing. Both medical and surgical treatment of coronary artery disease may be evaluated by such testing since effective treatment causes improved exercise endurance and longer exercise times, and such subjects may be expected to exercise a longer time before the appearance of ischemic type ST segment depression or other evidence of ischemia.[26] Deterioration of exercise tolerance in a patient who is being followed-up is usually a sign of therapeutic failure. The surgical patient in particular may represent multiple-

graft closure in such a setting. Arrhythmia control also benefits from exercise testing.[27] After the recognized arrhythmia has been suppressed in the resting state, the next step in most cases is to determine whether the suppression persists during exercise.

Exercise testing is used to evaluate the degree of improvement caused by correction of congenital heart disease. Such testing in the past has shown that "complete" surgical correction of most malformations does not result in normalization of functional capacity.[28] In many cases, the degree of improvement is directly related to the youth of the patient at the time of operation.[29] Exercise testing also aids in the comparison of one surgical technique with another in order to obtain the best long-term result. Exercise testing has the same utility in the heart valve surgery patient.

3. Cardiac toxicity of antineoplastic agents, such as Adriamycin, is being monitored by periodic exercise testing. Conventional regimens simply indicated a total maximum dose which could be given with relative safety from cardiac toxicity; however, individual susceptibility varies widely, and some patients develop cardiac toxicity at lower dosages.[30] Other patients would benefit from higher dosages of the medication and still not develop cardiac toxicity. At present, it appears that newly developed reduction in exercise test endurance is an early warning of cardiac toxicity before the appearance of cardiac enlargement or congestive failure. Unfortunately, discontinuation of antineoplastic agents does not always guarantee that cardiac toxicity will not progress.

4. Evaluation of physical disability claims. In connection with claims for compensation for disability or requests for retraining due to incapacity, physical examination with various special tests are requested to help these agencies determine whether individuals can safely perform certain levels of activity.[31] Exercise stress testing is an excellent source of information for this purpose provided the individual's reactions are adequately and objectively documented. In such cases, treadmill endurance time is very important, but it must be evaluated in the light of corresponding heart rate, respiration rate, and the postexercise time required to return these parameters to within 10 percent of control values. Whenever the possibility of reverse motivation exists in the subject, objective exercise test observations are essential and subjective ones—such as apparent degree of cooperation, whether or not the subject appeared to put forth a good effort, and similar considerations—should be minimized.

Rehabilitation

1. Baseline functional capacity measurement is essential in order to gauge subsequent progress.[32]
2. Detection and evaluation of potential complications to exercise training may be accomplished by stress testing. This would include the detection of exertional arrhythmias, stress-induced congestive heart failure, and musculoskeletal problems.
3. The stress test provides an essential basis for devising an exercise prescription individualized to each subject.

Secondary Prevention

This is a logical extension of the rehabilitation process, and may be thought of as beginning after the rehabilitation process has clearly reached a plateau in terms of functional capacity. The realistic aim at this point is to conserve the gains already accomplished, continue the beneficial risk-lowering effect of exercise, and to continue to enjoy the feeling of well-being and personal accomplishment which derives from pursuit of a physical activity program.[33] During secondary prevention activities, periodic exercise testing is appropriate:

1. if there are exercise-induced complications which should be followed, such as exertional arrhythmias controlled by therapy;
2. when symptoms or exercise tolerance change noticeably;
3. to reassure the participant of the value of the program if he or she tends to become discouraged or lose motivation.

STRESS TESTING METHODOLOGY

Subjects will have been referred to the stress testing laboratory because of one or more indications for this procedure (Table 3). Although possible contraindications to the procedure will have been considered by those who refer subjects for testing, it is the ultimate responsibility of those actually performing the test to assure that no serious contraindications to exercise testing exist in each subject (Table 4). Adherence to appropriate contraindications is probably the single most valuable means of assuring subject safety.[34] In addition, there are some circumstances that only temporarily contraindicate exercise stress testing. Having eaten a meal within the last 2 hours is the most frequently encountered reason for rescheduling, but there are a few others (Table 5). It is desirable at the time of scheduling a subject for exercise testing to provide a brief, printed explanation of the test, which would include the instruction to have only a light meal within 4 hours before the test and nothing to eat or drink within 2 hours of testing.

Table 3
Indications for Exercise Stress Testing

1. Chest pain diagnosis.
2. Evaluate severity of coronary artery disease.
3. Evaluate prognosis after infarction.
4. For exercise prescription in a cardiovascular rehabilitation program.
5. Assess efficacy of cardiovascular therapy or progress of cardiac rehabilitation.
6. Evaluation of risk factors for coronary heart disease.
7. Evaluate functional capacity in other heart disease.
8. Early detection of cardiac toxicity during treatment with a cardiotoxic agent.

Table 4
Contraindications to Exercise Testing

1. Possible unhealed myocardial infarction.
2. Uncontrolled ventricular arrhythmia.
3. Acute general illness.
4. Known ominous coronary artery obstruction pattern.
5. Obviously too weak to exercise at lowest level.
6. Locomotion problem: consider arm exercise test.
7. Patient does not wish to be tested.

Table 5
Reschedule Exercise Stress Test

1. Not fasting for two hours before test.
2. Suffering from acute, temporary musculoskeletal problem.
3. ECG suggests infarction of uncertain age, no other clinical data available.
4. Subject donated blood in last 24 hours.
5. Subject under influence of psychoactive medication.
6. Not all monitoring and safety equipment functioning properly.

The explanation can also include the suggestion to bring jogging shorts and shoes for the test, although these are not required (Form 1).

The technician completes the explanation of the test to the patient, answers any questions the subject may have, and assures the subject that any medical questions can be dealt with by the supervising physician. The subject is requested to give informed consent to be tested at this time.

Form 1
Graded Exercise Test

You have been scheduled to have a graded exercise test on _____ at ____ (a.m.) (p.m.). This is a test of the efficiency of your heart and circulation. It is used to aid the diagnosis and evaluate the treatment of several kinds of heart disease and heart rhythm disturbances, and is also used as a screening test before an individual begins a physical activity program.

The test involves the application of several electrocardiogram electrodes to your chest, attachment of a blood pressure measuring cuff to your arm, and then walking on a motorized treadmill. The walk is very slow at first. Every three minutes the speed and slope of the treadmill are increased slightly so that the walking gradually becomes more vigorous. You are requested to continue walking until symptoms or fatigue cause you to stop, or the physician supervising the test may interrupt it earlier if a reason is discovered for doing so. *You may stop the exercise any time you choose to.* You should bear in mind however that too early termination of the test may prevent a useful test result.

Please avoid food or drink for at least two hours before the test, and if there is a mealtime just before that, make the meal a light one. If you are taking any medications regularly, ask the staff whether you should continue to take them right up until your test. You may inquire at this phone number (_____). Please have your prescription packages handy when you call.

If you regularly use sports shorts and shoes (no cleats!) you are encouraged to bring them. Otherwise wear low-heeled shoes. Appropriate garments will be furnished.

Any questions you have about the test will be answered to your satisfaction by technicians or physicians before you exercise, and you will be expected to give your informed consent to undergo the procedure.

Measurements and observations of you will continue for a few minutes after you stop exercising. Then all the gear will be removed from you and you may don your street clothes. We request that you relax in the reception area ten minutes or so afterward. When your breathing and heart beat have settled down and you feel entirely o.k. to leave, please check with one of the staff so we can be sure that it is all right for you to go.

Thank you for your cooperation!

In the exercise lab, the subject is requested to strip to the waist and women are supplied with an examination jacket with front opening. The blood pressure is taken and the supervising physician is notified so cardiac auscultation can be performed prior to the application of the electrodes. A skin-marking pencil is then used to mark the locations of each of the six precordial electrodes and the torso translocations of the limb electrodes,[35] i.e., the lateral aspect of each infraclavicular fossa and each antero-superior iliac spine. A no. 6 spherical dental burr rotated by a Dremel motorized hobby tool or similar tool is touched with about 5 grams of force to the middle of each skin mark and held there for about 1 second. This should cause the removal of skin-marking pigment in a circle of about 1 mm radius, along with removal of underlying cornified epithelium.[36] The exposed dermis should never be penetrated. Reusable or disposable fluid-column electrodes with self-adhesive circular disks are applied with adequate electrolyte at each electrode site.* Alternatively, the Quinton Quick-Prep disposable electrode system may be used with its intrinsic dermabrasion system. In each case, the special skin preparation results in electrode contact impedance of approximately 2,000 ohms, five to ten times lower than the contact impedance of unprepared skin. An ECG patient cable especially manufactured to be long enough for exercise testing is connected by short and preferably shielded wires to each electrode. The cable is draped over the subject's shoulder, and the lead wires, electrodes, and underlying soft tissue are stabilized by means of an elastic vest or an overwrap of 8-inch-wide elastic bandage.

When the left breast overlies the locations of the V_3, V_4, and V_5 electrodes, the breast is raised and the electrodes are applied directly to the chest wall in the proper location or as close as possible.

If subjects have brought running shorts and shoes, these may be worn, otherwise street trousers are worn and scrub pants are worn instead of skirts. Subjects who have not brought jogging shoes may walk barefoot or wear their flat-heeled street shoes. High heels should not be worn on the treadmill.

---

*Profuse sweating caused by vigorous exercise may loosen some electrodes. To prevent this, the skin contacted by the electrode adhesive (but not the central electrode itself) may be painted with tincture of benzoin which is dried thoroughly (hair drier) before the electrodes are applied.

The technician tests each electrode by tapping and shaking it while observing its ECG signal. When all are providing satisfactory noise-free signals, 12-lead ECGs are recorded in the recumbent, sitting, and standing positions. These are presented to the supervising physician for interpretation and freedom from contraindications prior to beginning exercise. The treadmill is demonstrated to the subject, and if the subject has never been on a treadmill before, this demonstration would appropriately include about 30 seconds of actual walking on the treadmill by the subject.

The Exercise Period: The stress testing team make last-minute assurance that no contraindications to testing exist, that informed consent has been given (either written or verbal is satisfactory), and that the defibrillator and other safety equipment are in satisfactory condition (Table 6). A decision is made as to whether to start the subject at Stage 1 or to use Stage 0 or one-half because of anticipated patient weakness. This choice is based on the appearance and demeanor of the subject, and in particular, on the response to the treadmill demonstration earlier. The treadmill is started, the subject begins walking on the belt, assisted at first by the supervisor if necessary. The subject continues to exercise under close observation and the treadmill is set to succeeding stages every 3 minutes.

Table 6
Safety Measures for Exercise Stress Testing

1. Have a definite plan of emergency action in case of misadventure. This will include the duties of each member of the team. In addition to direct patient care, they will include notification of appropriate individuals, commandeering of an elevator and other necessities for patient transfer.
2. Prearrangement for admission of subject to a CCU without "red tape."
3. All members of team trained in CPR.
4. Defibrillator within cable reach of treadmill, on and charged (200 J) during test. (Full tube of electrode paste on top of unit.)
5. Emergency drug kit stocked and maintained by pharmacist (antiarrhythmics, pressor agents and miscellaneous).
6. Intravenous solutions, administration sets, needles and syringes.
7. Oropharyngeal airways, laryngoscope, endotracheal tubes, ventilation bag, and suction machine.
8. Oxygen administration equipment.

Electrocardiography

Heart Rate

The ECG is the most convenient and practical means for determination of heart rate. Ideal heart rate recording and display are provided by exercise ECG computer systems which display the time course of heart rate as a continuous line graph so that the rate of change of heart rate in each stage and after exercise is readily appreciated. In the absence of such a computer, a simple strip chart recorder connected to the heart rate meter can serve the same purpose.

Cardiac Rhythm

Cardiac rhythm is best monitored on a multichannel CRT display. Typically V_5, V_1, and lead 2 are displayed continuously except when a 12-lead ECG is being recorded one or more times per 3 minutes stage. V_5 and V_1 are best for recognizing aberrant ventricular complexes, while V_1 and II are best for displaying P waves. When a rhythm disturbance is suspected, a continuous hard copy of the monitored leads is recorded until sufficient data has been acquired for accurate evaluation. A paper speed of 25 mm/sec is ideal for wave recognition and interval measurement.

QRST Changes

In the majority of cases when left ventricular ischemia develops, it is best seen in lead V_5 with progressively decreasing frequency in the adjacent leads V_6, V_4, and V_3.[37] In a minority of instances, ischemic ST segment depression is seen only in lead 2 or lead 3. Ischemia affecting a major fraction of the left ventricle, such as might be caused by multivessel disease, has the same vectorial direction as the R wave. This accounts for its maximal expression in lead V_5 which also typically shows greatest R wave voltage. On the other hand, when most of the ventricle is normally perfused and only a localized area is ischemic, such as might occur with single vessel disease of the left anterior descending coronary, ST depression may be maximal in a lead other than V_5 (in this case, lead V_2). Chaitman and others have demonstrated the increased diagnostic yield provided by multilead ECG recording during exercise testing.[19] A convenient way to achieve this diagnostic yield is by using an automatic lead switching three-channel recorder for exercise testing, and recording a complete 12-lead ECG near the end of each stage of exercise (or whenever ischemia is suspected). The Mason-Likar torso modification of the limb leads is recommended.[35] The shoulder electrodes should be applied as distally as possible along the clavicle, since applying the shoulder electrodes too close together causes serious distortion of the frontal QRS vector. Some investigators record bipolar leads in addition to the conventional 12 leads for a small added measure of diagnostic sensitivity.[19] On the other hand, one or even three bipolar leads is not considered an adequate substitute for the recording of the conventional 12 leads for diagnostic exercise testing.

Promising but not yet sufficiently proved means of improving exercise ECG accuracy have been reported.[38] These involve combining multiple measurements of the ECG and other data. Thus computerized exercise ECG systems should be made which are adaptable to whatever methods of data combination prove most diagnostically useful.

Blood Pressure

Means of Recording

Most accurate exercise blood pressure recording is obtained by catheterization of the ascending aorta. A fine, short catheter in either the brachial or femoral artery would come next in order of accuracy. In either case, a variable degree of artifactual increase in measured peak systolic pressure would take place due to hydrodynamic pressure wave reflections which increase distal to the aortic valve. The indirect cuff method employing acoustic detection of the Korotkoff sounds just distal to the cuff is less accurate in both systolic and diastolic pressure measurements. This method is recommended for exercise testing, however, because of its noninvasive safety, painlessness, and ease of use.[39] Its accuracy is quite sufficient for exercise testing purposes. The blood pressure measurements before, during, and after the exercise can be performed entirely manually with a conventional sphygmomanometer and a stethoscope. Varying degrees of automation of the process are available, including automatic inflation and deflation of the blood pressure cuff, the addition of an amplified microphone to the cuff to permit recognition of the blood pressure sounds at a distance from the test subject, the detection of the distal arterial pulse by some other means such as ultrasonic or oscillometric recording, or in at least one case, the computerized recognition of the Korotkoff sounds with digital display of the measured systolic, diastolic, and mean arterial pressures. During vigorous exercise it is advantageous for the examiner to hold and gently stabilize the cuffed arm and thus prevent treadmill (or bicycle) mechanical noise from traveling up the arm from the handrail, handlebar, or from the legs and shoulders past the inflated cuff.

Exclusion from Testing

Contraindications to exercise testing are discussed in the section on Stress Testing Methodology. If the test subject is not known to be normotensive, the blood pressure should be checked prior to other preparation for exercise testing. If an initial blood pressure is greater than 220 mmHg systolic or 120 mmHg diastolic, the subject should be questioned about activities just prior to entering the testing laboratory, and invited to lie down in a quiet place and relax prior to a second blood pressure determination.

For Termination of Exercise

On beginning the first stage of the exercise test, the typical subject will have a rapid rise of systolic pressure which tapers off after a minute or two as the subject settles down into the test procedure. Thereafter the blood pressure usually rises from 5 to 10 mmHg systolic with each 3-minute exercise stage (Bruce protocol). Since a fall in systolic pressure is a reason for terminating exercise, the last previous blood pressure reading should be kept in mind when taking the pressure so one can listen with particular care during the expected pressure range. Any suspected fall should quickly be confirmed by another reading and then acted upon without delay.

For Prognostic Interpretation

Although any fall in systolic blood pressure during the exercise test is an indication for stopping the exercise—and even failure of pressure to rise with succeeding stages of exercise is abnormal—the prognostic implication of a blood pressure drop is closely related to the stage of exercise at which it occurs.[13] For this reason, the time of observation should be carefully recorded on the exercise test work sheet in addition to repeating any dubious or abnormal values for confirmation of these findings.

Symptoms

All symptoms elicited by the procedure should be recorded on an appropriate work sheet in order of their occurrence. The time for any possible editing and deletion of unimportant symptoms is after the exercise and postexercise recovery if at all. As the amount of objective information available from exercise testing increases, there is a natural tendency to deemphasize the subjective data generated by exercise testing. This should be avoided not only because of the very high benefit/cost ratio of symptom analysis, but also because of the beneficial effect it has on the test subject who appreciates the interest and concern of the testing staff for his or her symptoms. This improves subject cooperation during the test and may have a lasting influence on long-term adherence to a prescription.

Preparation of Patient

While the ECG electrodes are being attached, the patient should be instructed to report all symptoms and feelings as they occur, without regard to their presumed importance. The subject should be reassured that such reporting will not be considered complaining, but on the contrary will in fact aid in the interpretation of the test for the patient's benefit. Establishing a cooperative attitude toward the reporting of symptoms prior to treadmill exercise is an important part of symptom detection and analysis.

Repeated Questioning

After the subject has begun exercise, a running conversation should take place between the test supervisor and the subject. Such questions as "Do you have any unpleasant feeling in your chest? Is your breathing all right? Does anything bother you?" should be woven into the conversation repeatedly. Whenever any symptom is reported for the first time, this should be entered in the exercise test record and followed up later.

Receptive Attitude

The test subject must be convinced that the supervisor is sincerely interested in the exercise-induced symptoms and has an open-ended attitude toward replies to all the questions. The best way to accomplish this is by giving the subject adequate time to reply to each question without interruption and without any sign of impatience. Questions should be asked in an encouraging, sympathetic tone of voice with entries written on the work sheet demonstrating to the subject that the supervisor considered the symptom worth recording.

Time Course of Symptoms

The pattern of change of any symptom with respect to time is likely to be very important. In an exercise test of progressively increasing work load, angina pectoris gradually increases in severity until after the termination of exercise. This is a crucial difference from many kinds of musculoskeletal pain which appear early in the course of the test and remain constant in severity or even improve as the exercise progresses. The time course of other symptoms is also important, including breathlessness, dizziness, and leg discomfort. Finally, whenever a subject admits having chest discomfort, this symptom should be followed up thoroughly to establish the location, quality, intensity, and radiation. If the subject has had chest pain in the past, it should be established whether the present discomfort is the same as that previously experienced. A judgment should always be made as to whether the discomfort is considered to be angina pectoris or not, and a degree of confidence of this judgment (such as "possible" or "definite") should be recorded.

Perceived Exertion

In addition to the total treadmill endurance time, a regular series of questions concerning the subject's perceived exertion will aid in evaluating the subject's physical fitness. This can be done informally by asking at each stage how difficult the exercise seems to be, and recording the responses as a series of plusses; or perceived exertion may be based on a standardized wall chart with a scale of 6 through 20. With such a perceived exertion scale "6" corresponds to a gentle walk and "20" indicates maximal or sprint intensity.[40] If the test record reveals a gradual increase of subjective difficulty until the point of stopping is reached, there is assurance that the patient was adequately motivated and cooperated well. On the other hand, an abrupt and premature report of severe exertional difficulty might raise doubts about the adequacy of the subject's cooperation.

Reasons for Stopping Exercise

Ingenious tests have been developed for predicting maximal oxygen consumption in exercise from the physiologic response, typically of the heart rate, to a fixed submaximal work load.[41] Other tests, such as the original graded exercise test (GXT), aim at 90 percent of maximal exercise heart rate in order to obtain good diagnostic sensitivity for detecting ischemia with slightly less time and effort than that required for maximal exercise.[11] However, in recent years, the safety of subjective maximal exercise has become established,[42] and the maximal exercise endurance time has been found to be a powerful prognostic measurement. It now appears that the best end-point for exercise testing under most circumstances is the subjective maximal response.

Subjective maximal exercise implies exercise to maximal endurance if no abnormality has appeared, or exercise to maximal tolerance of an abnormal symptom, such as chest pain. In addition, exercise should be interrupted in the interest of patient safety upon recognition of certain ominous findings, especially electrocardiographic abnormalities (Table 7). Finally, there are some reasons for stopping exercise which will render an otherwise normal test response incomplete because insufficient exercise has been performed. These include equipment problems, lack of patient cooperation, and other factors.

When the treadmill is stopped, the subject is gently hurried to a sitting position on the examining table, since standing still and upright directly after vigorous exertion is likely to cause postural hypotension and possible syncope. Postexercise auscultation is performed immediately after exercise with particular emphasis on the development of a ventricular or third sound gallop, the development of a murmur of mitral incompetence possibly due to papillary muscle ischemia, the development of an aortic systolic ejection murmur produced by subclinical idiopathic hypertrophic subaortic stenosis, or the development of a click and murmur secondary to mitral valve prolapse. If murmurs or extra sounds were present prior to exercise, the immediate intent is to determine the effect of exercise on their intensity and distribution. The time course of any new or preexisting sounds or murmurs

---

Table 7
Reasons for Terminating Exercise

A. Subjective maximal
    I. General fatigue
    II. Leg fatigue
    III. Dyspnea
    IV. Unable to keep up with the treadmill without holding on
B. Evidence of ischemia
    I. Progressive chest discomfort typical of angina
    II. Excessive ST segment shift or other waveform change
    III. Blood pressure drop at low exercise level
C. Test interruption. Exercise possibly insufficient for confident interpretation of normal result
    I. Staggering gait (otherwise not near maximal)
    II. Ventricular premature complexes
    III. Ventricular couplets or tachycardia
    IV. Supraventricular tachycardia
    V. Intracardiac block
    VI. Leg discomfort (claudication)
    VII. Orthopedic problem
    VIII. Equipment problem
    IX. Physician's discretion
    X. Subject's discretion

should be followed during the postexercise period, likewise the time course of any symptoms brought on by exercise. This information is appropriately noted in the exercise test record for optimal interpretation of the overall test results.

It is recommended that postexercise recordings and observations be continued for 6 minutes after exercise, provided recovery has taken place by then and any abnormality provoked by exercise has resolved. Otherwise the subject should remain under observation until after any such abnormalities have resolved. Further, the subject should wait in a nearby reception area for an additional 15 minutes, and a member of the testing team should make sure that the subject looks, acts, talks, and feels well before leaving the facility.

INTERPRETATION AND PROGNOSIS

Detection of Ischemia

Electrocardiogram

1. For many years the development of transient exertional ST segment depression (or more rarely, ST elevation) has been the hallmark of objective evidence of myocardial ischemia.[43] In evaluating ST segment shifts, any ST deviation in the resting electrocardiogram should be subtracted from the value measured during or after exercise.[44] ST changes must be evaluated in an ECG strip of consecutive cardiac complexes which are alike in terms of QRS and ST-T voltage and contour. In particular, the ST segment slopes of successive beats should be the same. When there is flat or nearly flat ST segment depression, the amplitude of the ST segment shift is measured 60 msec (3 mm, at 50 mm/sec chart speed) after the end of the QRS complex. The measurement is made with respect to the PR segment at the onset of the QRS complex (Qo). When the ST segment is downsloping, it is considered to represent significant depression only if the J point is depressed 0.1 mV below Qo. The amplitude of the ST depression is measured to 60 msec after the J point. When the ST segment is depressed with an upsloping contour, measurement is again made at 60 msec after J (Fig. 1).

For the unipolar chest leads and conventional limb leads of the recommended 12-lead ECG, 2 mm of ST segment shift during

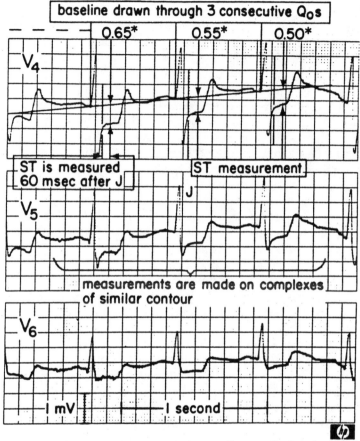

baseline drawn through 3 consecutive Q₀s

| 0.65* | 0.55* | 0.50* |

ST is measured 60 msec after J

ST measurement

measurements are made on complexes of similar contour

I mV I second

*when measurements vary, the median value is considered true, e.g., -0.55 mV

Method of ST Segment Measurement

Figure 1.

exercise and 1 mm ST segment shift in the postexercise ECG are recommended criteria for ischemia (0.2 and 0.1 mV, respectively). If bipolar chest leads are used, the recommended criteria are 3 mm and 2 mm, respectively.

To be considered characteristic of ischemia, ST segment changes should progress with exercise. An ST segment shift which is the same at the ends of two successive exercise stages is not at all characteristic of ischemia. To be characteristic of "significant" ischemia, ST abnormalities should persist for at least 1 minute post exercise. ST depression which vanishes immediately after exercise, especially if the exercise was continued up to Stage 3 or higher, is considered a minor finding. On the other hand, ST depression which persists longer than 4 minutes post exercise, or which undergoes "evolution" with transient T wave inversion as well as ST segment depression, is considered a major index of exertional ischemia (Table 8). Kansal and co-workers have found that diagnostic accuracy of the exercise ECG is improved if ST changes are combined with other test measurements to yield a diagnostic treadmill score.[45] Hollenberg et al. have developed a treadmill test score based upon computerized ECG measurements which may be able to predict not only the presence of CAD, but the number of diseased vessels as well.[38]

2. Another electrocardiographic finding which has been shown associated with exertional ischemia is transient post exercise U wave inversion. McHenry and colleagues find this to be an infrequent but highly specific indication of coronary artery disease.[48]

3. Augmentation of R wave amplitude after exercise has been found by Ellestad and others to be an indication of coronary artery disease.[47] Since there are hemodynamic and electrophysiologic reasons for both increase and decrease of the R wave amplitude with ischemia, the sensitivity of this finding is variable. It does seem, however, to be fairly specific when it is present.

Table 8
Prognostic Exercise Test Findings

A. Major
  1. Significant ST segment depression beginning at low exercise intensity
  2. Angina pectoris during exercise, typical, convincing
  3. Blood pressure drop early in exercise
  4. Short treadmill exercise time (less than 66% of predicted normal)
  5. Low exercise heart rate index (less than 80% of predicted normal)
B. Minor
  1. Minor ST segment depression
  2. Ventricular arrhythmia provoked by exercise
  3. Negative U wave appearing postexercise
  4. R wave augmentation, unequivocal, postexercise
  5. Transient ventricular gallop postexercise
  6. Transient mitral regurgitation postexercise

Angina Pectoris

Angina pectoris which develops in the course of treadmill exercise is a highly valuable indicator of ischemia. Since its characteristics can be examined as they are actually being experienced, the description is likely to be more accurate than that obtained from recollection of past episodes. The great value of this finding during the exercise test depends upon the symptoms being characteristic and convincing, in contrast to other types of chest pain of different origin. To qualify as typical angina, the discomfort should originate in the substernal region, in either of the shoulders or upper arms, in the lower jaw or in the lateral aspect(s) of the neck between the angle of the mandible and the deltoid ridge, or in the interscapular region of the back. The discomfort should have a deep visceral quality, and not be sharply localized. It should be constricting or expanding in nature, and may also have a sensation of heat or cold. It should not be sharp, stabbing, or cutting. It may radiate from one of the regions mentioned above to another, but should not radiate to other areas such as the top of the head or one entire side of the body below as well as above the waist. The discomfort is typically not called pain, but subjects usually agree with the suggestion that it is an unpleasant, disagreeable, or uncomfortable sensation. It should develop gradually over several seconds or tens of seconds, rather than abruptly, and any change in intensity should have a similarly gradual time course. Inasmuch as the treadmill (or other exercise device) protocol is a progressive one, the discomfort should also increase progressively in severity. The walk-through phenomenon wherein the angina may stabilize, improve, and even disappear with continued walking cannot take place with the progressive protocol employed, and any such behavior of the chest discomfort makes it suspect of not being real angina pectoris. Although increasing progressively in severity during exercise, true angina will usually (but not always) begin to improve immediately after stopping exercise, and will have disappeared completely within 2 minutes postexercise.

Early Blood Pressure Drop

In 1975 Thomson and Kelemen reported that drop of systolic blood pressure during exercise testing corresponded with severe multivessel coronary artery disease.[13] They went on to point out that in order to carry this diagnostic significance, the drop must involve the systolic blood pressure irrespective of the diastolic pressure response, and it must follow an earlier increase in systolic blood pressure from resting control level to a higher level at the beginning of exercise. Finally, the drop in systolic pressure must occur at a low level of exercise, Stage I or II of the Bruce test, rather than at a higher level which would be considered normal peak exercise for the individual's age and sex. They correctly pointed out that normal individuals exhibit a drop in systolic blood pressure at maximal exercise (Stage III or higher for adults depending on age). Since their report, this finding has been confirmed by others, but the normality of blood pressure drop at peak exercise tends to be overlooked. Failure to increase the systolic blood pressure above 130 mmHg during the exercise test is also a major abnormality (Fig. 2).

Short Exercise Duration

McNeer and colleagues have reported that failure to complete Stage II of the Bruce protocol corresponds with the presence of significant coronary artery disease.[4] Actually, it would seem that the percentage of normal exercise capacity for age and sex would be a more specific indicator of coronary artery disease than an absolute figure, such as 6 minutes of exercise. In terms of percentage of exercise capacity, values below about 66 percent of normal for age and sex would correspond with a 6-minute treadmill time for a 50-year-old man, and thus a low percentage of normal exercise capacity is recommended as one indicator of coronary artery disease (Figs. 3 and 4).

Low Heart Rate Index

Failure to develop a normal degree of tachycardia upon exercise testing has also been shown to correlate with significant coronary artery disease. In the Duke study, peak heart rates under 150 beats per minute were a strong indication of coronary artery disease.[4] As in the case of exercise duration, it would seem that the relative percentage of predicted maximal heart rate achieved during exercise testing would be more specific than a fixed figure for heart rate, such as 150 per minute. The heart rate index—the

NORMAL & ABNORMAL SYSTOLIC BLOOD
PRESSURE RESPONSES TO EXERCISE TESTS

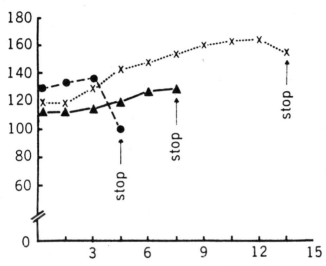

x – Normal response – subject able to exercise
13½ minutes, drops blood pressure at peak
of normal exercise capacity.

● – Abnormal – subject increases systolic pressure
initially, but pressure drops early in exercise
before normal exercise capacity is reached.

▲ – Abnormal – subject fails to raise systolic
pressure to 130 mmHg or higher, even though
exercise duration may be nearly normal.

Figure 2.

quotient maximal attained heart rate divided by age-predicted
maximal exercise heart rate—is recommended for evaluating this
response. A heart rate index of .80 corresponds with an achieved
heart rate of 150 beats per minute for a 50-year-old man, and it is
suggested that heart rate indices below .80 be considered abnormal and an indicator of probable coronary artery disease (Table 9).

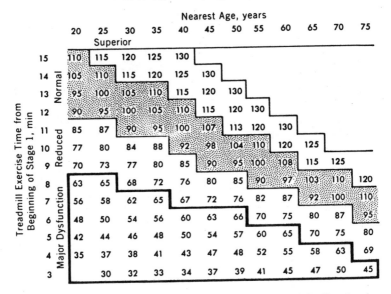

RELATIVE EXERCISE CAPACITY
Percentages of Average Normal

Percentage of average normal men's exercise capacity (functional aerobic capacity) determined by minutes of exercise endurance on the Bruce treadmill protocol when exercise is continued until the subject can no longer keep up with the treadmill without holding on to the handrail.

Figure 3.

Ventricular Arrhythmias

The development of ventricular premature complexes, bigeminy, couplets, or runs of ventricular tachycardia is not a specific indicator of CAD, but rather a more general disturbance which can be due to diverse causes.[46,47] Epidemiologically, however, the likelihood of having CAD is approximately doubled when an exertional ventricular arrhythmia is detected. Therefore the development of ventricular arrhythmia should be considered a weak although not specific sign of CAD.

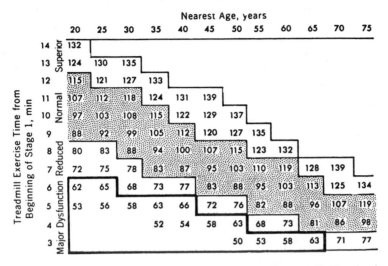

RELATIVE EXERCISE CAPACITY
Percentages of Average Normal

Percentage of average normal women's exercise capacity (functional aerobic capacity) determined by minutes of exercise endurance on the Bruce treadmill protocol when exercise is continued until the subject can no longer keep up with the treadmill without holding on to the handrail.

Figure 4.

Table 9
Heart Rate Index*

Attained heart rate		110	115	120	125	130	135	140	145	150	155	160	165	170	175
Predicted maximal heart rate	170	.65	.68	.71	.74	.76	.79	.82	.85	.88	.91	.94	.97	1.00	1.03
	175	.63	.66	.69	.71	.74	.77	.80	.83	.86	.89	.91	.94	.97	1.00
	180	.61	.64	.67	.69	.72	.75	.78	.81	.83	.86	.89	.92	.94	.97
	185	.59	.62	.65	.68	.70	.73	.76	.78	.81	.84	.86	.89	.92	.95
	190	.58	.61	.63	.66	.68	.71	.74	.76	.79	.82	.84	.87	.89	.92
	195	.56	.59	.62	.64	.67	.69	.72	.74	.77	.79	.82	.85	.87	.90

*Heart rate index (HRi) = attained heart rate ÷ age predicted maximal heart rate.
The shaded zone indicates an abnormally low exercise heart rate range (in absence of heart-slowing medication).

Ventricular Gallop

The development of a third heart sound or ventricular gallop after exercise, when not previously heard, and its later gradual disappearance in the postexercise period indicates transient exertional ventricular dysfunction. In the United States and most industrialized countries the most likely cause is CAD, although this is strictly speaking a nonspecific finding and might be due to other less common causes of heart disease.

Mitral Incompetence

Transient mitral valve incompetence precipitated by exercise and disappearing with rest may be due to CAD, and it has been speculated that its mechanism is transient ischemic dysfunction of the papillary muscles, permitting some mitral valve prolapse and consequent mitral incompetence.

Prognostic Classification of Stress Test Results

The exercise stress test interpretation should not be limited to the electrocardiographic ST segment, but also includes heart rate and rhythm response, other ECG wave form responses, blood pressure regulation, functional capacity evaluation, and symptom analysis. Exercise stress testing is a broad field indeed, and on occasion may include thallium perfusion scintigraphy, wall motion studies determined by technetium-labeled ventricular blood pool scintigraphy, or wall motion studies detected by two-dimensional echocardiography.

ST segment interpretation depends on finding a significant degree of depression, namely greater than 1 mm (0.1 mV) of ST segment change from the resting value, which persists over 1 minute after exercise.[48] The ST segment depression abnormality can then be classified as major if it began in Stage 2 or less of the Bruce protocol or if the depression continues to be of diagnostic degree at least 4 minutes after exercise. The ST depression may be classified as minor if it began in the third or higher Bruce stage and did not persist as long as 4 minutes postexercise. Exertional ST segment depression when properly classified has great prognostic significance.[49]

Angina pectoris, when typical and convincing in nature, likewise has major prognostic significance.[12] These two findings are both rather specific for myocardial ischemia, whereas blood pressure drop early in exercise, short treadmill exercise time, and low heart rate index although strongly prognostic are not as inherently specific for ischemia (Table 7).

Exercise test findings that correlate with the presence of CAD but do not carry the severe prognostic implication of the preceding major findings include minor ST segment depression abnormality, exertional ventricular arrhythmia, negative U waves postexercise, R wave augmentation postexercise, and ventricular gallop or mitral regurgitation immediately postexercise.[50]

Ellestad et al, McNeer et al., and Goldschlager et al. have shown that the prognosis of CAD can be quantitated by combination of exercise test findings.[4,5,50] The Duke study in particular showed that the presence of two major exercise test abnormalities classified a chest pain patient as high risk, and the absence of major exercise test abnormality classified chest pain patients as low risk, irrespective of their coronary angiographic findings.[4] These findings have had additional confirmation by findings of the cooperative Coronary Artery Surgery Study (CASS), in which patients with proved coronary artery disease who were not operated had a good survival rate and their treadmill test showed good exercise capacity and not over 1 mm of ST depression. Survival was poor if exercise capacity was low and significant ST depression occurred.[53] Clearly the aim of prognostic exercise test interpretation should be to identify high risk subjects who should be considered promptly for coronary bypass surgery, but also to identify the large group of patients who do not require such drastic treatment and who can safely and properly be treated by medical, dietary, and hygienic means with the assurance that although some subjects will fail to improve or will even deteriorate, these patients can be crossed over into surgical treatment while leaving a large successfully managed group who have avoided needless coronary bypass surgery. Prognostic interpretation can also identify a mild degree of abnormality which indicates risk of future clinical coronary disease justifying life-style modification but not requiring medical treatment. Finally, it can identify a group of subjects showing no evidence of ischemia or other abnormality who are free of detectable risk of clinical CAD in the immediate future. The suggested schema for such classification is not the work of a single coordinated study, but rather is the rational synthesis of available

Table 10
Prognostic Classification of Exercise Test Findings

Classification	Exercise Test Abnormalities (from Table 7)
Grave or urgent	Two major abnormalities or one major abnormality and two minor abnormalities (or worse)
Definite but moderate risk	One major abnormality or two minor abnormalities
Minor or borderline increase in CAD risk	One minor abnormality
Incomplete/nondiagnostic	Unconvincing effort but no abnormalities
Normal/no evidence of CAD risk	Normal treadmill time or heart rate index plus satisfactory effort, no abnormal findings either major or minor

CAD = Coronary artery disease.

knowledge on this subject at the time of writing (Table 10). The schema has the advantages of being readily understood and easy to employ. It contains sufficient stratification to operate synergistically with clinical judgment in selecting the optimal course for each individual, and it permits ready comparison of degrees of normality or abnormality when exercise tests are conducted sequentially for follow-up studies.

REFERENCES

1. Gould KL, Lipscomb K: Effects of coronary stenoses on coronary flow reserve and resistance. Am J Cardiol 1974;34:48−55.
2. Froelicher VF Jr: The detection of asymptomatic coronary artery disease. Ann Rev Med 1977;28:1−12.
3. Weiner DA, Ryan TJ, McCabe CH, Kennedy JW, Schloss M, Tristani F, Chaitman BR, Fisher LD: Exercise stress testing. Correlations among history of angina, ST-segment response and prevalence of coronary-artery disease in the coronary artery surgery study (CASS). N Engl J Med 1979;301:230−235.
4. McNeer JF, Margolis JR, Lee KL, Kisslo JA, Peter RH, Kong Y, Behar VS, Wallace AG, McCants CB, Rosati RA: The role of the exercise test in the evaluation of patients for ischemic heart disease. Circulation 1978;57:64−70.
5. Ellestad MH, Wan MKC: Predictive implications of stress testing.

Follow-up of 2700 subjects after maximum treadmill stress testing. *Circulation* 1975;51:363–369.

6. Bruce RA, Blackmon JR, Jones JW, Strait G: Exercising testing in adult normal subjects and cardiac patients. *Pediatrics* 1963;32 (Suppl):742–756.

7. Sheffield LT, Roitman D: Stress testing methodology. *Progr Cardiovasc Dis* 1976;19:33–49.

8. Dalke B, Ware RW: An experimental study of "physical fitness" of Air Force personnel. *US Armed Forces Med J* 1959;10:675–688.

9. Lester FM, Sheffield LT, Reeves, TJ: Electrocardiographic changes in clinically normal older men following near maximal and maximal exercise. *Circulation* 1967;36:5–14.

10. Sheffield LT, Maloof JA, Sawyer JA, Roitman D: Maximal heart rate and treadmill performance of healthy women in relation to age. *Circulation* 1978;57:79–84.

11. Sheffield LT, Holt JH, Reeves TJ: Exercise graded by heart rate in electrocardiographic testing for angina pectoris. *Circulation* 1965; 32:622–629.

12. Cole JP, Ellestad MH: Significance of chest pain during treadmill exercise: correlation with coronary events. *Am J Cardiol* 1978;41: 227–232.

13. Thomson PD, Kelemen MH: Hypotension accompanying the onset of exertional angina. A sign of severe compromise of left ventricular blood supply. *Circulation* 1975;52:28–32.

14. Zaret BL, Stenson RE, Martin ND, Strauss HW, Wells HP Jr, McGowan RL, Flamm MD: Potassium-43 myocardial perfusion scanning for the noninvasive evaluation of patients with false-positive exercise tests. *Circulation* 1973;48:1234–1241.

15. Schelbert HR, Verba JW, Johnson AD, et al: Nontraumatic determination of left ventricular ejection fraction of radionuclide angiocardiography. *Circulation* 1975;51:902–909.

16. Ascoop CA, Simoons ML, Egmond WG, Bruschke AVG: Exercise test, history, and serum lipid levels in patients with chest pain and normal electrocardiogram at rest: Comparison to findings at coronary arteriography. *Am Heart J* 1971;82:609–617.

17. Enos WF, Holmes RH, Beyer J: Coronary disease among United States soldiers killed in action in Korea. *J Am Med Assoc* 1953;152: 1090–1093.

18. Mitrani Y, Karplus H, Brunner D: Coronary atherosclerosis in cases of traumatic death. In *Medicine and Sport*, Vol 4: *Physical Activity and Aging*, Brunner D, Jokl E (eds). Baltimore, University Park Press, 1970;4:241–248.

19. Chaitman BR, Bourassa MG, Wagniart P, Corbara F, Ferguson RJ: Improved efficiency of treadmill exercise testing using a multiple lead ECG system and basic hemodynamic exercise response. *Circulation* 1978;57:71–79.

20. Paffenbarger RS Jr, Wing AL, Hyde RT: Contemporary physical activity and incidence of heart attack in college men. *Circulation* 1977 (Suppl III); 55 & 56:111–115.

21. American College of Sports Medicine: *Guidelines for Graded Exercise Testing and Exercise Prescription*. Philadelphia, Lea & Febiger, 1976.

22. Erb BD, Fletcher GF, Sheffield LT: Standards for cardiovascular exercise treatment programs. American Heart Association Subcommittee on Rehabilitation. Target Activity Group. *Circulation* 1979; 59:1084A–1090A.
23. Andersen KL, Shephard RJ, Denolin H, Varnauskas E, Masironi R: Exercise tests in assessment of fitness for jobs and work activity. In *Fundamentals of Exercise Testing*. Geneva, World Health Organization 1971:113–118.
24. Master AM: The two-step exercise electrocardiogram: A test for coronary insufficiency. *Ann Intern Med* 1950;32:842–863.
25. Detry JR: *Exercise Testing and Training in Coronary Heart Disease*. Baltimore, Williams and Wilkins, 1973.
26. Lawrie GM, Morris GC Jr, Howell JF, Ogura JW, Spencer WH III, Cashion WR, Winters WL, Beazley HL, Chapman DW, Peterson PK, Lie JT: Results of coronary bypass more than 5 years after operation in 434 patients. Clinical, treadmill exercise and angiographic correlations. *Am J Cardiol* 1977;40:665–672.
27. DeMaria AN, Zakauddin V, Amsterdam EA, Mason DT: Disturbances of cardiac rhythm and conduction induced by exercise: diagnostic, prognostic and therapeutic implications. In *Exercise in Cardiovascular Health and Disease*. Amsterdam EA, Wilmore JH, DeMaria AN (eds). New York, Yorke Medical Books, 1977:209–217.
28. James FW, Kaplan S, Schwartz DC, Chou TC, Sandker MJ, Naylor V: Response to exercise in patients after total surgical correction of Tetralogy of Fallot. *Circulation* 1976;54:671–679.
29. James FW, Kaplan S: Systolic hypertension during submaximal exercise after correction of coarctation of aorta. *Circulation* 1974;49–50 SII:27–34.
30. Minow RA, Benjamin RS, Gottlieb JA: Adriamycin cardiomyopathy: An overview with determination of risk factors. *Cancer Chemother Rep* 1975;6:197.
31. Glasser SP, Clark RI: *The Clinical Approach to Exercise Testing*. New York, Harper & Row 1980;184–187.
32. Hellerstein HK, Hirsch EZ, Ader R, Greenblott N, Siegel M: Principles of exercise prescription for normals and cardiac subjects. In *Exercise Testing and Exercise Training in Coronary Heart Disease*. Naughton JP, Hellerstein HK (eds). New York, Academic Press 1973; 129–167.
33. Wilson PK, Fardy PS, Froelicher VF: Cardiac rehabilitation, adult fitness, and exercise testing. Philadelphia, Lea & Febiger 1981; 416–430.
34. Koppes G, McKiernan T, Bassan M, Froelicher VF: Treadmill exercise testing. Part II. *Curr Probl Cardiol* 1977;7:1–45.
35. Mason RE, Likar I, Biern RO, Ross RS: Multiple-lead exercise electrocardiography. Experience in 107 normal subjects and 67 patients with angina pectoris, and comparison with coronary cinearteriography in 84 patients. *Circulation* 1967;36:517–525.
36. Shackel B: Skin-drilling: a method of diminishing galvanic skin-potentials. *Am J Psychol* 1959;72:114–121.
37. Blackburn H, Taylor HL, Okamoto N, Rautaharju P, Mitchell PL,

Kerkhof AC: Standardization of the exercise electrocardiogram. A systematic comparison of chest lead configuration employed for monitoring during exercise. In *Physical Activity and the Heart*. Karvonen MJ, Barry AJ (eds). Springfield, Charles C. Thomas 1967;101–133.

38. Hollenberg M, Zoltick J, Go M, Yaney CA, Bedynek J: Quantitative treadmill score yields less than 1% false positive responders in young asymptomatic officers vs 12% by standard ECG criteria. *Circulation* 1984;70:II–158.

39. Hellerstein HK, Franklin BA: Exercise testing and prescription. In *Rehabilitation of the Coronary Patient*. Wenger NK, Hellerstein HK (eds). New York, John Wiley & Sons 1978;149–202.

40. Borg G: A simple rating scale for use in physical work tests. *Kgl Fysiogr Saellsk Lund Foerh* 1962;32:7–15.

41. Astrand PO, Rhyming I: A nomogram for calculation of aerobic capacity (physical fitness) from pulse rate during submaximal work. *J Appl Physical* 1954;7:218–221.

42. Stuart RJ Jr, Ellestad MH: National survey of exercise stress testing facilities. *Chest* 1980;77:94–97.

43. Selzer A, Cohn K: On the interpretation of the exercise test. *Circulation* 1978;58:193–195.

44. Kansal S, Roitman D, Sheffield LT: Stress testing with ST-segment depression at rest. An angiographic correlation. *Circulation* 1976;54:636–639.

45. Kansal S, Roitman D, Bradley EL, Sheffield LT: Enhanced evaluation of treadmill tests by means of scoring based on multivariate analysis and its clinical application: a study of 608 patients. *Am J Cardiol* 1983;52:1155–1160.

46. Gerson MC, Phillips JF, Morris SN, McHenry PL: Exercise-induced U-wave inversion as a marker of stenosis of the left anterior descending coronary artery. *Circulation* 1979;60:1014–1020.

47. Bonoris PE, Greenberg PS, Castellanet MJ, Ellestad MH: Significance of changes in R wave amplitude during treadmill stress testing: angiographic correlation. *Am J Cardiol* 1978;41:846–851.

48. McHenry PL, Morris SN, Jordan JW: Stress testing in coronary heart disease. *Heart and Lung* 1974;3:83–92.

49. Faris JV, McHenry PL, Jordan JW, Morris SN: Prevalence and reproducibility of exercise-induced ventricular arrhythmias during maximal exercise testing in normal men. *Am J Cardiol* 1976;37:617–622.

50. Goldschlager N, Selzer A, Cohn K: Treadmill stress tests as indicators of presence and severity of coronary artery disease. *Ann Intern Med* 1976;85:277–286.

51. Fletcher GF, Cantwell JD: Exercise stress testing: a review. In *Exercise and Coronary Heart Disease*. Springfield, Charles C. Thomas 1974;46–78.

52. Council on Scientific Affairs. Indications and contraindications for exercise testing. *JAMA* 1981;246:1015–1018.

53. Weiner DA, Ryan TJ, McCahe CH, Chaitman BR, Sheffield LT, Ferguson JC, Fisher LD, Tristani F: Prognostic importance of a clinical profile and exercise test in medically treated patients with coronary artery disease. *JACC* 1984;3:772–779.

3

The Exercise Prescription

J. Ronald Mikolich, M.D.
Gerald F. Fletcher, M.D.

INTRODUCTION

The recent popularity of a "fitness life-style" among both healthy and unhealthy segments of our society has resulted in a need for proper guidelines in the pursuit of regular exercise.[1] Physicians, both in hospitals and in private offices, are increasingly being called upon to prescribe programs of both supervised and nonsupervised exercise. Knowledge of the basic exercise prescription is rapidly becoming a "fundamental" for physicians dealing with patients on a daily basis, particularly in the current environment of a "wellness" oriented society.

In order to improve cardiopulmonary endurance and peripheral muscle conditioning, exercise activity should be defined specifically. Exercise means physical energy expenditure. The term does not always mean running, jogging, or high levels of physical activity. Prescribed exercise may be as little as "walking around the block" three times a week at a slow pace of one mile in 15 to 20 minutes or it may incorporate a higher levels of exercise of three to four miles in 25 to 30 minutes, three to five times a week. Alternatively, exercise may incorporate bicycling, swimming, racquetball, and in some instances, recreational sports such as tennis, if

From: Fletcher GF: *Exercise in the Practice of Medicine,* 2nd Revised Edition. Mount Kisco, NY, Futura Publishing Co., Inc., © 1988.

utilized properly at an effective level of oxygen consumption. Proper implementation of the multiple exercise activities for a given individual constitutes an "exercise prescription." Utilizing physiological principles, the exercise prescription specifies not only the type of activity, but also the intensity, frequency, and duration for any given subject. In addition, the potential dangers of an an exercise program should be delineated,[2] especially among those individuals who plan to exercise, regardless of their physician's opinion.

This chapter will discuss how exercise is prescribed for the benefit of both healthy and unhealthy individuals. The physiological principles involved in writing the exercise prescription will be explained. Categories of patients will be defined. The role of exercise testing in formulating the exercise prescription will be discussed and followed by examples of writing the exercise prescription utilizing the concept of target heart rate. The more general approach of using metabolic equivalents and rate of perceived exertion will also be discussed. The various phases of inpatient and outpatient exercise using both individual and group programs will be detailed. The role of the physician in writing the exercise prescription should be emphasized, especially for subjects with known heart disease. The execution of an exercise prescription should be conducted under medical supervision by allied health personnel who are familiar with and involved in exercise activities.

PHYSIOLOGICAL PRINCIPLES

The oxygen requirement of the myocardium, whether at rest or during periods of exertion, is defined by the physiologic term "myocardial oxygen consumption" (MVO_2). This term quantitates the amount of oxygen utilized by each 100 grams of myocardium per minute. Precise measurement of myocardial oxygen consumption requires simultaneous sampling of arterial and coronary sinus blood for oxygen content, as well as determination of coronary sinus blood flow. This invasive means of monitoring myocardial oxygen consumption is not always applicable in the clinical setting, particularly for repeated measurements. Therefore, one must evaluate the determinants of myocardial oxygen consumption in order to find an easily obtainable clinical index of myocardial oxygen consumption. The major determinants of myocardial oxygen consumption are heart rate, state of myocardial contractility, and left ventricular wall tension.[3,4] Since heart rate is the only determinant that is easily recorded during exercise, it has become the traditional method of assessing myocardial oxygen consumption with respect to exercise.

The most extensive investigation of the hemodynamic correlates of myocardial oxygen consumption during exercise was done by Kitamura et al.[5] This study assessed easily measurable hemodynamic indices which were reliably predictive of coronary blood flow and myocardial oxygen consumption for a clinically pertinent range of exercise levels in the upright position. Regression equation analysis substantiated a good correlation (coefficient = 0.88) between heart rate and myocardial oxygen consumption. Furthermore, it was determined that calculation of indices such as "rate-pressure product" (coefficient of correlation = 0.90) added little to the correlation with coronary blood flow and myocardial oxygen consumption. This excellent correlation between heart rate and myocardial oxygen consumption is not unexpected since heart rate is a reflection of the number of times per minute myocardial tension is developed. Furthermore, an increase in the rate of myocardial contractions increases the state of myocardial contractility (Bowditch effect) which in its own accord is a determinant of myocardial oxygen consumption.

It should be noted that the correlation between heart rate and myocardial oxygen consumption may not be acceptable in the presence of significant left ventricular dysfunction. This discrepancy occurs because of an increase in myocardial wall tension resulting in an increase in myocardial oxygen consumption above that reflected by a change in heart rate. Therefore, reliable assessment of myocardial oxygen consumption by heart rate monitoring can be done only when left ventricular dysfunction is compensated.

The ability to assess myocardial oxygen consumption noninvasively during exercise by monitoring heart rate is clinically pertinent with regard to coronary artery disease. When atherosclerotic lesions limit coronary arterial blood flow (i.e., limit oxygen supply), angina pectoris may occur when demand (myocardial oxygen consumption) exceeds supply. In most cases, angina is reproducible at a given heart rate (i.e., level of myocardial oxygen consumption) in a given patient.

When a subject exercises, oxygen supply to peripheral muscles increases usually by an increase in cardiac output. Cardiac output is a function of heart rate and stroke volume. Because the ability to increase stroke volume during exercise is limited to a degree, the increase in cardiac output and oxygen supply to peripheral muscles is accomplished primarily by an increase in the heart rate. Peripheral muscle utilization of oxygen becomes more efficient with physical training and the oxygen demand decreases. As a result of the peripheral changes that occur with physical training, the heart rate response to a given work load decreases. Thus, since heart rate is a reflection of myocardial oxygen consumption, the net effect of physical training is to reduce myocardial oxygen consumption for any given level of physical activity or work.

This beneficial effect of physical training may be documented by the change in heart rate to a standardized work load on a treadmill or a bicycle ergometer. The corollary effect is that physical training increases the amount of work which can be performed at a given heart rate. Knowledge of the relationship between increasing heart rate and increasing myocardial oxygen consumption during physical training is essential to the understanding and formulation of the exercise prescription as it is used clinically.

CATEGORIES OF EXERCISE SUBJECTS

In prescribing exercise, several groups of subjects must be considered. The *allegedly healthy* group is comprised of subjects who are often involved in their own personal exercise program and rarely see a physician. Young, urban professionals constitute a large portion of this group, who wish to embark on a regular exercise program. Although usually healthy, this group may have underlying disease—perhaps silent myocardial ischemia. An exercise test and cardiac evaluation are usually recommended in this group if the subject is more than 40 years of age. Repeat exercise testing and medical supervision is usually not necessary unless symptoms or signs of cardiac or pulmonary disease develop. Both individual and group-structured programs may be employed. The latter is often more effective in promoting compliance because of companionship. A problem among the allegedly healthy group is that they often "over exercise." They may be under the false impression that running 25, 30, or 40 miles per week promotes better health. Such level of exercise may actually be harmful and may be associated with poor long-term compliance.[2]

The *coronary-prone* group has a greater predilection toward coronary atherosclerotic heart disease. These subjects include hypertensive patients, those who are overweight with lipid abnormalities, cigarette smokers, and those with arrhythmias and other risk factors which may predispose to the development of coronary atherosclerosis. This group also includes patients with angiographically documented coronary atherosclerosis who have stable angina, with or without medications. These subjects require exercise testing prior to the writing of an exercise prescription. They also need medical supervision for a period of time until a home exercise program is established. Follow-up exercise testing is recommended and the exercise program should incorporate education and risk factor modification intervention. This particular group of patients should be observed diligently for signs of progressive coronary atherosclerosis, i.e., development of unstable angina, ischemic electrocardiographic changes or Holter recording evidence of silent myocardial ischemia.[6]

The *myocardial infarction* group has, for the last decade, comprised the largest population of subjects in medically supervised exercise programs. The prescription in this group of patients is quite variable, taking into account the type of myocardial infarction, complications, and current drug therapy. Definition of coronary anatomy and extent of atherosclerosis is of tremendous importance in this group of subjects. An initial exercise test with follow-up testing as often as every 6 months is standard practice. Often an acute phase program is utilized in which patients enter exercise programs immediately after leaving the hospital for a very low level of directly supervised activity. Such a structured, supervised program may be appropriate for a period of 1 to 3 weeks, depending on clinical stability, signs of progression of atherosclerotic disease, and functional response. These patients should be monitored carefully since often they do not admit their symptoms, and other manifestations of disease progression may go undetected.

The *myocardial revascularization* (coronary artery bypass) group is comprised of individuals who have undergone definitive surgical therapy for coronary atherosclerosis. During the last several years, medically supervised exercise and rehabilitation have been utilized to return these cardiac patients to the highest possible levels of occupational and physical activity. Several of these individuals have sustained a previous myocardial infarction. Coronary angiography data from these patients are vital to the formulation of prescriptive exercise with regard to knowing the basic integrity of the left ventricle and the native coronary circulation.

Patients with good left ventricular function may begin earlier and progress more rapidly with rehabilitation. Risk factor modification, especially abstention from cigarette smoking, is of utmost importance. Exercise testing is needed initially and should be repeated every 6 to 9 months. Surgical considerations, such as stability of the median sternotomy incision, healing of the saphenous vein donor sites, and potential for wound infection must be taken into consideration. Not only is anemia prevalent among this group of subjects, but rapid changes in intravascular volume status and cardiac rhythm can develop, requiring close hemodynamic monitoring during the exercise session and the time period immediately thereafter. The spectrum of this group ranges from the immediate postoperative period to a home maintenance program, well after the patient has returned to his usual occupation and life-style. The exercise prescription must be altered by the physician to meet the needs of this constantly changing group of individuals.[7]

The *post-interventional* (coronary angioplasty and thrombolysis therapy) group is comprised of individuals who have undergone a cardiac catheterization procedure to improve coronary blood flow, i.e., balloon dilatation angioplasty, streptokinase thrombolysis, tissue-activated plasminogen administration, or a combination of these procedures. Although extensive anatomic information is available by virtue of the patient's coronary arteriogram, hemodynamic status, and assessment of coronary flow reserve, these subjects require exercise testing prior to the writing of an exercise prescription. Although these cardiac patients usually return to the highest possible levels of occupational and physical activity after their intervention, previous myocardial events (e.g., myocardial infarction) and atherosclerosis in coronary vessels distant from the site of intervention must be considered. Because of the short hospital stay associated with most interventional procedures, a short-term, more intensive type of cardiac rehabilitation program may be appropriate for this group of patients.

EXERCISE TESTING

For ambulatory subjects, the most objective evaluation for prescribing a level of exercise training is the *exercise test*. A treadmill or bicycle ergometer may be used, although most programs favor use of the treadmill. The exercise test should be done under medical supervision with equipment available for cardiopulmonary resuscitation. A "submaximal" test, such as the modified Bruce protocol, is most appropriate for the immediate (up to 3 weeks) post-infarction and post-aortocoronary bypass patient. Four to 8 weeks after one of these cardiac events, a near maximal level test may be pursued.

The important data derived from exercise testing are seen in Table 1. The electrocardiographic ST segment, blood pressure, heart rate response, and duration of test time are all important as basic fundamentals of the test. ST segment flattening of > 2 mm for 0.08 seconds below the level of the preceding TP or PQ segment is considered to be positive for myocardial ischemia. Drugs and conditions known to cause false-positive and indeterminant tests must be considered and ST segment changes in these settings may be less significant. To the contrary, more extreme ST depression of $\geq 4-5$ mm, especially in association with angina pectoris, may be indicative of "critical" left coronary artery disease and may war-

---

Table 1
Data to be Obtained from the Exercise Test to be Used in Prescriptive Exercise

---

SUBJECTIVE
    Angina Pectoris   Leg Discomfort
    Dyspnea   Dizziness
    Fatigue-Weakness

OBJECTIVE
    Physical Examination
        Time on Treadmill
        General Appearance
        Cyanosis
        Blood Pressure Response
        Heart Rate Response
        Pulmonary Rales
        Peripheral Pulses
        Precordial Exam for Dyskinetic Areas, Murmurs, and Gallops—(Before and
          After Exercise)

    Electrocardiogram
        Repolarization Changes—ST segment and J point
        Rate Response
        Dysrhythmias
        Conduction Abnormalities—Atrioventricular and Ventricular

rant other studies including coronary angiography before a patient is allowed to exercise. Recent studies have supported the concern of obtaining an appropriate elevation in systolic blood pressure with exercise testing. In addition, the heart rate response for a given work load in testing is important. The lack of appropriate increase in heart rate (in absence of beta-blocking drugs) may indicate underlying myocardial or conduction system disease. To the contrary, extreme rate elevation, dysrhythmias, and conduction disturbances may warrant specific therapy before a subject enters an exercise program.

Palpation and auscultation of the precordium before and after testing to detect areas of dyskinesis, gallop rhythm, and murmurs are important. The general appearance of the patient and attitude on the treadmill provide additional information. Some laboratories measure oxygen consumption by analysis of expired air with exercise; however, this may be accurately estimated from the heart rate.[5] In addition, the lack of direct verbal communication with the patient during the collection of air may detract from the total evaluation of the patient's response to exercise.

More details on exercise testing are seen in Chapter 2.

PHASES OF CARDIAC REHABILITATION

Traditionally, cardiac rehabilitation programs have been divided into three phases: acute, therapeutic, and maintenance. An exercise prescription is required for successful implementation of all phases. The *acute phase* exercise prescription is a rigidly detailed inpatient program (see Table 2) which begins early in the patient's hospital course, usually in the Intensive Care Unit. Beginning with simple activities such as sitting in a chair for 20-minute periods, patients progress to daily walking routines and specific limb exercises in the later days of hospitalization. This type of exercise prescription usually incorporates electrocardiographic monitoring. Provided that no complications such as hypotension, cardiac arrhythmia, left ventricular failure, or pulmonary edema have occurred, the acute phase of cardiac rehabilitation may begin on the third hospital day. Progression through the various levels of activity must be tailored to the individual needs of the patient, and the rate of progression is highly variable depending upon motivation, socioeconomic background, previous level of physical fitness, and coexistent disease processes.

The *therapeutic phase* of exercise, as described in standards by the American Heart Association,[8] is formulated during hospitalization and may extend for 3 to 12 months after hospitalization under supervision of a physician. These programs frequently use monitored exercise with various stations such as rowing machines, bicycle ergometers, treadmills, and hand cranks (see Fig. 1). Such programs have the advantage of directly monitoring the heart rate and blood pressure in order to meticulously guide the patient through a precise exercise prescription. Alternatively, the therapeutic phase of exercise may involve a home walk program as seen in Tables 3 and 4. A more advanced or "intermediate" program is detailed in Table 5. These home programs, which do not utilize electrocardiographic monitoring, are best suited for those subjects who have been free of complications such as cardiac arrhythmias during the acute phase of cardiac rehabilitation. The ability of the patient to monitor his own pulse rate is crucial to the success of this type of exercise prescription. This phase of cardiac rehabilitation should include strict modification of risk factors. Patients usually demonstrate definable progress in this phase of exercise, thereby requiring frequent revision of the exercise prescription. Such revisions generally require objective re-evaluation of the patient's capacity for exercise, i.e., an exercise test.

The *maintenance phase*[9] of an exercise program is usually conducted without physician supervision, but initial and follow-up exercise testing is strongly encouraged. Except for the *allegedly healthy* group of patients, the maintenance phase follows a logical progression from a therapeutic exercise program. *Allegedly healthy* subjects may enter a *maintenance phase* program without having participated in a therapeutic program. This phase of cardiac rehabilitation encompasses the widest range of exercise programs including walking, bike riding, and group recreational activities. Such programs may be conducted on an individual basis or as a structured group utilizing an exercise leader or supervisor with a specific regimen of calisthenics, walk/jog activities, and competitive sports such as volleyball, tennis, basketball, and handball.

CONCEPT OF TARGET HEART RATE

The target heart rate is the most important single factor to be considered in writing the exercise prescription.[10] Target heart rate is the heart rate in beats per minute (BPM) at which a subject

Table 2
In-Patient Activity Protocol (Includes Physical Therapy Exercise)

Step/Day/Where	Post-Myocardial Infarction Activity (Noncomplicated MI)	Step/Day/Where	Post-Cardiac Surgery Activity
Step 1/Day 2	Bedside commode, feed self, self-grooming (brush teeth, comb hair wash hands & face) Dangle at bedside–if tolerated, increase to Chair 10–15 minutes b.i.d.	Step 1/Day 1 SICU	Feed self, self-grooming (brush teeth, comb hair, wash hands & face) Sit on side of bed in PM Chair 15–30 minutes in PM (as tol.) Diaphragmatic breathing Ankle dorsiflexion (10 ×)
Step 2/Day 3 CCU or Medical Floor if transferred	Chair 20 minutes t.i.d. Bed bath (staff to assist with back & lower legs) Active ROM 10 × supine q.d. BR privileges if bathroom in room	Step 2/Day 2 SICU Transfer to Surgical Nursing Area	BR with assistance, self-grooming Chair 20 minutes t.i.d. Walk 50–150′ as tolerated t.i.d. (Once with P.T. 50–150′) Active ROM 10 × supine q.d.
Step 3/Day 4 Medical Nursing Area	Bathe self (staff to assist with back & lower legs) BR privileges–may sit at sink to shave Chair 30 minutes q.i.d. Walk back & forth in room as tolerated Upper extremities long sitting (LS) in bed Lower extremities sitting P.T. to ambulate 50–100′ in hall	Step 3/Day 3 Surgical Nursing Area	Bathe self at bedside or basin Chair 30 minutes q.i.d. Walk 100–200′ as tolerated t.i.d. Upper extremities long sitting (LS) in bed Lower extremities sitting

Step/Day/Where	Post-Myocardial Infarction Activity (Noncomplicated MI)	Step/Day/Where	Post-Cardiac Surgery Activity
Step 4/Day 5 Medical Nursing Area	Bed bath or warm tub bath Walk 100–200' in hall t.i.d. Chair 45 minutes q.i.d. Active ROM 10 × sitting q.d.	Step/Day 4 Surgical Nursing Area	Chair q.i.d. & PRN Walk 200–400' q.i.d. & PRN with assistance Active ROM × 10 sitting q.d.
Step 5/Day 6–7 Medical Nursing Area	Up ad lib in chair Walk 200–400' q.i.d. Active ROM 10 × standing	Step 5/Day 5 Surgical Nursing Area	Up ad lib in room Walk 400' q.i.d. & PRN Active ROM × 10 standing Home Exercise Instruction
Step 6/Day 8–10 Medical Nursing Area	May shower Low level exercise test Climb one flight of stairs Walk 400' q.i.d. & PRN Exercises standing Home Exercise Instruction	Step 6/Day 6–8 Surgical Nursing Area	Walk 400' q.i.d. & PRN May tub bathe or shower after stitches removed-usually after 10th day
Step 7/after 10 days	Walk 400' q.i.d. & PRN	Step 7/Day 7	Walk 400' q.i.d. & PRN

CCU = Cardiac Care Unit
SICU = Surgical Intensive Care Unit
t.i.d. = three times daily
BR = bathroom

q.i.d. = four times daily
PRN = as needed
b.i.d. = two times daily
ROM = range of motion

q.d. = daily
× = repetitions
ex = exercise
LS = sitting up in bed with legs extended

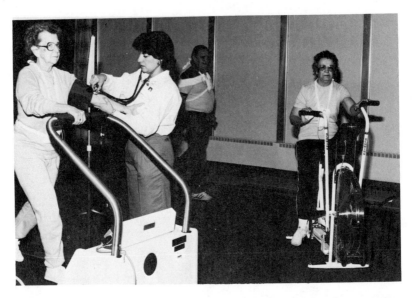

Figure 1A: Patients are shown in a monitored exercise program including a walk-jog program combined with individual exercise stations. Continued.

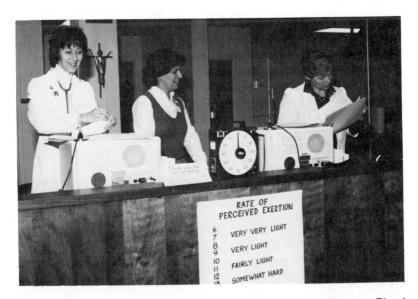

Figure 1B: The ECG rhythm is monitored continuously via telemetry. Blood pressure responses to exercise are also closely monitored. The total program incorporates both arm and leg exercises.

Table 3
Standard Home Walk Program
Cardiac Rehabilitation*

Week After Discharge	Distance	Allotted Time
Week 1	walk ¼ mile daily	Leisurely pace 5 minutes
Week 2–3	walk ¼ mile twice daily	Leisurely pace 5 minutes each time
Week 4	walk ½ mile daily or twice a day if tolerates the above	Leisurely pace 10 minutes
Week 5	walk ¾ mile daily	Leisurely pace 15 minutes
Weeks 6–7	walk 1 mile daily	Leisurely pace 20 minutes
Week 8	walk 1½ miles daily	Leisurely pace 30 minutes
Week 9	walk 2 miles daily	Leisurely pace 40 minutes
Week 10	walk 2 miles daily	Moderate pace 30 minutes
Weeks 11–12	walk 3 miles daily	Leisurely pace 60 minutes
Week 13	walk 3 miles daily	Moderate pace 50 minutes
Week 14	walk 4 miles daily	Moderate pace of 60 minutes (15 minutes per mile)

*Check your pulse rate immediately at the end of every walk. Do not advance to the next stage (as from week 3 to week 4) unless the immediate post-exercise rate is less than _____ beats per minute.

The key rule of thumb to remember is . . . "Listen to your body." If you get tired . . . stop walking for the day. Advance your distance as you feel ready.

Table 4
Accelerated Home Walk Program
Cardiac Rehabilitation

Week After Discharge	Distance	Allotted Time
**Week 1	¼ mile/day twice a day	Leisurely pace of 5 minutes
Week 2	½ mile/day twice a day	Leisurely pace of 10 minutes
Week 3	¾ mile/day	Leisurely pace of 15 minutes
Weeks 4 & 5	1 mile/day	Leisurely pace of 20 minutes
Week 6	1¼ miles/day	Moderate pace of 20 minutes
Week 7	1½ miles/day	Moderate pace of 25 minutes
Week 8	2 miles/day	Moderate pace of 30 minutes
Weeks 9 & 10	3 miles/day	Moderate pace of 45 minutes
Week 11	4 miles/day	Moderate pace of 60 minutes
Week 12	4 miles/day	Fast walk of 56 minutes
Continue Indefinitely		

**For the first few days after you get home, walk at a leisurely pace. If, after a few days, you don't feel challenged by walking ¼ mile, twice a day and you don't feel tired, you may increase your distance.

Check your pulse rate immediately at the end of every walk. Do not advance to the next stage (as from week 3 to week 4) unless the immediate post-exercise rate is less than _____ beats per minute.

The key rule of thumb to remember is . . . "Listen to your body." If you get tired . . . stop walking for the day. Advance your distance as you feel ready.

Table 5
Home Walk Program After Angioplasty
Cardiac Rehabilitation*

Week After Discharge	Distance	Allotted Time
Week 1	½ mile/day	Leisurely pace of 10 minutes
Week 2	½ mile twice a day	Leisurely pace of 10 minutes
	or	
	1 mile/day	Leisurely pace of 20 minutes
Week 3	1¼−1½ miles/day	Leisurely pace of 20−25 minutes
Week 4	1½−2 miles/day	Moderate pace of 25−30 minutes

After Week 4 - Continue to walk 2 miles per day (or 25−30 minutes of walking) at a moderate to brisk pace.

If you don't feel challenged by this, you may increase your walking by five minute intervals.

For example:
Walk 30 minutes and increase to 35 minutes for several days. If again you don't feel challenged increase to 40 minutes for several days.

You may increase to a total of 60 minutes of walking.
Try to walk a minimum of 6 days a week.
If you would like to begin a higher level of exercise, please discuss with your physician.

*For the first few days after you get home, walk at a leisurely pace. If, after a few days, you don't feel challenged by walking ½ mile and you don't feel tired, you may increase your distance.

Check your pulse rate immediately at the end of every walk. Do not advance to the next stage (as from week 3 to week 4) unless the immediate post-exercise rate is less than _____ beats per minute.

The key rule of thumb to remember is . . . "Listen to your body." If you get tired . . . stop walking for the day. Advance your distance as you feel ready.

should exercise on a regular basis to achieve a "training effect" (i.e., improved maximal oxygen consumption and decrease in rate-pressure product for the same work load). It represents the heart rate just below the "critical" rate at which myocardial oxygen consumption may exceed oxygen supply resulting in myocardial ischemia.

Although the heart rate is the clinical index by which changes in the state of physical training are measured, heart rate should not be regarded as an entity unto itself. In order for a "training effect" to occur, the target heart rate must be achieved in response to skeletal muscle work. Target heart rate is easily derived from the results of standard treadmill or bicycle ergometer exercise tests. Ordinarily, a patient performs continuous exercise according to one of a number of standardized exercise protocols until he reaches his maximal heart rate or an objective end-point such as angina pectoris, ST segment displacement, or ventricular dysrhythmia.

Target heart rate may be calculated by the following formula: maximal heart rate achieved on exercise testing × 0.85 = target heart rate.

From the practical standpoint, target heart rate (plus or minus 5 BPM) is acceptable during exercise. It is important to note that the formula is based on the heart rate actually achieved by a given patient and may not correlate with the age-adjusted maximal heart rate. The target heart rate should be recalculated at any time a patient's exercise tolerance would be expected to change—for instance, after coronary bypass surgery, with the addition of drugs such as beta-blocking agents, after physical conditioning occurs, or in instances when a subject must drop out of exercise for a period of time.

One of the clinical problems encountered in calculation of the target heart rate is adjustment for patients receiving beta-adrenergic blockade therapy, such as propranolol. Experience has revealed that fatigue often intervenes before target heart rate is achieved in patients on propranolol therapy. Difficulty in achieving target heart rate during the first few exercise sessions may discourage the patient, resulting in disinterest and discontinuance.

The study of Alderman et al.[11] provides objective data giving insight as to how the target heart rate might be adjusted. A portion of this study evaluated the heart rate response to exercise in patients who received *placebo, 80 mg, 160 mg,* and *320 mg of propranolol per day.* The authors determined that 80 mg of propranolol per day decreased the heart rate at the end-point of exercise by *14.6 percent* while 160 mg per day lowered it by *20.7 percent.* With the highest dosage studied (320 mg per day), the end-exercise heart rate decreased by *24.6 percent.*

On the basis of this study, recommendations for adjustment of the target heart rate for patients receiving propranolol can be made. By making such adjustments, an exercise program may be prescribed for the patient and a "training effect" achieved despite the negative chronotropic effects of propranolol.

An adaptation of the Karvonen formula[12] can also be used to calculate target heart rate for patients with impaired chronotropic responses to exercise testing. This method correlates closely with measured energy expenditure levels achieved on a standard exercise test, independent of beta-blocking agents which impair chronotropic responses. Utilizing the Karvonen formula, the target heart rate may be calculated by the following formula: target heart rate = resting heart rate + 85% (peak heart rate during exercise minus resting heart rate).

The calcium antagonists, verapamil and diltiazem, may exert a negative chronotropic effect and blunt the heart rate response to exercise. However, similar to the beta-adrenergic blockers, diltiazem does not alter the proportional relationship of heart rate and VO_2 max as demonstrated by the study of Chang et al.[13] Thus, use of verapamil and diltiazem as a part of the patient's drug regimen does not preclude the use of heart rate in the formulation of the exercise prescription. Furthermore, a "training effect" can also be achieved in these patients without apparent difficulty.

WRITING THE EXERCISE PRESCIPTION

The actual writing of the exercise prescription incorporates the following data:
1. The category of exercise subject (allegedly healthy, coronary prone, post-infarction, post-bypass surgery, post-angioplasty).
2. Exercise test results.
3. Phase of cardiac rehabilitation (acute, therapeutic, maintenance).
4. Target heart rate.
5. Type of exercise program (individual or group-structured, walk/run or station-exercise, monitored or nonmonitored).

Other specific clinical data such as patient profile, mental attitude, motivation, body weight, current medications, and history of previous exercise must also be considered. Careful evaluation of these data allow one to "prescribe" an exercise program.

The monitored, station-exercise program utilizing bicycle ergometers, arm ergometers, and treadmill is the most detailed type of exercise prescription. The active exercise time is composed of a 4-minute warm-up period, a 20–30 minute period at target heart rate, and a 4-minute "cool down" (Fig. 2). The work load on the

GRADED EXERCISE SESSION

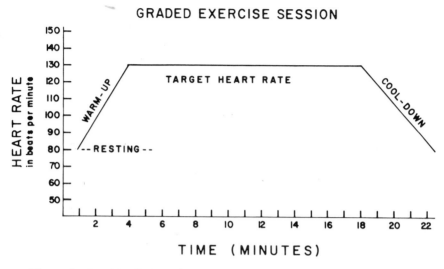

Figure 2: Graphic display of an individual response to a graded exercise session. This is applicable to most dynamic exercise sessions which should include a warm-up period followed by a 20 to 30 minute period of dynamic exercise at target heart rate attainment followed by a cool down period.

ergometers and treadmill is adjusted at regular intervals to achieve an increase, plateau, and decrease in the heart rate response of the patient. Although the most crucial portion of the exercise session is maintenance of target heart rate for a 20–30-minute period, difficulty may initially be encountered in producing a smooth progression from resting heart rate to target heart rate. Experience with bicycle ergometry has revealed that smooth progression to target heart rate can be achieved by setting the initial work load at 300 kilopond-meters (or the equivalent) lower than the maximum work load achieved during the initial exercise test (when done by bicycle ergometry). The work load is then increased by increments of 75 kilopond-meters per minute (or the equivalent) over the 4-minute warm-up period until target heart rate is achieved. This method serves as a guideline for determining the work load necessary to achieve an adequate warm-up period. Since each patient responds differently, this approach is empiric rather than absolute. A similar approach can be utilized for patients who have had exercise tests on a treadmill. For example, a patient may be started at Stage 1 of a Bruce protocol and advanced over a 4-minute period to a speed and inclination known to produce the desired heart rate.

Two to four exercise sessions may be required until a smooth heart rate response is obtained. Once target heart rate is achieved, work load is altered every minute to maintain it in the range of target heart rate (plus or minus 5 beats per minute). During the first six to eight exercise sessions, there will likely be a decrease in work load over the 10-minute plateau. However, as a "training effect" occurs, the required work load during the plateau phase will tend to remain at the 4-minute level, or may actually increase. The "cool down" period should be a smooth transition from target heart rate down to resting heart rate. This is accomplished by rapidly decreasing the work load to a zero resistance level over a 4-minute period. Following completion of exercise, the patient should be seated in a chair and oscilloscopic rhythm may be monitored for 10 or more minutes as necessary.

Although Thompson et al.[14] suggested that recommendations for including arm exercise in cardiac rehabilitation programs may not be justified, other studies[15] have documented a beneficial effect of arm exercise for cardiac patients, particularly those with occupational necessity of the upper extremities. Review of available data[14-16] suggests that approximately 25 to 50 percent of the training effect benefits untrained limbs, i.e., a "crossover" effect. Consequently, most cardiac rehabilitation centers incorporate some type of arm training into the exercise prescription. Franklin et al.[16] note that a lower maximal heart rate is achieved with arm ergometry as compared to leg ergometry (max heart rate with arm training = approximately 94 percent of max heart rate with leg training). Furthermore, 50 percent of the prescribed work load with leg training is sufficient for arm training. Accordingly, the exercise prescription must be altered appropriately when some form of arm training is implemented.

The group walk/run program is probably the most widely used method of executing the exercise prescription and is popular in many areas of the country.[17] These programs are usually medically supervised and involve patients who are post-infarction and post-bypass. These group-structured programs are designed to incorporate a warm-up period of 5 to 10 minutes, followed by a walk/run session of about 20–30 minutes and a 15-minute recreational session of volleyball, ping-pong, badminton, or pool games. Afterwards, there is a cool-down phase appropriate to the needs of the patient. Such programs have a physician supervisor and specialized personnel such as exercise program directors, exercise physiologists, nurses, occupational therapists, and physical therapists. Depending upon the patient's clinical status and available facilities, electrocardiographic monitoring via telemetry may or may not be utilized in such group-structured programs.

The individual home program is usually a progressive walk/jog/run protocol in which the subject monitors his or her own pulse rate. Such a program may incorporate calisthenics and recreational activities. The intensity of such an exercise program is quite variable, ranging from low levels for post-myocardial infarction and post-coronary bypass patients to high levels of intensity for allegedly healthy subjects. Most commonly, such a program is prescribed for patients who are discharged from hospitals in areas where group-structured programs are not available or for subjects who are unable, for other reasons, to join the group program.

Due to the recent popularity of commercial exercise facilities utilizing mechanical devices with variable resistance such as Nautilus[R] equipment, increasing numbers of subjects from the allegedly healthy group are requesting exercise prescriptions based on weight-training machines. Vander et al.[18] have demonstrated the safety of such exercise in cardiac patients, but note that peak heart rate responses were only 64 percent of the maximum values achieved during treadmill exercise testing.

It would appear that an exercise prescription incorporating variable resistance machines for specific muscle groups should incorporate high repetition, lower resistance levels so as to achieve aerobic conditioning. Such programs appear safe for cardiac patients and should include some form of pulse rate monitoring. Although a target heart rate for such subjects can be established utilizing a standardized exercise test, the intensity of exercise is usually established by the individual in an empiric manner.

In addition to intensity, duration, and mode of activity, frequency is the last component of an exercise prescription. *Acute phase* cardiac rehabilitation programs with low levels of progressive activity are generally conducted on a daily basis, whereas therapeutic and maintenance programs yield optimal results when pursued three times per week with rest intervals of 48–72 hours. More frequent exercise sessions usually result in "over training" and do not result in higher levels of conditioning. Emphasis should be placed on regularity of exercise sessions, avoiding sporadic attempts that frequently result in skeletal muscle injury. A minimum of two sessions per week appears to be required to maintain a training effect.

RATE OF PERCEIVED EXERTION (RPE) SYSTEM

A subjective method of assessing the intensity of exercise is the rating of perceived exertion (RPE) devised by Borg.[19] Exercise intensity is rated numerically on a scale from 6 to 20 (i.e., "very, very light" to "very, very hard"). A physiological basis for the RPE system has been documented,[20] but because of its subjective nature, the RPE may be difficult to apply in specific, individual cases. Increases in RPE give routine feedback to the individual pursuing an exercise program, allowing subjective signs of progress to be more apparent. Generally, RPE is used as an adjunctive parameter with target heart rate, rather than as an alternative to target heart rate. An exercise prescription based on RPE would be best suited for individuals from the allegedly healthy group.

THE METABOLIC EQUIVALENT (MET) SYSTEM

The MET (metabolic equivalent) is equal to 3.5 ml/kg/min of oxygen consumption. The MET is recommended as the unit of energy cost related to work load, since it is easily understood by both patient and physician, making it applicable to various tasks.[8] One MET is the approximate energy expenditure while quietly sitting in a chair. This unit, which corresponds essentially to the basal metabolic rate while sitting, may be used for all patients since it is expressed in terms of basal rate. Two METS is twice the energy expenditure of resting, while three METS is three times the energy expenditure of resting, and ten METS is ten times the energy expenditure of resting. A healthy 40-year-old male in the United States can function at ten METS at maximum capacity.

Recently, Fletcher et al.[21] have utilized the MET system as the basis for an exercise prescription, utilizing oxygen consumption determinations during the precardiac rehabilitation exercise test. Utilizing the Bruce protocol, the maximal oxygen consumption (VO_2 max) achieved at peak exercise was converted to METS ($VO_2 \div 3.5$ = maximal MET level). Utilizing a six-level protocol (see Table 6), an exercise prescription was written for subjects at levels ranging from 30 to 75 percent of the maximum MET level attained on exercise testing. A treadmill, arm ergometer, bicycle ergometer, and arm-leg bicycle ergometer were used in the six-level protocol. Continuous electrocardiographic monitoring was accomplished by telemetry. By prescribing exercise levels according to percentages of maximal MET levels on precardiac rehabilitation testing, patients successfully achieved their designated 50 to 75 percent target heart rate (Table 7). Completion of such a six-level protocol, based on metabolic equivalents, allows the patient to graduate into a nonmonitored exercise program more rapidly, while safely determining the patient's early response to various exercise procedures. In a nonmonitored setting, an exercise prescription may be written in a general manner for a given MET load. Table 8 displays a classification of various physical activities by MET units.

Table 6

Level	Arm Ergometer (60–75 rpm)	Treadmill*	Bicycle Ergometer Air Dyne (arm-leg)	Body Guard (leg only)
1	30% MM 100 turns 2 sets	50% MM	50% MM 8 min	35% MM 50 rpm 8 min
2	35% MM 125 turns 2 sets	60% MM	60% MM 8 min	40% MM 50 rpm 8 min
3	40% MM 125 turns 2 sets	70% MM	70% MM 8 min	45% MM 60 rpm 8 min
4	45% MM 150 turns 2 sets	75% MM	75% MM 12 min	45% MM 65 rpm 4 min
5	45% MM 150 turns 2 sets	75% MM	75% MM 15 min	No resistance 50 rpm 4 min Cool-down Do last
6	Repeat level 5			

*Each level consists of 1 minute of warm-up, 12 minutes of exercise and 1 minute of cool-down (warm-up and cool-down = 1.2 mph at 0% grade).

MM = maximal MET level achieved on exercise test; Turns = revolutions.

Table 7
Results of Exercise in the Six-Level Protocol (n = 31)

Variable	Mean 50–75% Target Heart Rate = 112 – 129 beats/min Session					
	1	2	3	4	5	6
Cal PE	11 ± 2	11 ± 2	10 ± 2	10 ± 2	10 ± 2	9 ± 2
HR achieved	104 ± 22	103 ± 24	101 ± 28	106 ± 25	105 ± 23	102 ± 21
Bicycle Erg						
MET level (Rx)	3 ± 1	4 ± 1	4 ± 1	5 ± 1	5 ± 1	5 ± 1
PE achieved	10 ± 2	11 ± 2	11 ± 2	12 ± 2	12 ± 3	12 ± 2
HR achieved	103 ± 23	107 ± 25	115 ± 25	121 ± 27	113 ± 36	123 ± 25
Arm Erg						
MET level (Rx)	2 ± 0.4	2 ± 1	2 ± 1	2 ± 1	2 ± 1	3 ± 1
PE achieved	10 ± 2	12 ± 2	12 ± 2	12 ± 2	12 ± 2	12 ± 2
HR achieved	104 ± 30	113 ± 27	115 ± 25	122 ± 24	117 ± 23	125 ± 35
Treadmill						
MET level (Rx)	4 ± 1	4 ± 1	5 ± 1	5 ± 1	6 ± 2	6 ± 1
PE achieved	11 ± 2	11 ± 2	12 ± 2	12 ± 2	13 ± 2	11 ± 2
HR achieved	112 ± 21	111 ± 24	118 ± 27	123 ± 41	125 ± 24	125 ± 24
Arm Erg R						
MET level (Rx)	2 ± 1	2 ± 1	2 ± 0.4	3 ± 1	3 ± 1	3 ± 1
PE achieved	11 ± 2	12 ± 2	12 ± 2	12 ± 2	12 ± 2	12 ± 2
HR achieved	109 ± 26	110 ± 27	119 ± 24	123 ± 26	120 ± 23	127 ± 24
Bicycle Erg R						
MET level (Rx)	3 ± 1	3 ± 1	4 ± 1	4 ± 1	2 ± 0.4	2 ± 0.4
PE achieved	11 ± 2	11 ± 2	12 ± 2	10 ± 2	7 ± 1	7 ± 1
HR achieved	105 ± 24	109 ± 28	117 ± 26	114 ± 26	96 ± 19	99 ± 21
Total ET (min)	39 ± 2	40 ± 1	40 ± 0.3	41 ± 1	44 ± 1	43 ± 3
Blood Pressure						
Rest SBP	130 ± 15	132 ± 21	123 ± 18	125 ± 16	123 ± 35	126 ± 16
Rest DBP	81 ± 11	81 ± 11	79 ± 11	81 ± 9	77 ± 10	80 ± 10
Peak SBP	141 ± 23	139 ± 21	138 ± 19	147 ± 21	146 ± 27	143 ± 39
Peak DBP	80 ± 11	78 ± 10	80 ± 11	82 ± 12	80 ± 11	79 ± 10
Rest HR	83 ± 19	84 ± 22	80 ± 20	83 ± 19	83 ± 21	79 ± 18

Values are mean ± standard deviation.
Cal = calisthenics; DBP = diastolic blood pressure (mm Hg); Erg = ergometry; ET = exercise time; HR = heart rate (beats/min); PE = perceived exertion; R = repeat set; Rx = prescribed; SBP = systolic blood pressure (mm Hg); TM = treadmill.

GENERAL COMMENTS REGARDING THE EXERCISE PRESCRIPTION

In writing an exercise prescription for an individual home program, monitored station program, or supervised group-structured program, there is constant need for updating of the prescrip-

Table 8
Classification of Activity by MET Units*

3–4 METS
 Walking (3 MHP)
 Cycling (6 MPH)
 Softball (excluding pitcher)
 Dancing (moderate)
 Pitching horse shoes
 Golf (pulling cart)
 Volleyball (6-man, not vigorous)
 Badminton (doubles)
 Steps (24 steps/minute, 12 cm,
  height) 4 METS
 Treadmill (2 MPH, 3.5%
  grade) 3 METS

4–5 METS
 Tennis (doubles)
 Walking (3½ MPH)
 Cycling (8 MPH)
 Ping-Pong
 Golf (carrying clubs)
 Raking leaves
 Calisthenics (in general)
 Rowing (noncompetitive)
 Dancing (vigorous)
 Step-up (24 steps/minute, 18
  cm height) 5 METS
 Treadmill (2 MPH, 7% grade)
  4 METS

5–6 METS
 Walking (4 MPH)
 Cycling (10 MPH)
 Ice skating
 Roller skating
 Horseback riding (trot)
 Swim (1 MPH)
 Step-up (24 steps/minute, 25
  cm height) 6 METS
 Treadmill (2 MPH, 10.5%
  grade) 5 METS

6–7 METS
 Walking (5 MPH)
 Cycling (11 MPH)
 Water skiing
 Lawn-mowing (hand mower)
 Skiing (towing or easy downhill)
 Square dancing

6–7 METS (continued)
 Tennis (singles)
 Badminton (competition)
 Swimming (1.6 MPH)
 Step-up (24 steps/minute, 32 cm
  height) 7 METS
 Double Master's test

7–8 METS
 Jogging (5 MPH)
 Cycling (12 MPH)
 Swimming (side stroke, 1 MPH)
 Treadmill (3 MPH, 10% grade)
  7 METS
 Basketball (moderate)
 Touch football
 Skiing (hard, downhill)
 Horseback riding (gallop)
 Mountain hiking (without back pack)
 Step-up (24 steps/minute, 35 cm
  height) 8 METS

8–9 METS
 Jogging (5½ MPH)
 Cycling (13 MPH)
 Fencing
 Basketball (vigorous)
 Handball
 Paddleball
 Step-up (30 steps/minute, 28 cm
  height) 9 METS

10–11 METS
 Running (6 MPH) 10 METS
 Handball (vigorous)
 Swimming (back stroke, 1.6 MPH)
 Step-up (30 steps/minute, 36 cm
  height) 11 METS
 Treadmill (3.4 MPH, 14% grade)
  10 METS

12 + METS
 Running (8 MPH) 13½ METS
 Rowing (11 MPH) 13½ METS
 Step-up (30 steps/minute, 40 cm
 height) 12 METS
 Treadmill (3.4 MPH, 18% grade)
  12 METS

*From S.M. Fox III et al., Physical activity and the prevention of coronary heart disease, *Annals of Clinical Research*, 1971, 3:404–432.

tion. This is important as a given patient progresses and stabilizes in the exercise program. In most experiences, updating is done every 2 to 3 weeks by the physician director based on the progress or lack of progress of the patient. Often the patient will relate that he needs more exercise or perhaps he cannot do that which was prescribed in the initial prescription. In such instances, the prescription can be appropriately changed.

Exercise testing should be done with regularity. This is done in many programs every 3 months for 9 months after the patient is entered and then every 6 months thereafter. Perhaps in some instances this is too often and in some not enough. At any time the patient's clinical course seems to change or regress, an exercise test or other evaluation may be indicated. In many programs, if the patient drops out of the program for 3 weeks or more, repeat exercise testing is mandatory. The importance of the exercise test is not to establish a diagnosis but to assess functional capacity and the progress of disease.

Interventions with medications such as digitalis, beta-blocking agents, and antiarrhythmic drugs usually cause need for reassessment of the exercise prescription. It is most important that the patient inform the program staff of drug changes since often a communication from the private physician is not available. A beta-blocking agent (added or increased in a patient's regimen) may, of course, alter the baseline and the target heart rate for exercise as previously discussed.

EXAMPLES OF EXERCISE PRESCRIPTIONS

With regard to specific exercise prescriptions, the following examples with a description of each case is most illustrative. Most examples discussed are actual patients enrolled in currently active programs. The number of brisk walks and jogs are in "laps." A lap is defined as one rotation around the outside of a basketball court in the gymnasium (1/18 mile). Each example is classified according to the parameters defined in this text.

Example #1
(Outpatient, therapeutic, group-structured, nonmonitored)

A 50-year-old male with hypertension was referred to the therapeutic phase of an outpatient exercise program after sustaining an anteroseptal myocardial infarction. During his initial exercise test, he completed 7 minutes of the standard Bruce treadmill protocol with no significant ST segment changes, a normal blood pressure response, no arrhythmias, and a maximal heart rate of 160 beats per minute. He joined the exercise program with the prescription noted in Figure 3, participating three times per week. He progressed from eight laps walking to 14 laps walking and 10 laps jogging during the 3-month period. Subsequent exercise testing demonstrated a treadmill exercise time of 12 minutes. He continued to demonstrate a normal training response and his exercise prescription was gradually increased as noted in Figure 3 (20 laps jogging with fewer brisk walks). Because his blood pressure continued to be a clinical management problem, it was felt that this level of exercise with a target heart rate of 138 beats per minute was sufficient for a training effect. This patient has remained in the exercise program for 5 years without further changes of the exercise prescription. He chose to remain in the

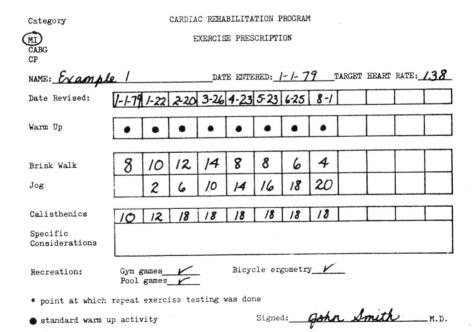

Figure 3: Example of a post-myocardial infarction patient exercise prescription for a fairly high level of exercise. The patient has maintained long-term status in the program. Detailed explanation in the text.

therapeutic program in order to pursue careful monitoring of his
blood pressure.

Example #2
(Outpatient, maintenance, individual, monitored)

The subject was a 36-year-old high level runner at intensity of
15 to 20 miles per week. He had previously completed a local road
race. Because of interest in preventive health, he had an exercise
test which revealed high grade ventricular ectopy with several,
nonsustained bursts of ventricular tachycardia. He was placed in a
monitored exercise program after being started on metoprolol 100
mg twice daily. This antiarrhythmic agent has controlled his ventricular ectopy and he has been able to progress as seen in Figure 4,
initially starting with 15 jogging laps and progressing in five

Category   CARDIAC REHABILITATION PROGRAM

MI   EXERCISE PRESCRIPTION
CABG
CP-**arrhythmia**

NAME: **Example 2**   DATE ENTERED: **3-17-80**   TARGET HEART RATE: **146**

Date Revised:	3-17-80	3-24	4-23	5-23	7-7	8-1					
Warm Up	●	●	●	●	●	●					
Brisk Walk	15	12	8	6	4	2					
Jog	15	20	30	34	38	40					
Calisthenics											

Specific
Considerations   Do instant ECGs

Recreation: Gym games ✓   Bicycle ergometry ✓
             Pool games ✓

* point at which repeat exercise testing was done

● standard warm up activity   Signed: **John Smith** M.D.

Figure 4: Example of the prescription of a young runner with ventricular
arrhythmias. Subject was escalated rapidly to a high level of exercise in the
supervised program. Details are outlined in the text.

months to 40 laps jogging. He has experienced no ventricular ectopy on ambulatory electrocardiography after institution of metoprolol. This is an example of an allegedly healthy subject with ventricular arrhythmia who has been able to participate in regular physical activity via a supervised exercise training program.

Example #3

A 65-year-old patient with a history of inferior myocardial infarction was referred for a therapeutic exercise program 1 week after hospital discharge. Predischarge treadmill testing demonstrated ST segment depression suggestive of myocardial ischemia at a heart rate of 113 beats per minute. No arrhythmias were detected and the blood pressure response was normal. He was placed in a group-structured gymnasium program as noted in Figure 5 with a target heart rate of 90 beats per minute.

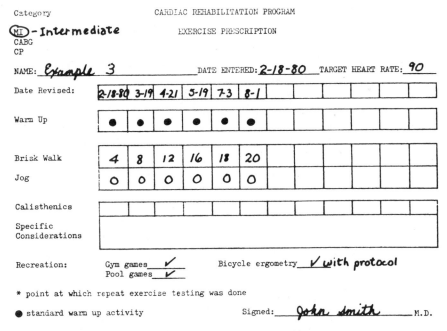

Figure 5: Example of a post-myocardial infarction patient who entered the exercise program in the early intermediate phase. His prescription was at a very low level of exercise. Details are outlined in the text.

He progressed with brisk walks as seen in Figure 5, but was not advanced to jogging because of severe coronary atherosclerosis documented by arteriography. He has done well in the program with low levels of exercise and is being followed by his private physician. Although he is not a candidate for aortocoronary bypass surgery by arteriographic criteria, he has derived an enhanced sense of "well-being" by participation in the above-noted exercise program.

Example #4

A 58-year-old male with multivessel coronary artery disease had been in an exercise program with a walking prescription for several years after a myocardial infarction. Because of recurrent angina, he underwent repeat catheterization which demonstrated the need for aortocoronary bypass surgery. Following surgery, he re-entered the exercise program at a very low level of walking because of moderately severe left ventricular dysfunction. During his exercise treadmill test, he completed 8 minutes of the Bruce protocol with no further ST segment deviation. Based on a maximal achieved heart rate of 130 beats per minute, his target heart rate was set at 110. Jogging activity was limited because of claudication of his lower extremities. This example demonstrates a low level of walking protocol that can be effective in a patient who is not only post-infarction but also post-bypass. This example also illustrates how other clinical data (claudication) must be considered when establishing an exercise prescription for an individual patient (see Fig. 6).

Example #5

A 38-year-old housewife purchased a membership at a commercial exercise facility which utilized a combination of calisthenics and circuit training on Nautilus^R equipment. She was approximately 40 pounds over her ideal body weight. Because of a family history of myocardial infarction, a "fitness" instructor requested that she be cleared by her physician prior to beginning an exercise program. She was able to complete only 5 minutes of the Bruce protocol because of generalized fatigue. Her maximal achieved

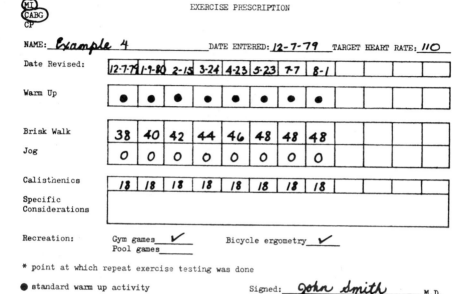

Figure 6: Example of the prescription of a coronary artery bypass graft patient who is also post infarction. The patient had been in the exercise program for some time post infarction, his angina had increased, and coronary angiography was done followed by bypass surgery. The prescription is an example of a very low level walking program that has been successful for this patient. Details are cited in the text.

heart rate was 150 beats per minute and there was no evidence of myocardial ischemia upon analysis of the ST segment. An exercise prescription was written beginning with brisk walking for a 5-minute period to raise her heart rate to 125–130 beats per minute. She was then advised to pursue high repetition, low resistance circuit training with the Nautilus[R] equipment with a regular program involving all major muscle groups. The subject was instructed to check her pulse between each exercise station and not to proceed if her heart rate exceeded 130 beats per minute. It was suggested that the number of repetitions or resistance be increased if her heart rate did not reach at least 120 beats per minute. Dietary counseling was also recommended.

Example #6

A 55-year-old Caucasian male underwent aortocoronary by-pass graft surgery. Following an uneventful inpatient hospital course, he was discharged and had an exercise treadmill test utilizing the standard Bruce protocol. At a weight of 220 pounds, his VO$_2$ max was 23.1 ml/kg/min, which is a maximal MET level of 6.6 metabolic equivalents. For purposes of prescribing a six-level protocol for cardiac rehabilitation, his 30 percent maximal MET level (30% of 6.6) was two metabolic equivalents and his 75 percent maximum MET level (75% of 6.6) was five metabolic equivalents. Utilizing standard guidelines which correlate MET levels with work load (see Table 9), an initial six-level exercise prescription for cardiac rehabilitation was written (Fig. 7). For arm ergometer exercise, a resistance of 25 watts (1 Bel) for a subject weighing 220 pounds was required to achieve a two MET level. This prescription meets the 30 percent maximal MET requirement established at level one of the six-level protocol. For treadmill exercise, a 50 percent maximal MET expenditure was required, i.e., 3.3 metabolic equivalents (50% of 6.6). A Bodyguard leg ergometer was used for this patient, with level one requiring 35 percent of the maximal MET level, i.e., 2.3 METS. At a body weight of 220 pounds, the resistance on the Bodyguard bicycle ergometer was set at 50 watts to accomplish this goal. Subsequent exercise prescriptions for this patient were written for levels two through six depicted in Table 10.

RECAPITULATION

The basis for an individual exercise prescription has been presented. The target heart rate, individualized for each subject, forms the basic guideline for the prescription. Other pertinent data, clinical profile, type of medical disease, current medications, and the extent of disease influence the intensity, duration, frequency, and type of exercise.

Initial and follow-up exercise testing is of paramount importance in exercise programs, both individual and group-structured. The input and follow-up of the primary physician is essential, as the exercise program is only one of several modes of management and should be integrated into the total care of the patient.

Table 9
Guidelines for Prescribing MET Levels

Arm Ergometry*

Body Weight (lbs)	Work loads (60 rpm) 25 / 1.0	37.5 / 1.5	50 / 2.0	Watts Bel
110	3.7	5.0	6.3	
132	3.1	4.2	5.3	
154	2.6	3.6	4.5	MET
176	2.3	3.1	3.9	levels
198	2.1	2.8	3.5	
220	1.9	2.5	3.2	

Walking-Slow Jog or Treadmill**

% Grade	1.2	1.7	2.0	2.5	3.0	3.4	3.8	5.0	mph
0%	1.9	2.3	2.5	2.9	3.3	3.6	3.9	8.6	
2.5%		2.9	3.2	3.8	4.3	4.8	5.2	9.5	MET
5.0%		3.5	3.9	4.6	5.4	5.9	6.5	10.3	levels
7.5%		4.1	4.6	5.5	6.4	7.1	7.8	11.2	

Bicycle Ergometry

Bodyguard** (leg work) Work loads (50 rpm)

Schwinn Air-Dyne† (arm and leg work)

Body Weight (lbs)	50 / 1	75 / 1.5	100 / 2	Watts kp	MET level	Work load
					3.0	0.5
					4.1	1.0
					5.3	1.5
110	5.1	6.9	8.6		6.4	2.0
132	4.3	5.7	7.1		7.6	2.5
154	3.7	4.9	6.1	MET	8.7	3.0
176	3.2	4.3	5.4	levels	9.9	3.5
198	2.9	3.8	4.8			
220	2.6	3.4	4.3			

*Adapted from Franklin[22] (used with permission).
**Adapted from ACSM Guidelines[23] (used with permission of ACSM).
†Adapted from Hagan [24] (used with permission).
Bel = 1 Bel is 25 watts; Kp = kilopond; MET = metabolic equivalent (see text).

Exercise should not be utilized alone in the patient with known coronary artery disease but should be part of a total program of risk factor modification. The latter should emphasize dietary modification with calorie and saturated fat restriction, cessation of cigarette smoking, and control of high blood pressure.

EXAMPLE PATIENT PRESCRIPTION

Name_____DB_____/_QL__Diagnosis____CABG_____/__4/84_Date__7-18-84_
                        (#)   (Date)

Weight __220lbs_Max MET__6.6___30% Max MET___2.0____75% Max MET___5.0_____

Level __l_ Session __l_ Total Exercise Time _40"_ Target Heart Rate_117-131__
                                                                    (50%-75%)

		BLOOD PRESSURE	RPE	(HR)
EXERCISE PRESCRIPTION		___/___	NA	( )

METS						
3.0	Calisthenics	All	repetitions			( )
2.3	Bicycle Ergometer	8	minutes			
	Bodyguard	50 rpm	speed			
		¾Kp	resistance			( )
1.9	Arm Ergometer	100	turns			
		18el	resistance			( )

3.3	Treadmill Stage	MPH	Grace	Minutes		
	1	1.2	0.0%	1		
	(2.9) 2	2.5	0%	4		
	(3.8) 3	2.5	2.5%	4		
	(3.2) 4	2.0	2.5%	4	___/___	( )
	5	1.2	0.0%	1		

1.9	Arm Ergometer	100	turns		
		18el	resistance		
2.3	Bicycle Ergometer	8	minutes		( )
	Bodyguard	50rpm	speed		
		¾Kp	resistance		( )
	Rate of Perceived Exertion for entire session	___/___		( )

Additional Comments: Monitoring Interpretation:

Figure 7: Sample of a patient exercise prescription.

Prescriptive exercise often serves as an effective catalyst for provoking risk factor modification in addition to its individual effects.

The exercise prescription when properly formulated and executed, serves as a tool to implement the appropriate frequency, intensity, duration, and type of physical activity for a given subject. The misuse and abuse of exercise are prevalent today and the proper prescription for each subject tends to avoid such problems. In doing so, it provides a life-style of physical activity that is safe and effective, even for the more restricted patients with sequelae of coronary artery disease.

Table 10
Patient Example (DB)

Weight 220 lbs — *Target HR* 117–131 beats/min
VO_2 23.1 ml/kg/min — *Max MET level* 6.6
MET range 2.0–5.0 (30–75%)

Session	Cal PE (HR)	Bicycle Erg	Arm Erg	Treadmill	Arm Erg	Bicycle Erg R
1	13(128)	9(119)* 2.3 METs 8′/50 rpm ¾ kp	9(120) 1.9 METs 100T @ 1 B	13(128) 3.3 METs 2.5 mph/0% G 2.5 mph/2.5% G 2.0 mph/2.5% G	11(121) 1.9 METs 100T @ 1 B	11(123)* 2.3 METs 8′/50 rpm ¾ kp
2	11(105)	13(113) 2.6 METs 8′/50 rpm 1 kp	11(114) 2.1 METs 125T @ 1⅛ B	12(110) 4.0 METs 2.5 mph/2.5% G 2.0 mph/5.0% G 3.0 mph/2.5% G	13(103) 2.1 METs 125T @ 1⅛ B	12(116) 2.6 METs 8′/50 rpm 1 kp
3	12(123)	14(123) 3.0 METs 8′/60 rpm† 1¼ kp	12(120) 2.3 METs 125T @ 1¼ B	12(127) 4.6 METs 3.0 mph/2.5% G 2.5 mph/5.0% G 3.4 mph/2.5% G	13(127) 2.3 METs 125T @ 1¼ B	14(125) 3.0 METs 8′/60 rpm† 1¼ kp
4	12(144)	13(140) 3.0 METs 12′/65 rpm† 1¼ kp	12(131) 2.5 METs 150T @ 1½ B	3(129) 5 METs 3.4 mph/2.5% G 3.0 mph/5.0% G 3.4 mph/2.5% G	13(132) 2.5 METs 150T @ 1½ B	12(131) 3.0 METs 4′/65 rpm† 1¼ kp
5	11(119)	13(131) 3.0 METs 15′/65 rpm 1¼ kp	12(125) As above	11(128) As above	12(132) As above	9(114) 4′/50 rpm 0 kp (cool-down)
6	12(116)	13(129) As above	12(127) As above	11(125) As above	11(127) As above	9(105) As above

*Performed both sets of bicycle activity on Bodyguard ergometer.
†Patient actually working at 4 MTSs with 60 rpm and 4.5 METs with 65 rpm.
B = Bel (1 Bel = 25 watts); Cal = calisthenics; Erg = ergometry; G = grade; HR = heart rate; ′ = minutes; PE = perceived exertion; R = repeat; T = turns.

REFERENCES

1. American College of Sports Medicine: *Guidelines for Graded Exercise Testing and Exercise Prescription,* 3rd ed. Philadelphia, Lea & Febiger, 1986.
2. Fletcher GF: Dangers of exercise. In *Current Problems in Cardiology.* Vol. IV (3), June 1979:60.
3. Sarnoff SJ, Braunwald E, Welch GF Jr., et al: Hemodynamic determinants of oxygen consumption of the heart with special references to the tension time index. *Am J Physiol* 1958; 192:148–156.
4. Monroe RG, Frence GN: Left ventricular pressure-volume relationships and myocardial oxygen consumption in the isolated heart. *Circ Res* 1961; 9:362–374.
5. Kitamura K, Jorgensen CR, Gobel FL, Taylor HL, Wang Y: Hemodynamic correlates of myocardial oxygen consumption during upright exercise. *J Appl Physiol* 1972; 32:516–522.
6. Cecch AC, Dovellini EV, Marchi F, et al: Silent myocardial ischemia during ambulatory electrocardiographic monitoring in patients with effort angina. *J Am Coll Cardiol* 1983; 1:934–939.
7. Metier CP, Pollock ML, Graves JE: Exercise prescription for the coronary artery bypass graft surgery patient. *J Cardiopulmonary Rehabil* 1986; 6:85–103.
8. Erb BD, Fletcher GF, Sheffield LT: Standards for cardiovascular exercise treatment program. *Circulation* 1979; 59:1084A–1090A.
9. Erb BD, Fletcher GF, Sheffield LT: Standards for supervised cardiovascular exercise maintenance programs. *Circulation* 1980; 62: 669A–673A.
10. Hellerstein HK, Franklin BA: Exercise testing and prescription. In *Rehabilitation of the Coronary Patient.* Wegner NK, Hellerstein HK (eds). New York, John Wiley & Sons, Inc. 1978, 149.
11. Alderman EL, Davis RO, Crowley JJ, Lopes MB, Brooks JZ, Friedman JP, Graham AF, Matlof HJ, Harrison DC: Dose response effectiveness of propranolol for the treatment of angina pectoris. *Circulation* 1975; 51:964–975.
12. Karvonen M, Kentala K, Mustala O: The effects of training heart rate: A longitudinal study. *Ann Med Exp Biol Fenn* 1957; 35:307–315.
13. Chang K, Hossack KF: Effect of diltiazem on heart rate responses and respiratory variables during exercise: Implications for exercise prescription and cardiac rehabilitation. *J Cardiac Rehabil* 1982; 2: 326–332.
14. Thompson PD, Cullinane E, Lazarus B, Carleton RA: Effect of exercise training on the untrained limb. *Am J Cardiol* 1981; 48:844–850.
15. Clausen JP, Trap-Jensen J, Lassen NA: The effects of training on the heart rate during arm and leg exercise. *Scand J Clin Lab Invest* 1970; 26:295–301.
16. Franklin BA, Scherf J, Pamatmat A, Rubenfire M: Arm exercise testing and training. *Practical Cardiol* 1982; 8:43–70.

17. Fletcher GF: Survey of current cardiac exercise programs. In *Exercise and Coronary Heart Disease*. Fletcher GF, Cantwell JD (eds). Springfield, Charles C. Thomas, 1979, 250.

18. Vander LB: Presented at the annual meeting of the American College of Sports Medicine. 1985.

19. Borg G: Perceived exertion as an indicator of somatic stress. *Scand J Rehabil Med* 1970; 2:92–98.

20. Williams MA, Fardy PS: Limitations in prescribing exercise. *J Cardiovasc Pulmonary Technol* 1980; 8:33–36.

21. Fletcher BJ, Thiel J, Fletcher GF: Phase II intensive monitored cardiac rehabilitation for coronary artery disease and coronary risk factors: A six-session protocol. *Am J Cardiol* 1986; 57:751–756.

22. Franklin BA, Vander L, Wrisley D, Rubenfire M: Aerobic requirements of arm ergometry. Implications for exercise testing and training. *Phys Sports Med* 1983; 11:81–90.

23. Guidelines for graded exercise test administration. In *Guidelines for Graded Exercise Testing and Exercise Prescription* (American College of Sports Medicine). Philadelphia: Lea & Febiger, 1980, p. 11–32.

24. Hagan RD, Gettman LR, Upton SJ, Duncan JJ, Cummings JM: Cardiorespiratory responses to arm, leg, and combined arm and leg work on an air-braked ergometer. *J Cardiac Rehabil* 1983; 3:389–695.

4

Primary Prevention of Coronary Disease: The Role of Exercise and Risk Factor Modification

Gerald F. Fletcher, M.D.

INTRODUCTION

The concept of prevention goes back many years in the practice of medicine. In about the year 2550 B.C., the Chinese Yellow Emperor's Classic of Internal Medicine was finalized and reflected many of these philosophies[1,2] The Yellow Emperor is thought to have lived for one century, and in those days health was "a way of life." *The physician's role was not to cure but to prevent disease,* and it was felt that curing disease would be undertaken only by a poor physician, one who did not know his business well enough to have avoided the problem in the first place. The emperor was reported to have paid his physician a regular retainer and stopped paying when he stopped feeling well. The wise people (the sages) did not treat those who were already ill; they instructed those who were not yet ill. In these early writings, there were essentially five modes of therapy. Four of these were concerned largely with preventive measures, namely, nourishment, rest, exercise, and sleep.

From: Fletcher GF: *Exercise in the Practice of Medicine,* 2nd Revised Edition. Mount Kisco, NY, Futura Publishing Co., Inc., © 1988.

As Parker has related in a recent review,[3] millions of dollars are spent annually on interventional and corrective procedures in cardiovascular disease, while fewer sources are directed toward prevention. In accord with this, physicians often overlook opportunities to help patients modify coronary risk factors. As further stated, it seems that in large part (although there is a considerable trend toward prevention) we in the practice of medicine are in the "repair business." In particular, those of us in cardiovascular medicine are often called upon to repair the damage our patients have inflicted upon themselves. In so many words, we have returned to our "tool kits" for solutions, such as drugs to lower blood pressure and relieve angina, and skills in the catheterization laboratory or operating room.

In discussing physical activity in coronary disease, one must consider the role of exercise as part of a multidisciplinary approach in primary prevention. It is one of the most important modalities we have with which to catalyze efforts in coronary risk factor modification—that is, cessation of cigarette smoking, control of high blood pressure, and correction of abnormal blood lipids, especially serum cholesterol.

Current data remain astounding with regard to the prevalence of myocardial infarction—the coronary disease event our primary preventive efforts will hopefully eventually eliminate. In the United States approximately 1,000,000 people have infarctions yearly and there are 7,000,000 people living who have had a myocardial infarction. Of the infarction patients who live and are discharged from a hospital, 31 percent are dead within 5 years. Such data should be unacceptable in our current health care system, especially since the subjects involved are usually productive individuals in the 50 to 60 year age range. Certainly efforts in the primary prevention of this disease are a more logical and workable approach. In recent years this has certainly been the trend as reflected by improved health habits of the public especially with regard to exercise and recreation. Often as a byproduct of this, there are better dietary habits, weight loss, and less substance abuse (i.e., cigarettes, alcohol, and drugs).

ANIMAL EXPERIMENTAL DATA

Multiple studies[4-7] reflect that the animal heart responds to long-term exercise by enlarging. Wild animals, for instance, have larger heart-body ratios than do less active domestic animals.[8] An age factor seems to be important, however, in that although exercise induces cardiac hypertrophy in younger animals, there is actually a decrease in cardiac size and weight in older animals.[9] Most feel that exercise-induced cardiac enlargement reflects hypertrophy of myocardial cells and fibers; however, several studies suggest that hyperplasia (an increased number of fibers) may also occur.[10]

At least three types of investigations have dealt with enhancement of the coronary microcirculation following exercise training. Leon and Bloor[9] studied the age factor in detail and evaluated the exercise of three age groups which corresponded to the human brackets of teens, 20's to 40's, and 50's to 70's. Each age bracket contained a control group, a group that swam for 1 hour per day, and a group that swam for 1 hour 2 days per week. The results indicated increased capillary numbers, capillary/fiber ratios, and coronary lumen areas in young adult rats but not in their older counterparts. Tomanek[10] exercised rats on a treadmill for 40 minutes per day over a 3-month period and demonstrated an increased ratio of coronary microvessels to myocardial fibers, implying an enhanced blood supply to the heart muscle. The study also revealed that the greatest increase in capillary development occurred in the younger rats.

The aforementioned studies suggest that the microcirculation of cardiac muscle in animals will be significantly increased only if exercise is started in youth. The luminal area of the larger coronary arteries will enlarge in the teen group and in the young adults who exercise on a daily rather than a twice-weekly basis.

The effect of exercise on the coronary collateral circulation of animals has likewise been evaluated by multiple research groups. The most widely quoted study of this type was performed by Eckstein in 1957.[11] Using a precise surgical technique, he narrowed the large coronary arteries in 100 dogs. Those who developed signs of a myocardial infarction on subsequent electrocardiograms were divided into two groups. The dogs in group A were exercised on a treadmill for 5 hours per week over a 1½ to 2-month period. Dogs in group B were isolated in small cages over a similar time period. The collateral circulation around the narrowed vessels was markedly enhanced in the exercise group as compared to the nonexercised control group. Cobb et al.[12] attempted to duplicate Eckstein's work by studying the collateral vessel development radiographically in 50 dogs, half of whom were in an exercise group and half in a control group. The former ran on a treadmill for 40 minutes daily over a 3-month period. When the coronary arteries in both groups were then injected with radiographic dye, there was no enhancement of collateral growth in the exercise group. One weakness of such a study, however, is that small collateral vessels cannot be demonstrated by angiographic technique. Burt and Jackson[13] evaluated whether or not an animal could develop collateral vessels through exercise without first having had a large coronary artery partially occluded. Using a technique that was otherwise similar to Eckstein's, they were unable to demonstrate any exercise-induced collateralization, implying that one needed the ischemia of a narrowed vessel to stimulate the growth of the collateral vasculature. Kaplinsky et al.[14] studied the effects of total occulsion of a major coronary artery in 40 dogs. Twenty-six of the dogs survived the insult and were subsequently equally divided into exercise and control groups. Coronary arteriograms were performed at the end of the study, the animals were sacrificed, and pathologic studies were then made of the coronary arteries. Both groups developed extensive networks of collateral vessels, but the exercise group had no better development than the control group. This study suggests that if a vessel is suddenly totally occluded, as opposed to the partial occlusions induced by Eckstein, exercise does not enhance collateral formation.

The effect of exercise on the size of the large coronary arteries was studied by Tepperman et al.[15] and Stevenson et al.[16] The former conducted an experiment in which they compared two exercise groups of rats with two control groups. One exercise group ran 1 mile per day for 36 days, while the other swam for 30 minutes on a daily basis for 10 weeks. The animals were sacrificed at the end of the study, and all heart tissue except the coronary arteries was experimentally digested. Both exercise groups had significantly greater weights of the remaining coronary arteries compared to the control groups. Stevenson et al.[16] studied rats in a similar fashion, analyzing different frequencies and intensities of treadmill and swimming activities. They were able to show increases in coronary arterial tree sizes in all exercise groups compared to the nonexercise groups. However, rats who swam for 8 hours per week actually developed larger coronary artery diameters than those who swam 16 hours per week. This study provokes concern with regard to possibilities of a maximum exercise tolerance, beyond which no significant increases in the size of large coronary arteries occur.

Exercising rats, when compared to controls, are able to perform greater amounts of cardiac work and have an enhanced stroke volume.[17] When heart rates in both groups are artificially increased by cardiac pacing, the hearts of physically trained rats utilize more oxygen and produce less lactic acid than do the control hearts.

Holloszy[18] has described an increase in both size and number of skeletal muscle mitochondria after exercise training and a quantitative increase in the respiratory enzymes per gram of muscle tissues. In another study, the mitochondria of rat heart muscle were examined after various intensities of exercise.[19] While most of the exercised rats increased both size and number of myocardial mitochondria (similar to skeletal muscle), some mitochondrial degeneration occurred in the intensively exercised rats, suggesting that overexercise might have harmful effects. Banister et al.[7] showed that the degeneration of mitochondria is more noticeable shortly after exhaustive exercise is begun and is much less once a training effect is achieved.

The best, most current data in animals is by Kramsch et al.[20] on the reduction of coronary atherosclerosis by moderate exercise in monkeys on an atherogenic diet. Twenty-seven young adult male monkeys were randomly divided into three groups of nine animals each and studied for 36 months. One of the groups studied received a control diet of ground Purina Monkey Chow blended with banana mash during the entire period of 36 months and the other group received this diet for 12 months and was then fed an isocaloric, atherogenic diet consisting of the control diet mix with an added 0.1 percent cholesterol and 10 percent butter (by weight) for another 24 months. The physical activity of both groups was limited to that permitted by housing in a single cage. They were therefore designated "sedentary." The third group of monkeys consumed the control diet for 18 months; during this period, the monkeys were gradually conditioned by exercise on a treadmill within the first 12 months and then kept in the physically trained state for 6 additional months. Thereafter, the animals were given the atherogenic diet for 24 more months while the exercise program was continued. The level of exercise in the conditioned monkeys was comparable to jogging in human beings. The physical training effect in these monkeys was demonstrated by slow heart rates.

Results revealed that although serum cholesterol was the same in the exercising and nonexercising monkeys, there was significantly higher high density lipoprotein cholesterol and much lower triglyceride and low density lipoprotein, plus very low density lipoprotein triglyceride in the exercise group. Ischemic electrocardiographic changes, angiographic size of the coronary artery narrowing, and sudden cardiac death were observed only in the nonconditioned monkeys, in which the post-mortem examination revealed coronary atherosclerosis and stenosis. Exercise was therefore associated with substantially reduced overall atherosclerotic involvement, lesion size, and collagen accumulation. The data suggest that moderate exercise in monkeys may prevent or retard coronary heart disease. Benefits derived from such moderate exercise for 1 hour three times per week in the presence of hypercholesterolemia were less atherosclerosis in wider coronary arteries, supplying a larger heart that functioned at a slower state. Whether more strenuous exercise may influence atherosclerotic cardiovascular disease in a similar manner remains uncertain.

In an overview of animal experimental data, several concepts are apparent. First, the evidence is substantial that exercise seems to have a beneficial effect on the animal heart, based on an increase in the coronary macro- or microcirculation, in the mitochondria, or the cardiac performance. Comparing young and old animals, it appears that exercise produces more impressive changes in the former. If one can extrapolate this to the human, it would seem best to develop proper exercise habits at an early age. The animal data also poses the question as to whether overexercise can actually be harmful.

EPIDEMIOLOGICAL STUDIES IN MAN

Retrospective

A retrospective study evaluates a population after the development of coronary disease, seeking factors in the past which might have predisposed to the disease. One of the most often quoted studies of this type is that of the London transport employees. In this study, Morris et al.[21] reviewed the records of 31,000 men (ages 35 to 64) and noted that the more sedentary bus drivers had an incidence of coronary disease 1.5 times that of the more active conductors who spent most of their day going up and down the steps of double-decked buses. Moreover, the sudden death rates and the death rates during the first 2 months after a myocardial infarction were twice as high in drivers. This study, though often the basis for the "hard sell" of exercise benefits, had certain weaknesses. For instance, there was no attempt to actually substantiate the total activity differences between the two groups, nor was consideration given to specific off-the-job activities. Subsequent reviews of the data revealed that the drivers had higher blood pressure and cholesterol levels than did the conductors, even when they first applied for the job.[22] Such differences could have made the drivers a higher risk for coronary disease for reasons other than the proposed difference in physical activity levels.

Taylor studied the mortality rates of white men employed by the United States Railroad Industry.[23] Death certificates for the years 1955 and 1956 were analyzed, and revealed that the more active sectionmen had less than half the death rates from coronary disease as that of the sedentary clerks. Thus, it could be assumed that men in sedentary occupations have more coronary disease than do those engaged in moderate to heavy physical activity. However, additional questioning of relatives and associates and detailed quantitations of on-the-job energy expenditure revealed that certain clerks actually expended as much caloric energy per day as did the presumably more active sectionmen. Also, the men with coronary disease symptoms either retired or withdrew from the position of sectionman and entered into that of a sedentary clerk. The death rates could, therefore, be explained by a bias in job transfers and retirement tendencies rather than by any protective influence of exercise.[24]

Another interesting retrospective study was that of Frank et al.[25] who evaluated 55,000 men (ages 25 to 64) enrolled in the Health Insurance Plan of New York. Over a 16-month period, 301 had experienced myocardial infarctions. Questionnaires and personal interviews with either the patient or his widow as to on-the-job and leisure time activity revealed death rates after infarction to be 49 percent in the light activity group as opposed to only 13 percent in the heavy activity group. Thus, it appears that even if physical activity does not prevent a coronary event, it might greatly enhance one's chances of survival.

Hames et al. structured a coronary epidemiological study[26,27] in Evans County, Georgia, after observing that black patients appeared to have much less coronary disease than whites, despite a greater tendency toward hypertension and high saturated fat dietary intake in the former. Analysis of the data confirmed the clinical suspicion that indeed the black males had a much lower prevalence of coronary artery disease than the white males. After assessing the various risk factors through the use of the multiple logistics equation, it was concluded that low social standards and relatively intense physical activity habits appeared to account for at least some of the protective effect among the blacks.

A number of studies are available in college athletes. Pomeroy and White[28] studied former Harvard football players and found no harmful cardiovascular effects from their prior strenuous activity. In addition, those who continued to exercise in later life had fewer myocardial infarctions than the nonactive or formerly active groups. Schnohr[29] obtained information on 297 male athletic champions who were born in Denmark between 1880 and 1910 and compared their mortality with that of the general Danish male population. Although the causes of death were essentially the same among the athletes as among the general population, the mortality of the athletes was significantly lower under the age of 50 years. A more recent study by Polednak[30] compared longevity and cardiovascular mortality among 681 former Harvard lettermen. Subdivision of the athletes by the type of sport revealed no significant differences in longevity. A unique finding was that men who earned three or more varsity letters had significantly higher coronary mortality rates than did the one- to two-letter athletes. These data are again somewhat restricted in view of the inaccuracy of death certificate data and by the lack of follow-up knowledge as to exercise habits after graduation.

A retrospective study of coronary deaths in New Mexico[31] showed a serial decline in deaths from the lowest to the highest altitude. One of their speculations was that "adaptation to reduced oxygen tension at higher altitudes is never complete and, therefore, that exertions associated with the activities of daily living represent increased physical exercise."

Prospective Studies

In this type of study, a population group is evaluated and then closely followed for a period of time. Those persons developing coronary disease in the follow-up are compared with those who are free of clinical disease, utilizing the initial screening data.

One of the most widely publicized prospective studies in the medical literature is the Framingham study reported initially by

Kannel et al.[32] Over 5,000 men and women initially free of coronary disease have been followed since 1949. While those with sedentary life habits had significantly more coronary disease than their more active counterparts, there are certain limitations to the analysis. The level of physical activity was not precisely ascertained, and the physiological measurements (level of obesity, vital capacity, handgrip strength, etc.) used to assess the degree of physical activity are somewhat arbitrary.

Paffenbarger et al.[33] reported a 16-year follow-up study on San Francisco longshoremen. The study initially encompassed over 300 men, ages 35 to 64 years. It was possible to separate the workers into two levels of work activity, differing by over 900 calories in energy expenditure per day. During the follow-up period there were 291 deaths attributed to coronary disease. The less active group had a 33 percent higher coronary death rate than their more active colleagues. The differences due to activity were sustained even when blood pressure levels and smoking habits were taken into consideration. Unfortunately, serum cholesterol levels were not available, leaving a big question as to whether or not this important risk factor could have accounted for the group differences.

The Seven Countries study is an ongoing prospective study[34] involving a population of over 12,000 men, ages 40 to 59, from Japan, Greece, Yugoslavia, Italy, the Netherlands, Finland, and the United States. When the data were tabulated at the 5-year point, Japan had the lowest rate of coronary disease, while the United States and Finland had the highest rates. Physical activity levels could perhaps explain the low rate in the Japanese (who tend to be very active) and the high rates in the Americans (noted for escalators and motor-driven bicycles), but certainly not the high rates for the Finns (the ultimate in physical fitness orientation). By using the multiple logistics equation, wherein all other measure factors were held constant while a single risk factor was being assessed, physical inactivity was considered a much less significant coronary risk factor than was hypertension and hypercholesterolemia.

The Goteborg, Sweden, study[35] involved 834 men who were all born in the year 1913. In 1963, when the men were 50 years old, there were no clinical signs of coronary heart disease. Four years later, myocardial infarction was diagnosed in 23 of the men, angina pectoris in 18, and new electrocardiographic abnormalities in nine others. The incidence of myocardial infarction was significantly less in those whose occupations involved "heavy" physical activity than those in "medium" and "sedentary" job classifications. Unfortunately, leisure time activities were not considered in this study.

In an update of the Goteborg study, Tibblin et al.[36] described 19 deaths from ischemic heart disease and 31 survivors. Cigarette smoking and alcohol abuse were more common in the coronary patients than in the remaining subjects; similarly, systolic blood pressure, serum cholesterol, and triglycerides were higher in the coronary group. There was no relationship between physical inactivity during work and coronary disease.

Exercise habits during leisure hours were, however, carefully reviewed by Morris et al.[37] Between 1968 and 1970, these investigators obtained weekend activity questionnaires on 16,882 men, ages 40 to 64 years. In the follow-up period to date, 232 of the men developed clinical evidence of coronary disease. Each of the latter was matched with two colleagues. Those who reported vigorous activity during the single 2-day weekend assessed had about one-third the risk of developing coronary disease than the less active group. The shortcomings of this study were apparent to the authors, in that misclassifications could easily occur when assessing the activity of only a single weekend. Another deficit was that some of the forms of arduous exercise such as "vigorously getting about" are extremely difficult to determine and more so to quantitate.

Pathological Studies

Of the pathological studies, that of Morris[38] has been widely cited. In the mid-1950s, these investigators performed autopsies on 3,800 men, ages 45 to 70, who died of noncoronary causes. The last occupation of the deceased was estimated as involving light, moderate, or heavy physical exertion. An independent assessment as to the degree of coronary atherosclerosis was made, and the results indicated that so-called "silent" complete occlusions of a major coronary vessel (i.e., a complete occlusion without clinical awareness), were more common in those of the light activity group. However, all occupational groups had an equally high prevalence of less extensive coronary atherosclerosis, somewhat clouding the issue.

Another interesting single autopsy study was that of Clarence

DeMar.[39] DeMar was a remarkable man who competed in over 1,000 distance races over a 60-year period. He competed in over 100 marathons, including 34 in Boston. His record of seven wins in the Boston marathon has never been equalled. When he died of metastatic bowel cancer at age 70, his coronary arteries were found to be two or three times the diameter of the average man in his age category. Although he had some atherosclerosis, the overall vessel diameter was such that it was of little consequence. While it is possible that DeMar inherited larger-than-average coronary vessels, there is nothing in his family history to suggest unusual physical development. Studies by Hutchins et al.[40] suggest a direct linear relationship between heart weight and the cube of the normal coronary artery diameter. Hence, it seems likely that DeMar's large arteries were indeed related to his myocardial hypertrophy, produced by life-long exercise habits.

EXERCISE AND CORONARY RISK FACTORS

With the importance of the multi-risk factor modification approach in the prevention of coronary disease, it is pertinent to consider the effect of exercise on certain coronary risk factors in primary prevention. It has been difficult to assess the relative importance of a single factor in comparison to the others. Many of the factors are interrelated, such as blood lipid abnormalities, diabetes, heredity, and obesity. Individual studies taken alone can contribute to this confusion. For example, in a study comparing the relative importance of diet and physical inactivity, Irish men residing in their native country consumed more calories and saturated fat than did their blood brothers residing in the United States,[41] yet they had a significantly lower incidence of coronary heart disease. The latter was attributed by some to reflect their increased physical activity, which was mainly in the form of bicycle riding and manual labor.

Exercise could explain why the Masai tribesmen of East Africa have such a low incidence of atherosclerosis despite eating foods extremely high in saturated fats[42] and also the reason why farm laborers in Evans County, Georgia, have less coronary disease than their more affluent constituents, in spite of the fact that they consume more saturated fat.[43] To the contrary, certain studies have indicated that regular exercise is no panacea against premature coronary disease. The Rendille tribesmen of Africa exercise vigorously each day, walking up to 25 miles. However, they consume a diet high in saturated fat and have a high incidence of atherosclerosis, suggesting that diet is perhaps a more significant risk factor than physical activity.[44] Another negative point regarding the importance of physical activity was a report comparing 100 male military personnel (prisoners) who survived a myocardial infarction at age 40 or less with a control group.[45] There was no significant difference in physical activity levels between the two groups. It should be noted, however, that such reports may be "misleading" in that the accustomed degree of physical activity was determined by questionnaires rather than by direct interrogation.

Coronary heart disease is no doubt multifactorial in etiology as the exercise effect is also multifactorial. It is therefore of value to review the *effect of exercise on individual major coronary risk factors.*

Blood Cholesterol – Hypercholesterolemia

Lipoprotein electrophoresis techniques have enhanced our knowledge of the different types of hyperlipidemias.[46] Despite such techniques, the serum cholesterol level remains the most practical screening test.

Considerable data from numerous *animal studies* suggest that exercise has a beneficial effect in reducing serum and tissue cholesterol levels. Myasnikov[47] and Kobernick et al.[48] found that exercising rabbits had lower serum cholesterol levels and lesser degrees of coronary atherosclerosis than did the sedentary groups. In the latter study, 36 rabbits were placed on a cholesterol-rich diet for 2 months. Half were kept sedentary, while the others exercised for 10 minutes per day on a rotating drum device, a level of exercise which was sufficient to produce the cholesterol-lowering effect. Several investigators have used chickens as their study model.[49] In general, the exercised birds (some of which walked 4 miles per week) had reduced serum cholesterol levels and lesser degrees of large vessel atherosclerosis than did the matched controls. Gollnick[50] found that vigorous exercise could decrease the concentration of cholesterol in rat livers. Watt et al.[51] also studied rats and recorded several interesting observations. The rats were exercised on a motor-driven wheel over an 8-week period, and then underwent detraining over a similar time period. Training had a significant lowering effect on serum cholesterol and serum and adipose triglyceride levels in the rats, but did not significantly affect the adipose levels in the heart or skeletal muscle. The decreased lipid levels persisted during the 8-week detraining period, despite the fact that the body weight loss during training was regained.

In humans, decreases in serum cholesterol following an active physical conditioning program have been noted by many investigators. These include studies on prisoners,[52] Air Force officers,[53] postcoronary patients,[54,55] and the general population.[56] The latter study indicated that the decrease was related to the percent of exercise sessions attended over a 6-month period. The duration of individual exercise sessions and of the total physical conditioning period was quite variable.

Siegel et al.[57] reported a mean decrease in serum cholesterol from 247 to 210 mg/dl in nine blind men who were exercised for only 12 minutes, three times per week, over a 15-week period. This was independent of any weight change. Berkson et al.,[58] Mann et al.,[59] and Golding[60] reported similar weight-independent changes in other studies.

Other studies have shown an exercise-related lowering of serum cholesterol levels. Johnson et al.[61] found that 11 swimmers had significantly lower cholesterol levels during training than at other times and Karvonen et al.[62] found that Finnish skiers had lower cholesterol levels than did nonathletes. Chailley-Bert et al.[63] studied middle-aged men and found lower cholesterol levels in those who were more physically active. Unlike the rat study of Watt et al.,[51] Rochelle[64] found that the decrease in human cholesterol levels during intensive physical training returned to pretraining levels within 4 weeks after the exercise regimen. Phillips[65] had a similar experience with six study patients. The serum cholesterol levels fell from an average of 298 mg percent to 195 mg percent during the 8 weeks of running and handball activities but increased to baseline levels during the detraining period (also 8 weeks). When retrained, the levels fell as before.

The effect of exercise frequency, duration, and intensity upon serum cholesterol levels has been studied in several centers. Daniel[66] divided male faculty members into control, mild, and moderate-to-heavy exercise groups. The exercise consisted of variable speed treadmill work, 5 days per week, for 7 weeks. While all exercise groups had significantly lower cholesterol levels than the controls, there were no significant differences among the exercise groups. Pollock et al.[67] likewise found that there was no greater cholesterol-lowering effect in four exercise sessions per week than in two sessions. Konttinen[68] divided 187 Finnish military recruits into light and heavy exercise groups. Both showed significant decreases of serum cholesterol. Although the heavy exercise group did not have a greater decrease in serum cholesterol, they consumed more calories, which added a variable factor to the interpretation.

Few studies have dealt with exercise and serum cholesterol levels in women. Pohndorf[69] followed a married couple (both of whom were physicians) for a 10-week period during which both swam 1,000 yards daily. The husband then underwent periods of detraining and retraining, while the wife remained active, though at a decreased frequency of exercise activity. Cholesterol levels decreased in both during detraining. Metivier[70] compared the effects of stationary bicycle, vibrating table, and free exercises in college women. Significant decreases in cholesterol levels occurred only with the latter type of exercise.

There have also been negative studies regarding exercise and cholesterol levels. Despite 16 hours of vigorous daily physical activity over a 22-week period in one study, there was no significant decrease in the serum cholesterol of 101 Marine trainees.[71] Holloszy et al.[72] studied 27 subjects over a 6-month period of vigorous training and found no change in serum phospholipids. Studies comparing cross-country skiers[73] with matched nonathletes detected no difference in cholesterol levels. Skinner[74] reported no significant decrease in the serum cholesterol levels of 14 middle-aged men who exercised 30 minutes per session, five times weekly, for 6 months. Olson[75] randomly assigned 31 faculty members to sedentary and exercise groups. After a 3-month period, there was no significant difference in serum cholesterol levels between the two groups. The active group participated in "recreational" swimming, however, and one can question the intensity of such activity. Brumbach[76] divided college men into two groups of 20 each. The groups were matched for initial cholesterol levels, relative physical conditioning, weight, and age. The exercise group met three times weekly for 10 weeks, participating in calisthenics, weight-lifting, and running sessions. No significant cholesterol-lowering effect could be demonstrated in the latter group. Zauner and Swenson[77] trained 10 middle-aged men over an 8-week period, using activities similar to Brumbach's.[76] After 14 days of training, significant reduction of serum cholesterol was demonstrated. As training continued, however, the cholesterol level drifted upward toward the initial values.

It appears then that there is no uniform agreement as to whether exercise alone has a significant effect on the serum cholesterol level. Many of the preceding studies are difficult to interpret because true control groups were not mentioned, seasonal variations in lipid levels were not considered, and details of concomitant weight and dietary alterations are lacking.[78,79] Furthermore, as Mirkin[80] described, there may be a marked fluctuation in serum cholesterol levels on a day-to-day basis during a long-distance running program.

With regard to more current data on cholesterol and the lowering effects of exercise, Craig et al.[81] in South Australia studied the effects of a 12-week exercise program on serum lipid levels in men and women. They found a decrease in low density lipoproteins and cholesterol in both men and women, and suggest a beneficial effect of readily achievable exercise programs in both males and females.

Williams et al.[82] have also looked at the effect of exercise intensity and duration on plasma lipoprotein cholesterol levels. They found that low density lipoprotein decreases did not occur in runners until after 9 months of exercise, and only when a certain mileage threshold was exceeded. This suggests a rather high level of exercise must be maintained to alter serum cholesterol positively. Ballantyne et al.[83] have reviewed the effect of physical training per se on plasma lipids and lipoproteins. They concluded, after review of a number of reports, that regular exercise appears to "produce possibly beneficial changes in the plasma lipids and lipoproteins." Recently Tran and Weltman[84] have summarized results of 95 studies measuring changes in blood lipid levels in response to exercise training. The summary results suggest that reduction in cholesterol levels were greatest when exercise training was combined with body weight losses.

High Density Lipoproteins

More current data continue to support the role of physical activity in the alteration of high density lipoprotein (HDL) levels. Haskell et al.[85] reported in 1980 the results of lipid analysis in 2,319 men and 2,067 women. They found that the more active men and women had significantly higher ($p < 0.05$) values of HDL cholesterol than those with less activity. Hartung et al.[86] reported the effects of exercise on plasma HDL levels. They found that vigorous physical training can contribute to increases in HDL-C in patients with coronary disease without change in total cholesterol or body weight.

Sopko et al.[87] studied in a controlled fashion the effect of mild exercise and diet modification on total cholesterol and HDL. The exercise consisted of walking on a treadmill for 1 hour, 3 days a week. The exercise diet group had significant increases in HDL and significant decreases in both low density lipoprotein and body weight. They concluded that the beneficial effect of exercise on raising HDL levels and producing weight loss is well within the work capacity of most individuals.

Most currently, Nikkila et al.[88] have studied the effect of physical inactivity on plasma lipoproteins. They found a significantly lower HDL cholesterol in 30 patients who were immobilized because of traumatic fracture of the spine. They concluded that the low plasma HDL levels may account for the increase in the coronary heart disease in physically inactive people. Kleeman et al.[89] studied the impact of a lipid-lowering diet and aerobic exercise on HDL cholesterol. They found in 192 females and 147 males that diet was the most important factor and that exercise seemed to be less influential. A significant contribution was published in 1982 by Dressendorfer et al.,[90] who evaluated plasma HDL cholesterol and lipid levels in 12 male marathon runners who ran an average of 28 km/day for 10 days, rested 70 hours, and continued to run for 8 more days, covering a total distance for both running periods of 500 km. HDL-cholesterol levels increased 18 percent and triglyceride levels decreased 22 percent. However, the 3-day rest period reversed these changes. As running resumed, the HDL-cholesterol levels again increased and triglyceride levels decreased. There were no significant changes in total cholesterol, body weight, or skinfold thickness despite an average caloric intake of 4,800 kcal/day. Heavy beer drinking had no discernible effect on HDL-cholesterol. The study demonstrates that HDL-cholesterol levels increase with higher running mileage and decrease within days of stopping exercise when caloric and alcohol intake remain elevated. Herbert et al.[91] evaluated high density lipoprotein metabolism in five trained men who ran 16 km daily and in five inactive men. The mean HDL cholesterol was 65 mg/dl in the runners and 41 mg/dl in the controls. The lipid-rich HDL_2 species accounted for a much higher proportion of the HDL in runners. Tracer studies of radio-iodinated autologous HDL demonstrated that runners did not produce more HDL proteins but rather catabolized less. The activity of lipoprotein lipase was 80 percent higher in the post-heparin plasma of the runners, whereas the activity of hepatic triglyceride hydrolase was 38 percent lower. Thus, the prolonged survival of plasma HDL proteins in runners may result from augmented lipid transfer to HDL by lipoprotein lipase or diminished HDL clearance by hepatic lipase.

Other studies[92,93] have shown an inverse relationship between high density lipoprotein levels and coronary risk. Of particular interest is the data reported by Cohen et al.[94] supporting a beneficial role of vigorous leisure time activity on serum lipids, especially HDL.

More recently emphasized and probably the thrust of research for the future is the role of exercise in altering apolipoprotein AI levels. These proteins are the specific substrate "carrier" for the HDL particle and likely reflect a more accurate measurement of the "good" cholesterol component. Schwartz,[95] for example, has shown that aerobic exercise has a beneficial effect on both HDL and apolipoprotein AI levels. It is felt, therefore, that more sophisticated lipid evaluations in the future will add new dimensions to the evaluation of the effects of exercise.

Blood Pressure

Comparisons of resting blood pressure in active and inactive population groups have yielded varying results. Taylor[96] found lower systolic blood pressures in 416 active railroad switchmen as compared to 298 less active clerks. This difference was not present when the men were first hired for their respective jobs. Kang et al.[97] found similar results in Korean divers as compared to less active controls. Miall and Oldham[98] compared 60 heavy workers with 180 light workers and found that the former had significantly lower systolic and diastolic pressures. The differences could not be explained by social class standing. Karvonen et al.[99] showed that Finnish lumberjacks had lower systolic and diastolic blood pressures than did less active countrymen, and Morris[100] had similar findings in comparing active and inactive London transportation workers. In the Seven Countries study,[101] the more active men had lower systolic and diastolic blood pressures as compared to the less active men.

To the contrary, Chiang et al.[102] compared 100 pedicabmen with 1,346 less active Chinese and found no blood pressure differences between the two groups. Similarly, no differences were shown between the blood pressures of active and less active YMCA members,[103] Chicago utility workers,[104] professional men,[105] and civil servants.[106]

Considerable data has accumulated to indicate a modest blood pressure lowering effect of exercise both in normals[107] and in post coronary patients.[57] Mann et al.[56] found a decrease in both systolic and diastolic levels after physical training, as did Boyer and Kasch.[108] In the latter study, the mean systolic blood pressure fell 13.5 mmHg in 23 essential hypertensive patients who participated in a 6-month exercise program. The mean diastolic pressure fell 11.8 mmHg. Although the normotensive exercise group had no significant change in mean systolic blood pressure, there was a mean decrease of 6 mmHg in the diastolic blood pressure. Mellerowicz[109] noted that trained sportsmen had an average systolic blood pressure of 20 mmHg lower than the control group. Although Naughton et al.[110] and Clausen et al.[55] found a significant decrease in systolic blood pressure in nine cardiac patients who underwent 4 to 6 weeks of physical training, other investigators have reported no basic change in arterial pressure.[40,111] The evidence to date, therefore, suggests that exercise therapy may cause reductions in systolic and diastolic pressure in both hypertensive and normotensive persons. (Further data on the exercise effect on blood pressure are found in Chapter 7.)

Personality and Behavior Patterns

Exercise has been shown to cause changes in personality and behavior patterns.[112] Most of the latter are subjective; however, there are scattered reports containing more objective evaluations. Ismail and Trachtman[113] evaluated the effects of physical training on the personality traits of 60 middle-aged Purdue University faculty members, using the Cattell 16 Personality Factor Questionnaire. They found that those in the higher trained group were more imaginative, self-sufficient, emotionally mature, and self-satisfied of conquering a certain goal.

Blumenthal et al.[114] have shown that a supervised exercise program can modify the physiological and psychological variables associated with increased risk for coronary heart disease. In their study, they found that Type A subjects lowered their scores on the Jenkins Activity Type A scale after training, while scores of the Type B subjects remained unchanged.

A summary of the present knowledge concerning the effects of exercise on major coronary risk factors can be seen in Table 1. Beneficial effects are indicated with a plus (+). In other instances, exercise is either unrelated (U) to the factor or there is insufficient evidence (IE) to indicate a positive or negative effect.

Therefore, considerable evidence is present to support the beneficial effect of exercise on coronary risk factors. With this knowledge, we have in recent years utilized exercise more and more in the management of the coronary-prone individual. This was quite aptly stated by Friedman and Rosenman[115] when they wrote on the prudent management of the coronary-prone individual: "We believe that an hour or more of mild exercise daily is to be strongly recommended to every coronary-prone subject. On the other hand, we believe that strenuous activities such as jogging, tennis singles, handball, or *intensely competitive* exercise only too often might prove to be instantaneously fatal, not only for the coronary-prone subject but for any other American man over the age of 35, unless the latter's coronary angiogram reveals a relatively patent coronary vasculature."

Table 1
Effects of Exercise on Major Coronary Risk Factors

Risk Factor	Effect of Exercise
1. Blood lipids	
a. Cholesterol	IE, probably +
b. High density lipoproteins	+
2. Blood pressure	
a. Systolic	+
b. Diastolic	+
3. Physical inactivity	+
4. Overweight	+
5. Heredity	u
6. Personality and behavior patterns	IE, probably +

+ = beneficial effects; u = unrelated; IE = insufficient evidence.

REGRESSION OR RETARDATION OF ATHEROSCLEROSIS (A NEW THRUST IN PRIMARY PREVENTION)

In primary prevention, we are particularly interested in the atherosclerotic lesion and whether or not the atherosclerotic process can be delayed, stabilized, prevented, interrupted, or reversed. There is considerable *animal data* to document that atherosclerotic lesions do undergo recession. Fritz et al.[116] have shown this by the effects of moderate diet and clofibrate on regression of swine atherosclerosis, and Wissler et al.[117] have documented regression of severe atherosclerosis in cholestyramine-treated Rhesus monkeys. Kottke et al.[118] reported regression of established natural atherosclerotic lesions by intestinal bypass surgery in pigeons, and Bevins et al.[119] reported regression of lesions in canine atherosclerosis. In addition, Friedman and Byers[120] have reported observations concerning the evolution of atherosclerosis in the rabbit after cessation of cholesterol feeding.

In humans, femoral artery atherosclerosis has been shown to regress in treated Types II and IV hyperlipoproteinemic patients (Barndt, Blankenhorn et al.)[121] In addition, Basta et al.[122] have reported regression of atherosclerotic stenosing lesions of the renal arteries and spontaneous cure of hypertension through control of hyperlipidemia. In a study of coronary arteriography in patients with unstable angina, Rafflenbeul et al.[123] revealed that five of 25 patients exhibited regression of coronary artery stenosis over a 1-year period after what was felt to be optimal medical therapy. Using angiographic comparisons over a 7-year period, Kuo et al.[124] showed stabilization of coronary atherosclerotic lesions in 21 of 25 Type II hyperlipoproteinemic patients after achieving a satisfactory hypolipidemic response. In their study, however, they noted no examples of regression, only stabilization.

An isolated case reported by Roth and Kostuk[125] has aroused considerable interest. A 46-year-old man was admitted to a cardiac care unit with acute dyspnea and chest tightness. He had been a previous cigarette smoker with hyperlipidemia and had a family history of coronary artery disease. His serial ECGs and serum enzymes remained normal in the coronary care unit and he was discharged. An exercise test with thallium-201 radionuclear imaging caused chest discomfort radiating to the left arm, ECG ST segment depression of 5 mm, and evidence of an anterior perfusion defect.

The patient was discharged on a beta-adrenergic blocking agent which he only took for a short period of time. One month later, coronary angiography revealed a proximal left anterior descending artery stenosis at the origin of the first septal perforator that persisted even after the use of sublingual nitroglycerin. Coronary bypass surgery was advised, but the patient elected a nonsurgical approach after the pros and cons of the surgery were explained.

During the ensuing 6 months, the patient became *more physically active* and made a few changes in diet and life-style by eating less meat and dairy products, and reducing his law practice. Six months after his initial clinical presentation, his exercise chest pain resolved totally and 1 year later exercise testing with thallium-201 imaging was normal. Repeat coronary angiograms obtained a few weeks later revealed the proximal lesion of the left anterior descending coronary artery to be smaller. This case report represents an isolated instance of apparent regression of a coronary artery lesion in a patient who modified coronary risk factors by utilizing many of the interventions available today in primary prevention.

A number of therapeutic interventions may therefore prevent, stabilize, retard, or cause regression of atherosclerosis. As noted before, these include proper dietary management in the form of modified cholesterol and other fatty food intake, control of high blood pressure, and cessation of cigarette smoking. It is also felt that properly prescribed, moderate, regular, and *long-term physical activity* in the form of walking, running, bicycling, or swimming may also influence this change.

This physical activity may be quite "low-level" in intensity and still afford a beneficial effect. Such has recently been substantiated in studies by Paffenbarger et al. [126] who reported results of contemporary physical activity (emphasis on total weekly energy output) and incidence of heart attack as a manifestation of atherosclerosis in college men who were followed over a 6 to 10 year period. In these studies of 16,936 men in 112,000 person-year's observation, heart attack rates declined with increasing physical activity. Activity was measured as stairs climbed, blocks walked, or participation in strenuous sports (see Figure 1 for graphic display of this data). Further follow-up and analysis of this population has recently been reported.[127] In this analysis, exercise reported as walking, stair-climbing, and sports has related inversely to *total mortality*, primarily, however, to death due to cardiovascular or respiratory causes. By the age of 80, the amount of longevity

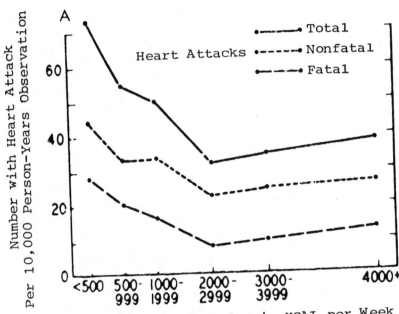

Figure 1: Age-adjusted first heart attack rates by physical activity index in a 6–10 year follow-up of Harvard male alumni. (From Paffenbarger RS, et al: Physical activity as an index of heart attack risk in college alumni. *Am J Epidemiol* 1978; 108:161. Used by permission.)

attributable to adequate exercise, as compared to sedentary life, was 1–2 years. This survey and its results emphasize the beneficial effects of long-term physical activity habits at all ages and all levels of energy expenditure.

Exercise training in primary prevention has many effects, most of which are relevant and beneficial to the cardiovascular system. The physiological effects include a decrease in resting and exercise heart rate and blood pressure with concomitant increase in arteriovenous oxygen difference and oxygen consumption. With regard to the coagulation process, there is a decrease in blood platelet aggregation activity and increased fibrinolysis in the trained state. In addition, exercise may cause beneficial changes in certain blood lipid fractions, decrease in body weight, and decrease in circulating catecholamines. Finally, exercise is associated with certain psychological benefits and a general state of well-being in the subjects involved.

In essence, there are many mechanisms in our medical armamentarium for provoking retardation, stabilization, or regression of atherosclerosis. The total impact of this approach in primary prevention of atherosclerosis is yet to be determined as it involves an intense educational and behavioral modification process for the public. This approach must obviously be utilized long before the overt clinical manifestations of coronary atherosclerotic disease, such as myocardial ischemia or infarction, are manifest. In accord with this, coronary risk factor modification interventions are often difficult to implement, as with many other "preventive health" measures, for allegedly healthy subjects often feel they are "immune" to disease.

As the public becomes more health-conscious with regard to prevention of disease and as atherosclerosis becomes more apparent as a public health problem, early preventive measures should become more popular and acceptable. With this, and a cautious but optimistic attitude, we in the health professions eventually may possibly witness a marked diminution and/or virtual nonexistence of the atherosclerotic process. This indeed should be the goal of our efforts in primary prevention.

CURRENT EXERCISE TRENDS

With the current interest in exercise and coronary disease, the issue of a causal relationship between physical activity levels and mortality from coronary disease continues to inspire debate and stir controversy. Emphasis on exercise over the past decade has focused attention on the role of physical activity in maintaining health, especially in relation to prevention of coronary disease. The "exercise boom," typified by the popularity of jogging and running, coincides temporarily with a progressive decline in age-adjusted mortality from coronary disease of 20 percent in the United States between 1968 and 1976 and has persisted into the 80's. Increased activity levels coincide with a variety of changes in life-style, reflecting a lower prevalence of known coronary risk factors such as hypertension, hypercholesterolemia, and cigarette smoking.[128] Findings from the Framingham study suggest an inverse relationship between activity levels and coronary mortality.[129] The effects of exercise cannot, however, easily be separated from the influence of other risk factors in more active individuals.

Special attention has focused on the relationship between strenuous exercise such as *marathon running* and altered cardiovascular mortality. Some epidemiologic studies have indeed shown a definite relationship between increasing energy expenditure and degree of protection from coronary disease.[126] An individual assertion (with no scientific basis) has been made that conditioning sufficient to complete the marathon distance of 26.2 miles (42.195 km), confers virtual immunity from death from coronary atherosclerosis.[130]

The strong circumstantial case for exercise as protection against coronary disease does not, however, prove a causal relationship. The possibility exists that persons who exercise on a regular basis have a lowered coronary risk to begin with and that continued activity reflects this state of cardiovascular health. Some contribution of self-selection may indeed exist, which does not exclude the strong circumstantial evidence that exercise provides a protective element against risk for coronary heart disease. This protective relationship (Paffenbarger) observed at a level of 2,000 kcal/wk[126] bears upon the issue of altered coronary risk with strenuous exercise. The work expenditure required to run 1 mile in 10 minutes (for a 150 pound person) is approximately 100 kcal, or 100 kcal/mile. This protective threshold translates into jogging approximately 5 miles four times a week, or 20 miles a week, which represents from 20 percent to 50 percent of the energy expended weekly by the average marathon runner.

These data[126] do not show a statistically significant decrease in coronary risk beyond the 2,000 kcal threshold, partly because the number of such individuals is too small for comparison. The lower reported incidence of paternal history of coronary heart disease among marathon runners compared with age-matched controls suggests that a component of selection bias may be operative in the apparent protection of such individuals.[131]

Siegel et al.[131] and Milvy[132] reported that there is now reasonably good evidence that physical inactivity is associated with an increased probability of coronary disease. There are several possible explanations for such an association. *First*, persons with symptomatic coronary artery disease may reduce their level of physical activity. While in some instances this may obviously be the total case, it is unlikely to be the whole explanation. Many epidemiologic studies have shown that such an association may be found in persons who are asymptomatic at the start of observation. *Second,* there may be factors that predispose to coronary disease on the one hand and athletic prowess on the other. But this possibility is also unlikely: Paffenbarger observed that the development of coronary disease in Harvard alumni depends not on the degree to which they exercise as undergraduates but on *whether or not they continue to exercise in later life.* [126] *Third,* exercise may exert a protective effect by influencing other risk factors such as blood pressure and serum cholesterol. Although available evidence suggests that the effects of exercise on blood pressure are comparatively small, there seems to be a definite effect on the cholesterol component. A *fourth* likely possibility is that exercise exerts a protective effect independent of the known major risk factors; the Paffenbarger study attempted to control for other risk factors and showed that the effects of exercise were independent (with the exception of serum cholesterol which was unknown).

Assuming that running and other forms of sustained dynamic exercise reduce the likelihood of developing coronary heart disease, what are the potential numbers of people who would be affected by this? The most accurate answer to this question probably comes from the Perrier Survey of Fitness in America,[133] conducted in 1978. In this survey, it was found that although 59 percent of a random survey of 1,510 adults profess to be engaged in some form of physical activity (including walking), only 15 percent spent more than 5 hours a week exercising—equivalent to an energy expenditure of around 1,500 kcal/week which is a figure somewhat less than the 2,000 kcal Paffenbarger estimated to confer a definite protective effect in his study of Harvard alumni. In the Perrier survey, running ranked sixth in popularity, after walking, swimming, calisthenics, bicycling, and bowling, not all of which are likely to improve cardiovascular fitness. Of the highly active 15 percent, 13 percent were runners, 1.5 percent swimmers, and .5 percent cyclists. These figures indicate that the total number of Americans who indulge in dynamic exercise to a degree that would significantly improve their cardiovascular fitness is still relatively small, perhaps 5 percent of the adult population. Nevertheless, this number is growing and is likely to continue to do so *if the benefits of exercise are acknowledged by the medical profession.* Respondents in the Perrier survey reported that the single factor most likely to increase their involvement in athletic activity was a physician's recommendation.

RECENT STUDIES

Current thoughts and insights into exercise and heart disease have been reflected by Eichner[134] who reviewed extensively the epidemiologic evidence for and against the "exercise hypothesis." The weight of evidence, he feels, supports the view that exercisers have a lower risk of coronary disease, but that vigorous exercise cannot always prevent progression of coronary atherosclerosis and may increase the risk of sudden death in patients with advanced coronary atherosclerosis. He concluded that the "exercise hypothesis" is plausible, even likely, but still unproven. Fried et al.[135] have studied exercise as a protective factor against coronary artery disease in women. The study population consisted of 231 white women (138 working women and 93 housewives). All had diagnostic coronary arteriography. Women who were sedentary or who had mild levels of exercise at leisure had significantly more coronary disease than those with moderate or heavy levels of exercise at leisure. The study suggests that *exercise at leisure* is protective against coronary disease in both housewives and working women, particularly those 50 years of age and older.

Leisure time activity relevant to mortality was also studied in the multiple risk factor intervention trial. Leon et al.[136] reported the relation of duration (minutes per year) and intensity of leisure time activity. In this large study, a significant inverse relationship was found between physical activity duration at baseline and coronary heart disease mortality in the special intervention group, which also received intensive hypertension, dietary and smoking intervention, as well as a group which received usual medical care. The most active quintile had about 0.6 the coronary heart disease mortality rate as the least active. Thus physical activity was associated with reduced coronary heart disease mortality in both the usual medical care and the special intervention group, but with reduced total mortality only in the special intervention group. This data is reflected in 9,000 men. Salonen et al.[137] reported on the effects of leisure time activity and occupational physical activity on the risk of death from ischemic heart disease. They found in 15,188 persons (age 30 to 59) that both lack of leisure time activity and sedentary occupations are associated with increased risk of death from ischemic heart disease.

Kannel et al.[138] from the Framingham study have summarized the *important role of physical inactivity in the development of cardiovascular disease*. Their data incorporates not just Framingham data but that of other centers, and their summary includes data from these other centers. In the Framingham study, there was a suggestion that the fraction of coronary heart disease deaths that are sudden increase with physical activity. However, evidence strongly suggests that endurance exercise protects against coronary disease. Overall mortality, cardiovascular mortality, and coronary heart disease mortality in particular have been found to be inversely related to level of physical activity in a host of epidemiologic studies discussed in the summary. This has been demonstrated prospectively and even after eliminating proximate mortality. Persons who are fat, breathless, and given to tachycardia at rest in the Framingham study had five times the risk of those who had none of these "sedentary traits" (see Fig. 2). According to the Framingham study, very active people live longer and suffer fewer cardiovascular catastrophes than the sedentary population. The authors feel there are a number of arguments, therefore, for assigning an independent, causal role of physical indolence on the rate of occurrence of coronary heart disease:

1. "There is a close relationship with average energy expenditure and an added effect of vigorous activity;
2. the effect seems to be specific for coronary disease and the protection applies to most of its clinical manifestations;
3. there is a beneficial effect on most risk factors;
4. the effect is independent, taking other risk factors into account;
5. reasonable pathogenic mechanisms can be discerned."

It is felt that there is also a rationale for recommending exercise despite the incomplete evidence to date for beneficial physiologic and metabolic changes. There is a need to incorporate physical activity back into daily living as regular physical activity helps to control obesity, hypertension, dyslipidemia, hypercoagulability, hyperglycemia, and hyperinsulinemia. The potential benefits, therefore, appear to strongly outweigh the hazards.

EXERCISE PROGRAMS IN PRIMARY PREVENTION

Groups in consideration for exercise in primary prevention are the healthy, or allegedly healthy, subjects and the coronary-prone individuals.

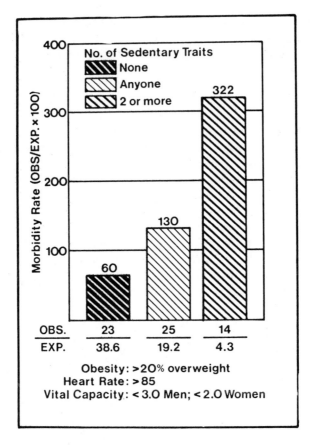

Figure 2: The risk of coronary heart disease mortality based on evidence of physical activity. From the Framingham study, William B. Kannel, et al.[138] in modified format.

The *allegedly healthy* person has no coronary risk factors recognized or documented. These subjects often exercise in local YMCA's or "on their own." They do not necessarily need an exercise test regardless of age unless they have a high coronary risk profile such as family history of coronary disease in early age.

The *coronary-prone group* includes individuals with a history of high blood pressure, cigarette smoking, early familial coronary disease, hyperlipidemia, diabetes mellitus, and being overweight. These persons should have a medically supervised exercise test and medically advised (and sometimes supervised) exercise program.

Effective cardiovascular training exercises are referred to as aerobic or dynamic exercises. Such exercise is not confined to running. Alternatives include cycling (both stationary and conventional), swimming, skipping rope, running, skiing, recreational sports such as volleyball or tennis, and weight training. Regular prescribed exercise should be at least three to four times weekly with a dynamic component of 20 to 40 minutes each time. An exercise prescription should be developed to attain a certain target heart rate during this dynamic sequence (see Chapter 3 for more details).

One of the more practical presentations of the role of exercise in the prevention of coronary disease was that discussed by Eliot et al.[139] in the Eleventh Bethesda Conference in late 1980. The emphasis was on the physician in the work setting, specifically in industrial and occupational medicine. The report is paraphrased and quoted subsequently:

> It was emphasized that *physical activity programs in occupational settings* are increasingly popular as a means to promote employee health. One explanation is that such programs offer a positive approach to cardiovascular health. Exercise can be done for participants in addition to what they already enjoy, whereas reducing weight, stopping smoking, and taking antihypertensive medications seem to be inhibiting and unattractive. A convenient mechanism for introducing health promotion programs may be to initiate an exercise program that incorporates group activities, divisional organization, leadership volunteers, and friendly rivalry among individuals and groups.

The purpose of advocating physical activity programs in industrial and occupational settings is to delay or prevent the development of coronary artery disease. Such programs may serve to eliminate cigarette smoking and control blood pressure, serum lipid levels, and obesity. They may also serve to enhance physical work capacity.

The objectives of such programs are to reduce the prevalence of cardiovascular disease, increase physical fitness through participation in vigorous recreational activities, improve psychological health, and reduce prevalence and severity of cardiovascular risk factors.

The likelihood that an exercise program will be successful and the measure for quantitating its success depends on thorough evaluation of employees and the occupational setting before the program begins. Demographic characteristics should be determined, health and illness data assembled, and summaries of health care service utilization prepared. Physical and laboratory data relevant to cardiovascular risk factors and coronary artery disease should be evaluated. The history of exercise programs and other health promotion programs currently or previously in operation should be reviewed. If possible, the attitudes of executives, middle managers, and white collar and blue collar employees toward exercise programs should be determined. Finally, a survey of community resources is useful to reveal what recreational facilities, physical conditioning programs, and physical educators are available. The attitudes and knowledge of local physicians and the existence of similar programs in other settings should also be determined.

It is felt that many mechanisms are available for establishing program visibility and spreading information. Newsletters, posters, mailers, lectures, and demonstrations all may be useful. Specific individuals known to be at high risk for coronary artery disease or individuals of special concern to the organization, such as executives and managers, may be targeted for special effort in recruitment. An ideal opportunity to develop social and environmental situations favorable for exercise programs is the targeting of specific operational divisions for intensive efforts in promotion and recruitment.

A special concern for promotion and recruitment in such exercise programs is involvement of other family members, especially spouses of employees. Recreational activities may take time away from the family and other family members may resent the loss of that time. If recreational activities can be shared, resentment may be lessened or avoided.

Individualized exercise recommendations should be prepared whenever there is no contraindication to increased physical activity. The type, intensity, duration, and frequency of exercise recommended should be based on the participant's health, estimated physical capabilities, physical activity interests and proficiency, and on the recreational facilities available. Guidelines to warm-up and cool-down periods as well as safeguards should also be specified for each participant.

Special attention should also be given to the manner of reporting results of health risk appraisals to personal physicians. A description of the program and its objectives, results of laboratory data obtained, physical measures made, and other information available should be provided to physicians. Copies of reports should also be given to the participants, and a description of the programs available in the corporation sponsoring the health promotion and disease prevention program should be provided. Success of the program ultimately is influenced strongly by the attitudes of the physicians in the community. Experience reveals that they respond well when informed about programs involving their patients.

Many corporations have provided physical conditioning facilities and have hired physical educators to conduct programs. Community resources should also be utilized whenever possible to broaden the scope of programs by making facilities more accessible to families. Sponsoring programs confined to walking are limited; every effort should be made to include calisthenics, dancing, bicycling, swimming, racquet sports, as well as team sports such as volleyball, basketball, and hockey. Even bowling and golf are a good beginning for sedentary individuals not accustomed to vigorous exercise. Use of community facilities can be monitored by attendance records and evidence of improvement in heart rate response to exercise, in strength and flexibility, body weight, and skinfold thickness. As many facilities and professional personnel as possible should be available to all participants. Practical experience reveals that if physical conditioning facilities are to be used, they must be close to work or home, pleasant and safe, and their use should be expedited by the sponsoring corporation on a cost-sharing and time-sharing basis with employees.

Corporations should also supply on-site facilities if at all possible. Showers and lockers for both men and women are desirable, especially for employees who walk, run, or bicycle to and from work. Recreational facilities such as gymnasiums, running tracks, circuit training rooms, swimming pools, and racquetball courts are much more expensive than other resources for health promotion and disease prevention programs. Consequently, great care must be taken not to spend all available money on elaborate facilities just because they are visible and fashionable. The purpose in establishing a physical activity program is to introduce other health promotion and disease prevention programs. Therefore, enough resources must be available to develop a balanced program.

Reliable professional personnel supervising the health programs are even more important than good facilities. Those concerned with physical activity programs must be capable of much more than leading conditioning classes and showing participants how to count their pulse rate. They must also be competent in nutrition, psychology, and health education. Nurses, physicians, psychologists, dietitians, and health educators should also be available as consultants. Employee volunteers are also valuable as leaders and organizers of employee groups. When these people are educated and supervised and their efforts channeled, they are an important source of spirit and enthusiasm for group recreational facilities.

The *components of an Occupational Physical Activity Program* include many services in addition to provision of recreational facilities:

Baseline measures and evaluations: With these measures it is possible to determine the health-related costs in a corporation, the epidemiology of health-related behaviors and measures, as well as the prospects for improving health and preventing disease.

Health risk appraisal: Present health status of employees can be determined and recommendations made to improve health and prevent disease. Detection of signs and symptoms caused by subclinical disease and referral for early care are valuable products of this service.

Facilities: These must be supervised, inspected, certified, and maintained to ensure a high quality physical activity program.

Professional personnel: These individuals must be recruited, certified, trained, and periodically evaluated to maintain quality programs.

Education: Attention must be paid to improving attitudes, knowledge, and skills of participants in exercise programs. Attention also must be paid to improving attitudes and knowledge of managers, decision makers, other employees, and the general public in contact with program participants.

Supervision: Initial appraisal, individual counseling, and periodic evaluation with feedback are essential parts of a physical activity program.

The impact of physical activity programs on coronary artery disease will take several years to evaluate. Fortunately, the effectiveness of health programs can be evaluated by using other measures. Comparisons of participants in a program should be made with comparison groups that are properly matched. Alternatively, comparisons with baseline measures of the same individuals can be made before and during the program. The measures may include:

Outcome measures:
1. Incidence of cardiovascular disease.
2. Physical conditioning, including physical working capacity and body weight.
3. Program costs computed on the basis of cost per participant and cost per employee eligible to participate.

Social benefits:
1. Employer-employee relations, including satisfaction with work.
2. Public relations, including recognition from local government, general public, other corporations, and customers.

Examples of occupational preventive maintenance programs of "wellness" are now seen in a number of United States firms.[140] For example, Control Data Corporation of Minneapolis, a computer and financial services company, markets to other American businesses three preventive medicine programs for employees. Offered through the Life Extension Institute (LEI), a subsidiary of Control Data, the programs are directed at:

Health insurance, wherein employees learn about how to lead healthier lives and possibly save money on health-care costs;

Employee assistance, a 24-hour per day service designed to aid employees in solving personal and work-related problems, such as alcoholism and drug and chemical abuse, before they become serious; and

Compliance assistance systems designed to monitor the health status of the employee and the work environment based on government regulations or criteria governing toxic substances.

The three programs, which are marketed individually or as a package, employ private physicians country-wide to perform examinations on employees. In instances where disease is diagnosed, the employee is referred to a private practitioner.

In the health maintenance type of program, participating employees complete a confidential questionnaire about the state of their health and their life-styles. They are asked about such things as hypertension, smoking, drinking, use of seat belts, exercise, their emotions, and family disease history. Combined with laboratory test results, this provides information about the presence or absence of disease precursors, such as smoking. Employees are given copies of the results and may consult a private physician.

Workers' spouses are invited to become involved to reinforce their family members' motivation and to help them change their lifestyles to lead healthier lives.

Support groups, such as Alcoholics Anonymous and TOPS (Take Off Pounds Sensibly), are formed at the worksite, and educational programs are provided to help employees lose weight, stop smoking, control blood pressure and diabetes, or make other health-related changes. The employees also organize clubs devoted to athletic activities, such as jogging and volleyball.

The belief is that when employees are involved in mutual support activities, the programs cease to be regarded as company activities and become employee programs. This better facilitates behavioral change. The employee assistance type of program provides a round-the-clock hot-line with professional help available at all times. Problems may range from financial and legal problems to finding a babysitter. Since few of these problems can be solved over the telephone, counselors refer those with psychological problems to psychiatrists, mental health facilities, and other sources of long-term assistance.

Compliance assistance involves a computer-based system that gathers and organizes medical and toxic substance exposure information for each employee and recommends any corrective action necessary. Not only is information about the workplace assessed against government standards, but the employee's own health risks are analyzed so that safety programs may be tailored for the individual. Such a computer-based system offers small companies the sophisticated services that they could not otherwise afford. At the same time, the system can be adapted to individual needs of particular companies, depending on the toxicity of chemicals involved in their operations.

A network of private practitioners across the country conducts physical examinations of the workers. Also under development is a parallel network of associate physicians interested in occupational health who will be data collectors for a national occupational health program.

Five data bases are included in the computer program: the level of hazard in the work environment, the substances to which workers are exposed, the level of exposure, each worker's habits, and the results of physical and laboratory examinations.

The computer also may be programmed to examine groups of workers at risk within a plant and compare them with a similar group working in a no-risk area. If a plant had 300 workers, for example, and 40 are found to have hypertension, the computer can relate job function to the laboratory findings. Likewise, blood chemistries may be compared for employees with possible various toxic substances.

Compliance assistance services also can interface health benefits, utilization of health care, and physician office visits with employee job function and location, thereby helping to reduce long-term health costs while aiding a company in meeting federal regulations.

With recent interest in and evidence for the benefits of cardiac rehabilitation after various cardiac events, business and industry have become more involved in the community phase of cardiac rehabilitation. This interest and activity have developed through programs of primary prevention, which have subsequently evolved into activities of both secondary and tertiary prevention.

Guidelines[141] have been proposed for physical fitness programs in business and industry, as reflected in a joint statement of the President's Council on Physical Fitness and Sports and the American Medical Association's Committee on Exercise and Physical Fitness. These guidelines address purpose and beliefs, medical provisions, administration and facilities. Prototype programs have been developed in various areas.

A number of businesses and industries in the United States have developed physical activity programs for employees, and have begun initial efforts at cardiac rehabilitation.[142] Those involved with cardiac rehabilitation are Coca Cola in Atlanta, and the Burlington, Reynolds, and Haines companies in North Carolina. The latter three have utilized referral programs to local community facilities in North Carolina, while the Coca Cola Company has developed an on-site program which will be subsequently mentioned. Other American firms that have sponsored employee programs are Xerox, Arco, Rockwell, General Foods, Boeing, Kimberly-Clark, Insurance of Wausau, and Lockheed.

The Coca Cola Company in Atlanta was one of the first to develop cardiac rehabilitation on site. The company contracts with a large urban medical center to provide staff to aid the local Coca Cola staff with the program. The Coca Cola Company program provides medically supervised exercise classes using existing American Heart Association standards and guidelines of other existing programs in the area. The purpose and goal of the Coca Cola program have been to insure participants' safety during exercise and manage cardiac problems and/or co-existing medical disorders through life-style intervention. They are specifically involved with the management of hypertension, improvement of blood chemistry profiles through exercise, nutrition practices, smoking cessation, increased physical activity levels, stress management, and weight control. There has been a specific thrust in managing coronary heart disease risk factors, and the company feels that through this they can reduce the risk of heart disease, improve exercise tolerance, and improve the quality of life. The medically supervised program incorporates a standard class schedule.

Blair et al.[143] have recently reported on a public intervention model for worksite health promotion and the resultant effects over a 24-month period. In this study, employees at four companies (n = 2,600) were exposed to a health promotion program of structured education and exercise while employees of three comparison companies (n = 1,700) had only annual health screening. Daily energy expenditure in vigorous activity increased 106 percent in employees who experienced a health promotion program compared to only a 33 percent increase in comparison companies without such programs. (See Figure 3 for graphic display of results.)

With existing efforts in business and industry towards health and wellness programs for participants and the recent early involvement in cardiac rehabilitation programs, it is felt that there will be continued interest through efforts of other companies, especially as the success of such programs becomes more apparent. As we move further into the 1980s and 1990s, we feel that the on-site occupational input into subjects' everyday life-style and behavior modification will be of great impact in both primary and secondary prevention. The value of such health–physical activity programs and other related activities can be assessed with standard assessment methods as those recently described in the report of a National Heart, Lung and Blood Institute Workshop.[144]

All in all, the use of physical activity–exercise programs is likely more appropriate, more beneficial and safe in the primary prevention of coronary disease. With recent emphasis by health organizations and the spontaneity of the public in leading more healthy lives, the implementation of exercise in the total program of coronary risk modification will be more effective and far-reaching. The end result of such programs will not be evident until 20 or more years in the future. However, with cautious optimism, it is felt that evidence for benefits will be apparent with a country-

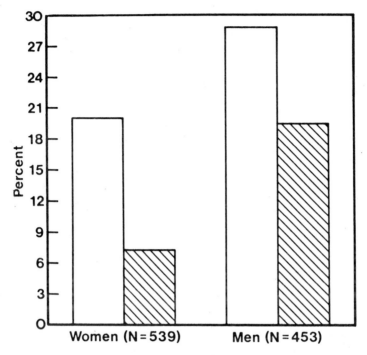

Figure 3: Bar graph showing percent of individuals who began vigorous exercise by the second year. Solid bars indicate health promotion program employees; slashed bars, health service only employees. Used with permission of Blair et al.[143] and JAMA.

wide orientation of the public to coronary risk modification with use of appropriate physical activity and exercise programs.

THE PEDIATRIC POPULATION

As we evolve more in the areas of prevention and health care, considerations must be focused on the early stages of life and the physical and behavioral attitudes that develop at that time. The specialty of pediatrics, in the last decade or so, has placed more emphasis on the importance of body weight control and physical activity in both preschool and early school years. This focus of prevention in childhood is long overdue and is felt to be most important in control of blood lipid abnormalities and high blood pressure, therein preventing atherosclerosis.

As one considers the life-style, including exercise habits of American children, we are often surprised at the *lack of preschool activity in the daily schedule of this age group*. This more sedentary life-style has likely evolved in conjunction with the "current state of the art" of home television and motorized vehicles. Parallel to this, of course, is the "overweight state" often seen in children who surprisingly lead a quite sedentary life. It is estimated that 20 percent of school age children are overweight.

Obesity in childhood has been considered in the past. Lowe[145] in 1967 demonstrated that childhood obesity is associated with an increased age-specific mortality rate in adult life. The majority of obese children remain obese. With intensive physical training, body weight may not change appreciably but the amount of subcutaneous fat decreases and lean body mass increases. Therefore, one may need to examine more than just the weight curves in these children and perhaps include objective data such as a triceps skinfold thickness. Lowe further relates that maintenance of the obese state does not require the same caloric intake as that of acquiring obesity; that is, one may eat less to maintain weight— the same weight that required a very large amount of food intake to acquire initially.

A decrease in physical activity is a most important factor in maintaining the state of obesity. Another important factor is that the "insulating" effect of adipose tissue may have an inhibitory effect on energy loss. Prophylaxis probably offers the most logical method of dealing with obesity, especially in childhood. Prevention is necessary in high risk families and counseling should be incorporated in families that tend to be overweight. Children should increase physical activity and maintain proper diets.

Bryan[146] reported on childhood obesity as a prelude to adult obesity. He concluded that there are several factors related to obesity:

Constitutional factors, such as heredity, are felt to be very significant. A child of normal-weight parents has a 10 percent chance of becoming obese. If one parent is overweight, however, the child has a 50 percent chance of becoming obese. If both parents are overweight, the child has an 80 percent chance of becoming obese.

Dietary factors, of course, also relate to obesity. Normally, the appetite regulates the intake of food for the body's needs to prevent excess storage of fat. This regulatory mechanism may be upset or offset by stress, boredom, frustration, or family customs.

Exercise is most important. An adolescent uses 300 to 400 calories per hour walking and 700 calories per hour while swimming or playing tennis. Studies show that obese children eat the same or less than their normal-weight friends. They are just *less active*. This certainly can lead to psychological problems and also continue on to a cyclic problem of inactivity and overeating.

Psychological factors may range from slight instability to marked disturbances. Psychic mechanisms seem to play a role in modifying one's subconscious operating reflexes that adjust food intake. Once one is obese, there appears to be a psychological effect of being obese. Obese girls have been found to exhibit personality features similar to those found in ethnic and racial minorities subjected to discrimination.

Hypothalamic factors are certainly of importance and paired satiety centers have been identified in the brain.

Environmental and social factors are also of importance. These include abundance of food availability, promotional advertisements, and "social urging" to "eat more."

All of Bryan's data may be related to physical activity or lack of it. The exercise habit, if dynamic and regular, may beneficially influence all of these factors.

Moore et al.[147] studied energy expenditure in preadolescent girls. They evaluated 12 girls at 10 to 12 years of age. They were advised to walk at a self-chosen speed. The energy used for walking surprisingly varied from 50 to 90 calories per square meter of body surface per hour. The difference was most likely due to the manner in which each individual walked. In accord with this data, it is advisable not only to suggest an activity for children but to specify how the activity should be done for each particular individual. For example, if we tell a child to walk, we should specify, "X" amount of feet in "X" amount of time.

Hansen[148] has presented data on abnormal serum growth hormone response to exercise in juvenile diabetics. He studied male, nonobese juvenile diabetics short term (1 to 8 years) or long term (12 to 30 years). Diabetics were compared to nondiabetic controls. The results revealed no change in serum growth hormone in the controls studied at a moderate level of exercise, although higher levels of exercise may cause increases. There was, however, an immediate increase in serum growth hormone in all juvenile diabetics at the end of exercise and this increase was not related to the duration of the diabetes. Abnormal serum growth hormone was noted whether the juvenile diabetic was well controlled or poorly controlled. However, this abnormal increase in growth hormone was diminished in the presence of strict control in these diabetics. Fasting serum growth hormone levels were also elevated in the juvenile diabetics. The fasting serum growth hormone levels, however, were decreased during regulation and there was also a significant correlation between blood glucose and fasting growth hormone concentration. A significant increase in serum insulin was also noted at the end of exercise in the diabetics.

Hagan et al. [149] studied the physiologic responses of juvenile-onset diabetic boys to muscular work. They found no difference between diabetics and controls in ventilatory volume, oxygen uptake, heart rate, and lactic acid. However, in the diabetic boys, maximal, light, and moderate work produced significant plasma glucose depression. It was concluded that juvenile diabetes with short duration insulin dependency and few vascular complications have aerobic work capacity similar to that of normal controls. However, caution is suggested with the exercise since progressive reduction in plasma glucose may cause hypoglycemic reactions.

Based on this information, it is important to emphasize that juvenile as well as adult diabetics' participation in exercise programs, whether supervised or individualized, should be done with special care. The subject should be followed closely and insulin regulated according to the intensity and type of activity chosen. In addition, the diabetic should be made aware of the influence of activity on insulin needs in order to better understand his/her disease.

With regard to hypertension, several studies have been reported in the pediatric population. Hagberg[150] has reported beneficial effects of endurance exercise training in adolescent hypertension. The authors studied the effects of 8 months of endurance exercise training on blood pressure in nine adolescents (mean age of $17 \pm .06$ years) with essential hypertension. They concluded that exercise training can lower blood pressure in children who have increased peripheral vascular resistance or an increased cardiac output.

Fixler et al.[151] have reported on the response of hypertensive adolescents to both dynamic and isometric exercise stress. In 109 hypertensives (compared with 74 normotensives), they concluded that the decision to restrict physical activity of an adolescent with high blood pressure should be based on the development of abnormal ECG ST segment depression, arrhythmias, or excessive blood pressure elevation at time of exercise testing.

With regard to exercise performance of hypertensive adolescents, Nudel et al.[152] studied ten subjects with sustained essential hypertension, eight with labile hypertension, and ten age-matched controls. The methodology incorporated progressive maximal exercise tests. The authors concluded that:

1. Maximal testing in hypertensive subjects is safe.
2. Exercise performance is normal.
3. In essential hypertension, systolic and diastolic pressures are significantly higher with exercise than in labile hypertension or in the normal state.
4. Exercise tests are recommended for all hypertensive adolescents to identify those with an excessive response in blood pressure.

Their data therefore re-emphasize the value of exercise testing in assessment of degree of high blood pressure and also in the adequacy of control in those subjects who are on treatment.

With such supportive data, one may advise activity programs for hypertensive children. However, it is felt, regardless of age, that such children should have exercise testing and specific activity advised, based on testing results. Strong has emphasized that the top normal systolic pressure response to exercise is 200 mmHg as a result of studies in healthy black children.[153] In accord with this, it is felt that pressures in excess of 100 mmHg with exercise likely identify individuals who have an abnormality of blood pressure due to increased systemic vascular resistance. Strong has further elaborated on the role of exercise testing in youths with elevated blood pressure[154] to determine the pressure response under conditions which are similar to those that occur in athletics. In youths whose blood pressure remains elevated with the routine exercise test, it is felt that both a dynamic and isometric exercise test be done to further evaluate the pressure response. This thorough testing may be of great importance in identifying persistent hypertension in a group in whom preventive techniques are quite appropriate.

Cumming and Friesen[155] have reported bicycle ergometry measurement of maximal oxygen intake in children. In this study, seven to 15 maximal exercise tests on a cycle ergometer were done on 20 boys (11 to 15 years of age). The work load was increased until it was sufficiently high that it could not be sustained for 3 minutes. The mean maximal heart rate was 202 beats per minute and the mean maximal oxygen uptake was 53.8 ml/kg/min. A plateau of the oxygen uptake curve occurred in only seven of the 20 subjects, whereas the pulse rate reached a plateau in 13 subjects. On the basis of the pulse rate-work load straight line relationship of submaximal exercise, the intensity of the work load that the subjects were able to complete was such that a mean predicted pulse rate of 247 beats per minute would have resulted. This information may be utilized carefully to obtain maximal oxygen uptake for a single test in children. Based on these data, it is important to realize that once the heart rate has reached maximum for the adolescent, there may still be further increments in oxygen uptake; however, such data must be individually assessed and utilized with caution in the clinical setting.

With regard to the effects of physical activity in children, it is general knowledge that decreased activity has been associated with childhood obesity.[156] Additional studies have revealed that physical activity for children is important for growth and development. As noted in the Saskatchewan Study,[157] school curricula in many communities have reduced the time available for physical activity and this factor may be the cause of decreased functional capacity. Of particular interest in this study was the finding that physical fitness as expressed by aerobic power decreased with age and coincided with the child's entry into school. Another interesting educational endeavor[158] has revealed that increasing the time devoted to physical activity during the routine school day improves academic performances despite a decrease in academic time. These latter data were derived from studies in France, Belgium, and Japan.

Therefore, data are available on both exercise testing and training in the pediatric population. Such data should be expanded and utilized for use in activity programs for normal children and especially for obese, diabetic, hypertensive, and atheroslcerotic-prone children. As the surging interest in exercise in adults continues, hopefully we will more often see children and parents walking, running, and biking together.

Current data in pediatrics have emphasized more the importance of blood lipid assessment and the effects and importance of correcting abnormal lipid patterns. This has been addressed with regard to the role of diet and weight loss as well as the specific role of exercise.

Sasaki et al.[159] reported on the effect of regular dynamic exercise on lipids and apolipoproteins in obese children (17 boys and 19 girls). The exercise program consisted of a 20-minute run twice daily with heart rate of 120–140/min for 2 years. The results after 2 years revealed a significant increase in apoprotein A-I, the major apoprotein of HDL along with weight reduction. Recently, much emphasis has been placed on primary prevention of atherosclerosis in the pediatric population by Glueck,[160] who feels it may be useful to broaden the guidelines for the diagnosis and management of hypercholesterolemia in children. It is emphasized that patterns of physical activity along with other coronary risk factors should be "tracked" into adulthood.

In contrast to adult practices of risk factor modification, those in children have been more conservative and less popular. It seems, therefore, that a major thrust in the future should be in the grade school level where *physical activity* should be regular and prescribed as *part of the school curriculum* along with weight control and dietary discretion.

REFERENCES

1. Veith I: *Huang Ti Nei Ching Su Wen.* Berkeley and Los Angeles, University of California Press, 1966, p. 97.
2. Veith I: Traditional Chinese medicine: historical review. In *Modern China and Traditional Chinese Medicine.* Risse GB (ed). Springfield, Charles C. Thomas, 1973, p. 18.
3. Parker BM: Case for preventive cardiology. *Cardio* April 1984; p. 31–35.
4. Froelicher VF: Animal studies of effect of chronic exercise on the heart and atherosclerosis. A review. *Am Heart J* 1972; 84:496–506.
5. Bloor CM, Pasyk S, Leon AS: Interaction of age and exercise on organ and cellular development. *Am J Pathol* 1970; 58:185–199.
6. Hakkila J: Studies of the myocardial capillary concentration in cardiac hypertrophy due to training; an experimental study with guinea pigs. *Am Med Exp Biol Fenn* 1955; 33(Suppl): 10:1–82.
7. Banister EW, Tomanek RJ, Cvorkov N: Ultrastructural modifications in rat heart: Responses to exercise and training. *Am J Physiol* 1971; 220:1935–1940.
8. Poupa O, Rakusan K, Ostadal B: The effect of physical activity upon the heart of vertebrates. In *Physical Activity and Aging.* Brunner E, Jokl E (eds). Baltimore, University Park Press, 1970; 4:202.
9. Leon AS, Bloor CM: Exercise effects on the heart at different ages (Abstr). *Circulation* 1970; (Suppl III) 41 & 42:50.

10. Tomanek RJ: Effects of age and exercise on the extent of the myocardial capillary bed. *Anat Rec* 1970; 167:55–62.
11. Eckstein RW: Effect of exercise and coronary artery narrowing on coronary collateral circulation. *Circ Res* 1957; 5:230–235.
12. Cobb FR, Ruby RL, Fariss BL: Effects of exercise on acute coronary occlusion in dogs with prior partial occlusion (Abstr). *Circulation* 1968; 37 & 38:104.
13. Burt JJ, Jackson R: The effects of physical exercise on the coronary collateral circulation of dogs. *J Sports Med* 1965; 5:203–206.
14. Kaplinsky E, Hood WB Jr, McCarthy B, et al: Effects of physical training in dogs with coronary artery ligation. *Circulation* 1968; 37:556–565.
15. Tepperman J, Pearlman D: Effects of exercise and anemia on coronary arteries of small animals as revealed by the corrosion-case technique. *Circ Res* 1961; 9:576–584.
16. Stevenson JA, Feleki V, Rechnitzer P, et al: Effect of exercise on coronary tree size in the rat. *Circ Res* 1964; 5:265–269.
17. Penpargkul S, Scheuer J: The effect of physical training upon the mechanical and metabolic performance of the rat heart. *J Clin Invest* 1970; 49:1859–1868.
18. Holloszy JO: Morphological and enzymatic adaptations to training: a review. In *Coronary Heart Disease and Physical Fitness*. Larsen OA, Malmbory RO (eds). Baltimore, University Park Press, 1971, pp. 147–151.
19. Arcos JC, Sohal RS, Sun SC, et al: Changes in ultrastructure and respiratory control in mitochondria of rat heart hypertrophied by exercise. *Exp Mol Pathol* 1968; 8:49–65.
20. Kramsch DM, Aspen AJ, Abramowitz BM, Kreimendahl T, Hood WB Jr: Reduction of coronary atherosclerosis by moderate conditioning exercise in monkeys on an atherogenic diet. *N Engl J Med* 1981; 305:1483–1489.
21. Morris JN, Heady JA, Raffle PA, et al: Coronary heart disease and physical activity of work. *Lancet* 1953; 2:1053–1057.
22. Morris JN, Kagan A, Pattison DC, et al: Incidence and prediction of ischemic heart disease in London busmen. *Lancet* 1966; 2:553–559.
23. Taylor HL, Klepetar E, Keys A, et al: Death rates among physically active and sedentary employees of the railroad industry. *Am J Public Health* 1962; 52:1697.
24. Taylor HL: Occupational factors in the study of coronary heart disease and physical activity. *Can Med Assoc J* 1967; 96:825–831.
25. Frank CW, Weinblatt E, Shapiro S, et al: Physical inactivity as a lethal factor in myocardial infarction among men. *Circulation* 1966; 34:1022–1033.
26. McDonough JR, Hames CG, Stulb SC, et al: Coronary heart disease among Negroes and Whites in Evans County, Georgia. *J Chronic Dis* 1965; 18:443.
27. Hames CG: Evans County cardiovascular and cerebrovascular epidemiology study: Introduction. *Arch Intern Med* 1971; 128:883–886.
28. Pomeroy WC, White PD: Coronary heart disease in former football players. *JAMA* 1958; 167:711–714.

29. Schnohr P: Longevity and causes of death in male athletic champions. *Lancet* 1971; 2:1364–1366.
30. Polednak AP: Longevity and cardiovascular mortality among former college athletes. *Circulation* 1972; 46:649–654.
31. Mortimer EA Jr, Monson RR, MacMahon B: Reduction in mortality from coronary heart disease in men residing at high altitude. *N Engl J Med* 1977; 296:581–585.
32. Kannel WB: Habitual level of physical activity and risk of coronary heart disease: The Framingham Study. *Can Med Assoc J* 1967; 96:811–812.
33. Paffenbarger RS, Laughlin ME, Gima AS, et al: Work activity of longshoremen as related to death from coronary heart disease and stroke. *N Engl J Med* 1970; 282:1109–1114.
34. Blackburn H, Taylor HL, Keys A: Coronary heart disease in seven countries. XVI. The electrocardiogram in prediction of five-year coronary heart disease incidence among men aged 40–59. *Circulation* 1970; (Suppl I) 41:154–161.
35. Werko L: Can we prevent heart disease. *Ann Intern Med* 1971; 74:278–288.
36. Tibblin G, Wilhelmsen L, Werko L: Risk factors for myocardial infarction and death due to ischemic heart disease and other causes. *Am J Cardiol* 1975; 35:514–522.
37. Morris JN, Adam C, Chave SP, et al: Vigorous exercise in leisure time and the incidence of coronary heart disease. *Lancet* 1973; 1:333–339.
38. Morris JN, Heady JA, Raffle PAD, et al: Coronary heart disease and physical activity of work. *Lancet* 1953; 2:1053–1057.
39. Currens JH, White PD: Half a century of running. Clinical, physiological and autopsy findings in the case of Clarence DeMar ("Mr. Marathon"). *N Engl J Med* 1961; 265:988–993.
40. Hutchins GM, Bulkley BH, Miner MM, et al: Correlation of age and heart weight with tortuosity and caliber of normal coronary arteries. *Am Heart J* 1977; 94:196–202.
41. Trulson MF, Clancy RE, Jessop WJ, et al: Comparisons of siblings in Boston and Ireland. *J Am Diet Assoc* 1964; 45:225–229.
42. Mann GV, Shaffer RD, Rich A: Physical fitness and immunity to heart disease in Masai. *Lancet* 1965; 2:1308–1310.
43. McDonough JR, Hames CG, Stulb SC, et al: Coronary heart disease among Negroes and Whites in Evans County, Georgia. *J Chronic Dis* 1965; 18:443–468.
44. Shaper AG, Jones KW: Serum-cholesterol in camel-herding nomads. *Lancet* 1962; 2:1305–1307.
45. Cantwell JD: Coronary heart disease in young prisoners. Unpublished data.
46. Fredrickson DS, Levy RI, Lees RS: Fat transport in lipoproteins: An integrated approach to mechanisms and disorders. *N Engl J Med* 1967; 276:215–225.
47. Myasnikov AL: Influence of some factors on development of experimental cholesterol atherosclerosis. *Circulation* 1958; 17:99–113.
48. Kobernick SD, Niawayama G, Zuehlewski AC: Effect of physical

activity on cholesterol atherosclerosis in rabbits. *Proc Soc Exp Bil Med* 1957; 96:623–628.

49. Montoye HJ: Summary of research on the relationship of exercise to heart disease. *J Sports Med* 1962; 2:35–43.
50. Gollnick PD: Cellular adaptation to exercise. In *Frontiers of Fitness*. Shephard RJ (ed). Springfield, Charles C. Thomas, 1971, p. 122.
51. Watt EW, Foss ML, Block WD: Effects of training and detraining on the distribution of cholesterol, triglyceride and nitrogen in tissues of albino rats. *Circ Res* 1972; 31:908–914.
52. Dalderup LM, Voogd N de, Meyknecht EA, et al: The effects of increasing the daily physical activity on the serum cholesterol levels. *Nutr Dieta* (Basel) 1967; 9:112–123.
53. Hoffman AA, Nelson WR, Goss FA: Effects of an exercise program on plasma lipids of senior Air Force officers. *Am J Cardiol* 1967; 20:516–524.
54. Hellerstein HK: The effects of physical activity: patients and normal coronary-prone subjects. *Minn Med* 1969; 52:1335–1341.
55. Clausen JP, Larsen OA, Trap-Jensen J: Physical training in the management of coronary artery disease. *Circulation* 1969; 40: 143–154.
56. Mann GV, Garrett HL, Farhi A, Murray H, Billings FT: Exercise to prevent coronary heart disease. An experimental study of the effects of training on risk factors for coronary disease in men. *Am J Med* 1969; 46:12–27.
57. Siegel W, Blomqvist G, Mitchell JH: Effects of a quantitated physical training program on middle-aged sedentary men. *Circulation* 1970; 41:19–29.
58. Berkson D, et al: Experience with a long-term supervised ergometric exercise program for middle-aged sedentary American men. *Circulation* 1967l 36: (Suppl II) 67.
59. Mann BV, et al: Exercise and coronary risk factors: the response. *Circulation* 1967l 36: (Suppl II) 181.
60. Golding LA: Effects of exercise training upon total serum cholesterol levels. *Res Q Am Assoc Health Phys Educ* 1961; 33:499.
61. Johnson TF, et al: The influence of exercise on serum cholesterol, phospholipids and electrophoretic serum protein patterns in college swimmers. *Fed Pro* 1959; 18:77.
62. Karvonen MJ, et al: Serum cholesterol of male and female champion skiers. *Am Med Int Fenn* 1958; 47:75–82.
63. Chailley-Bert, Libignette P, Fabre-Chevalier: Contribution A L'Tude des variations du cholesterol sanquin au corn des achivities physique. *La Presse Medicale* 1955; 63:415–416.
64. Rochelle RH: Blood plasma cholesterol changes during a physical training program. *Am Assoc Health Phys Educ* 1961; 32:838.
65. Phillips L: Physical fitness changes in adults attributable to equal periods of training, non-training and re-training. Doctoral dissertation, University of Illinois, 1960.
66. Daniel BJ: The effects of walking, jogging and running on the serum lipid concentration of the adult caucasian male. Doctoral dissertation, University of Southern Mississippi, 1969.

67. Pollock ML, et al: Effects of frequency of training on serum lipids, cardiovascular function and body composition. In *Exercise and Fitness*. Franks BD (ed). Chicago, Athletic Institute, 1969, p. 161.
68. Konttinen A: Physical activity and serum lipids. *Sotiaslaatietillinen Aikakauslchti* 1960; 35:169.
69. Pohndorf RH: Improvements in physical fitness on two middle-aged adults. Doctoral dissertation, University of Illinois, 1957.
70. Metivier JG: The effects of five different physical exercise programs on the blood serum cholesterol of adult women. Doctoral dissertation, University of Illinois, 1960.
71. Calvy GL, Cady LD, Mufson MA, Nierman J, Gertler MM: Serum lipids and enzymes. Their levels after high-caloric, high-fat intake and vigorous exercise regimen in Marine Corps recruit personnel. *JAMA* 1963; 183:1–4.
72. Holloszy JO, Skinner JS, Toro G: Effects of a six-month program of endurance exercise on the serum lipids of middle-aged men. *Am J Cardiol* 1964; 14:753–760.
73. Karvonen MW: Effects of vigorous exercise on the heart. In *Work and the Heart*. Rosenbaum FF, Belknap EL (eds). New York, Paul B. Hoebner Inc. 1959: p. 190.
74. Skinner JS: The effect of an endurance exercise program on the serum lipids of middle-aged men. Doctoral dissertation, University of Illinois, 1963.
75. Olson HW: The effect of supervised exercise program on the blood cholesterol of middle-aged men. *Phys Ed* 1958; 15:135.
76. Brumbach WB: Changes in the serum cholesterol levels of male college students who participated in vigorous physical exercise program. Doctoral dissertation, University of Oregon, 1959.
77. Zauner CW, Swenson EW: Physical training performance in relation to blood lipid levels and pulmonary function. *Am Correct Ther J* 1967; 21:159–165.
78. Rochelle R: Blood plasma cholesterol changes during a physical training program. *Res Am Assoc Health Phys Educ* 1961; 32:538.
79. Romanova D, Barbarin P: The influence of physical exercises on the content of serum protein, lipoprotein and total cholesterol in persons of middle and elderly age with symptoms of atherosclerosis. *Kardiologiia* 1961; 1:36.
80. Mirkin G: Labile serum cholesterol values. *N Engl J Med* 1968; 279:1001.
81. Craig IH, Brotherhood J, Hill G, D'Andrea R: Effects of 12-week exercise program on serum lipid and apolipoprotein A levels in men and women (Abstr). *Circulation* 1981; 64: (Suppl IV) 81.
82. Williams P, Wood P, Haskell W, Vranizan K, Vodak P: Effect of exercise intensity and duration on plasma lipoprotein cholesterol levels (Abstr). *Circulation* (Suppl IV) 1981; 64:185.
83. Ballantyne D, Clark RS, Ballantyne FC: The effect of physical training on plasma lipids and lipoproteins. *Clin Cardiol* 1981; 4:1–4.
84. Vu Tran Z, Weltman A: Differential effects of exercise on serum lipid and lipoprotein levels seen with changes in body weight. *JAMA* 1985; 254:7.

85. Haskell WL, Taylor HL, Woods PD, Schrott H, Heiss G: Strenuous physical activity, treadmill exercise test performance and plasma high-density lipoprotein cholesterol: The Lipid Research Clinics Program Prevalence Study. *Circulation* 1980; 62: (Suppl IV) 53–60.

86. Hartung GH, Squires WG, Gotto AM Jr: Effect of exercise training on plasma high-density lipoprotein cholesterol in coronary disease patients. *Am Heart J* 1981; 181–184.

87. Sopko G, Mittelmark M, Jeffery R, Lipchik R, Lenz K, Hedding B, Gerber W, Baxter J: Effect of exercise and/or diet modification and blood lipids in high risk population (Abstr). *Circulation* 1980; 62 (Suppl III) III–123.

88. Nikkila EA, Kuusi T, Myllynen P: Effect of physical inactivity on plasma lipoproteins: Decrease of high-density lipoproteins and apolipoprotein A-1 in immobilized patients (Abstr). *Circulation* 1980; 62: (Suppl III) 266.

89. Kleeman CR, Cobb L, Rock C, King K: The impact of a lipid lowering diet and aerobic exercise on high-density lipoprotein cholesterol. *Clin Res* 1981; 29:2.

90. Dressendorfer RH, Wade CE, Hornick C, Timmis GC: High-density lipoprotein-cholesterol in marathon runners during a 20-day road race. *JAMA* 1982; 247:12.

91. Herbert PN, Bernier DN, Cullinane EM, Edelstein L, Kantor MA, Thompson PD: High-density lipoprotein metabolism in runners and sedentary men. *JAMA* 1984; 252:8.

92. Rhoads GG, Gulbrandsen CL, Kagan A: Serum lipoproteins and coronary heart disease in a population study of Hawaii Japanese men. *N Engl J Med* 1976; 294:293–298.

93. Castelli WP, Doyle JT, Gordon T, et al: HDL cholesterol and other lipids in coronary heart disease. *Circulation* 1977; 55:767–772.

94. Cohen, JD, Davidson DM, Greenland P, Krakoff LR, Pearson TA, Riemenschneider TA, Van Citters, Stanford J: Vigorous exercise in young adults: Clustering of health habits do not explain beneficial effects on serum lipids (Abstr). *Circulation* 1985; 72: (Suppl III) 452.

95. Schwartz R: Apoprotein A-1 with diet or exercise (Abstr). *Circulation* 1985; 72: (Suppl III) 117.

96. Taylor HL: Occupational factors in the study of coronary heart disease and physical activity. *Can Med Assoc J* 1967; 96:825–831.

97. Kang BS, Song SJ, Suh CS, et al: Changes in body temperature and basal metabolic rate. *Am J Appl Phys* 1963; 18:483–488.

98. Miall WE, Oldham PD: Factors influencing arterial blood pressure in the general population. *Clin Sci* 1958; 17:409–444.

99. Karvonen MJ, Rautaharju PM, Orma E, et al: Heart disease and employment. Cardiovascular studies on lumberjacks. *J Occup Med* 1961; 3:49–53.

100. Morris JN: Epidemiology and cardiovascular disease of middle age: Part II. *Mod Concepts Cardiovasc Dis* 1960; 30:633–638.

101. Keys A, Aravanis C, Blackburn HW, et al: Epidemiological studies related to coronary heart disease: characteristics of men aged 40–59 in seven countries. *Acta Med Scand* 1966; (Suppl) 460.

102. Chiang BN, Alexander ER, Bruce RA, et al: Physical characteristics and exercise performance of pedicab and upper socioeconomic classes of middle-aged Chinese men. *Am Heart J* 1968; 76:760–768.
103. Doan AE, Peterson DR, Blackman JR, et al: Myocardial ischemia after maximal exercise in healthy men. One year follow-up of physically active and inactive men. *Am J Cardiol* 1966; 17:9–19.
104. Berkson DM, Stamler J, Lindberg HA, et al: Socioeconomic correlates of atherosclerotic and hypertensive heart disease. *Ann NY Acad Sci* 1960; 84:835–850.
105. Raab W, Krzywanek HJ: Cardiovascular sympathetic tone and stress response related to personality patterns and exercise habits. *Am J Cardiol* 1965; 16:42–53.
106. Rose G: Physical activity and coronary heart disease. *Proc R Soc Med* 1969; 62:1183–1188.
107. Harris WE, Bowerman W, McFadden RB, et al: Jogging, an adult exercise program. *JAMA* 1967; 201:759–761.
108. Boyer JL, Kasch FW: Exercise therapy in hypertensive men. *JAMA* 1970; 211:1668–1671.
109. Mellerowicz H: Vergleichende Untersuchungen uber das Oknoie-prinvip in Arbeit and Leistung des trainierten Kreislaufs and seine Bedeutung fur die praventive und rehabilitive Medizin. *Arch Kreislaufforsch* 1956; 24:70–176.
110. Naughton J, Shanbour K, Armstrong R, McCoy J, Lategola MT: Cardiovascular response to exercise following myocardial infarction. *Arch Int Med* 1966; 117:541–545.
111. Frick MH, Katila M: Hemodynamic consequences of physical training after myocardial infarction. *Circulation* 1968; 37:192–202.
112. McPherson BD, Paino A, Yuhasz MS, et al: Psychological effects of an exercise program for post-infarction and normal adult men. *J Sports Med* 1967; 7:95–102.
113. Ismail AH, Trachtman LE: Jogging the imagination. *Psychology Today* 1973; 7:79–82.
114. Blumenthal JA, Williams RS, Williams RB Jr, Wallace AG: Effects of exercise on the type A (coronary prone) behavior pattern 1. *Psychosomatic Med* 1980; 42:2.
115. Rosenman RH, Friedman M, Straus R, et al: A predictive study of coronary disease. *JAMA* 1964; 189:15–22.
116. Fritz K, Augustyn J, Jarmolych J, Daroud A: Effects of moderate diet and clofibrate on regression of swine atherosclerosis (Abstr). *Circulation* (Suppl II) 1975; 52:II–16.
117. Wissler DW, Vesselinovitch D, Borensztajin J, Hughes R: Regression of severe atherosclerosis in cholestyramine treated rhesus monkeys with or without a low-fat, low cholesterol diet (Abstr). *Circulation* (Suppl II) 1975; 52:II–16.
118. Kottke BA, Unni KK, Carlo IA: Regression of established natural atherosclerotic lesions by intestinal bypass surgery in pigeons: structure and chemistry. *Trans Assoc Am Phys* 1974; 87:263–270.
119. Bevins J, Dawson JD, Kendmi FE: Regression of lesions in canine atherosclerosis. *Arch Pathol* 1951; 51:228.

120. Friedman M, Byers SO: Observations concerning the evolution of atherosclerosis in the rabbit after cessation of cholesterol feeding. *Am J Pathol* 1963; 43:349–359.
121. Barndt R, Blankenhorn D, Crawford D, Brooks S: Regression and progression of early femoral atherosclerosis in treated hyperlipoproteinemic patients. *Ann Intern Med* 1977; 86:139–146.
122. Basta L, Williams C, Kioschos J, Spector A: Regression of atherosclerotic stenosing lesions of the renal arteries and spontaneous cure of systemic hypertension through control of hyperlipidemia. *Am J Med* 1976; 61:420–423.
123. Rafflenbeul W, Smith LR, Rogers WJ, Mantle JA, Rackley CR, Russell RO Jr: Coronary anatomy of patients with unstable angina pectoris re-examined one year after optimal medical therapy. *Am J Cardiol* 1979; 43:699–707.
124. Kuo PT, Kayase K, Kostis JB, Moreya A: Use of combined diet and colestipol in long-term (7–7½ years) treatment of patients with type II hyperlipoproteinemia. *Circulation* 1979; 59:199–211.
125. Roth D, Kostuk WJ: Noninvasive and invasive demonstration of spontaneous regression of coronary artery disease. *Circulation* 1980; 62:888–896.
126. Paffenbarger RS, Wing AL, Hyde RT: Physical activity as an index of heart attack risk in college alumni. *Am J Epidemiol* 1978; 108:161–175.
127. Paffenbarger RS Jr, Hyde RT, Wing AL, Hsieh CC: Physical activity, all-cause mortality, and longevity of college alumni. *N Engl J Med* 1986; 314:605–613.
128. Gordon T, Castelli WP, Hjortland MC, et al: Predicting coronary heart disease in middle-aged and older persons: The Framingham Study. *JAMA* 1977; 238:497–499.
129. Kannel WB, Sarlie P: Some health benefits of physical activity. The Framingham Study. *Arch Intern Med* 1979; 139:857–861.
130. Bassler TJ: Marathon running and immunity to atherosclerosis. *Ann NY Acad Sci* 1977; 301:579–592.
131. Siegel AJ, Hennekens CH, Rosner B, et al: Paternal history of coronary heart disease reported by marathon runners. *N Engl J Med* 1979; 301:90–91.
132. Milvy P: Statistics, marathoning and CHD. *Am Heart J* 1978; 95:538–539.
133. Perrier Survey of Fitness in America, study no. 92813. Louis Harris Associates, Inc. 1978.
134. Eichner ER: Exercise and heart disease epidemiology of the "exercise hypothesis." *Am J Med* 1983; 75:1008–1023.
135. Fried LP, Pearson TA, Achuff SC, Bulkley BH: Physical exercise: A protective factor against coronary artery disease in women. *Clin Res* 1983; 193; 31:2.
136. Leon AS, Connett J, Jacobs DR Jr, Taylor HL: Relation of leisure time physical activity to mortality in the multiple risk factor intervention trial (MRFIT). *Circulation* 1984; 70:(Suppl II).
137. Salonen JT, Slater JS, Tuomilehto J, Rauramaa R: Risk of death

from ischemic heart disease in relation to leisure-time and occupational physical activity (Abstr). *Circulation* 1985; 72: (Suppl III) 151.

138. Kannel WB, Wilson P, Blair SN: Epidemiological assessment of the role of physical activity and fitness in development of cardiovascular disease. *Am Heart J* 1985; 876–885.

139. Eliot RS, Bond MB, Brandenburg RO, et al: Eleventh Bethesda Conference, Prevention of coronary heart disease. *Am J Cardiol* 1981; 47:762–764.

140. Prevention maintenance for company employees. *JAMA* (Medical News) 1981; 245:1301–1303.

141. Thomas AS, Lee PR, Franks P, Paffenbarger RS: Exercise and health. The evidence and the implication. Cambridge, Mass. Oelgeschlager, Gunn & Hain Publishers, Inc. 1981; 191–196.

142. Fletcher GF: Role of business and industry in community phase of cardiac rehabilitation. Presented at Third World Congress of Cardiac Rehabilitation, Caracas, 1985.

143. Blair SN, Piserchia PV, Wilbur CS, Crowder JH: A public health intervention model for work-site health promotion. *JAMA* 1986; 255:921–926.

144. Wilson PWF, Paffenbarger RS Jr, Morris JN, Havlik RJ: Assessment methods for physical activity and physical fitness in population studies: Report of a NHLBI workshop. *Am Heart J* 1986; 111:1177–1192.

145. Lowe CU: Obesity in childhood. *Pediatrics* 1967; 40:455–467.

146. Bryan AM: Childhood obesity: prelude to adult obesity. *Can J Pub Health* 1967; 58:486–490.

147. Moore ME, Pond J, Korslund MK: Energy expenditure of preadolescent girls: Measurements taken in the basal state and while walking. *J Am Diet Assoc* 1966; 49:400–412.

148. Hansen AP: Abnormal serum growth hormone response to exercise in juvenile diabetics. *J Clin Invest* 1970; 49:1467–1478.

149. Hagan RD, Marks JF, Warren PA: Physiologic responses of juvenile-onset diabetic boys to muscular work. *Diabetes* 1979; 28:1114–1119.

150. Hagberg JM: Beneficial effects of endurance exercise training in adolescent hypertension. *Am J Cardiol* 1980; 45:489.

151. Fixler DE, Laird WP, Browne R, et al: Response of hypertensive adolescents to dynamic and isometric exercise stress. *Pediatrics* 1979; 64:579–583.

152. Nudel DB, Gootman N, Brunson SC, et al: Exercise performance of hypertensive adolescents. *Pediatrics* 1980; 65:1073–1078.

153. Strong WB, Miller MD, Striplin M, et al: Blood pressure response to isometric and dynamic exercise in healthy black children. *Am J Dis Child* 1978; 132:587.

154. Strong WB: Hypertension and sports. *Pediatrics* 1979; 64:693–695.

155. Cumming GR, Friesen W: Bicycle ergometer measurement of maximal oxygen uptake in children. *Can J Physiol Pharmacol* 1967; 45:937–946.

156. Voller RD Jr, Strong WB: Pediatric aspects of atherosclerosis. *Am Heart J* 1981; 101:815–836.

157. Bailey DA: Exercise, fitness and physical education for the growing child: A concern. *Can J Pub Health* 1973; 64:421–430.
158. Mackenzie J: The Vanberg experiment in education. Mesina Board of Education, 1972.
159. Sasaki J, Kitajima K, Tanaka H, Shindo M, Ando M, Jinriki H, Arakawa K: Effect of regular aerobic exercise on lipids and apolipoproteins in obese children. *Circulation* 1985; 72:Suppl III:111–258.
160. Glueck CJ: Pediatric primary prevention of atherosclerosis. *N Engl J Med* 1986; 314:3;175–177.

Chapter 5

Exercise in Rehabilitation of the Coronary Patient

Gerald F. Fletcher, M.D.

INTRODUCTION

Exercise in the rehabilitation of patients with coronary artery disease has been in widespread use for many years. Data are now available regarding the effect of early exercise intervention in *animal studies*. One of the more important is that of Kloner et al.[1] on the effect of early exercise on myocardial infarction scar formation. This involved 18 rats that underwent coronary artery occlusion experimentally. One member of each pair of rats was randomized to a nonswimming group and the other to graded swimming. Twenty-one days after the coronary occlusion, the rats were examined for changes in the myocardium. The data show that the exercise during the healing phase of acute infarction caused thinning of the transmural scar. This might have specific applications to exercise that is too intense and too early post infarction.

Another study by Hochman et al.[2] was on the effect of early exercise on expansion of acute infarction in the rat model. In this study, the authors evaluated early exercise after infarction on infarct expansion in 129 rats. Within 4 hours after ligation of the left coronary artery, the rats were exercised on a treadmill. No

From: Fletcher GF: *Exercise in the Practice of Medicine,* 2nd Revised Edition. Mount Kisco, NY, Futura Publishing Co., Inc., © 1988.

hearts had complete rupture, and the instance of intramural hemorrhage (a finding that has been associated with cardiac rupture) was similar in 39 unexercised rats as opposed to the exercising rats. These findings suggest that moderate, early exercise after myocardial infarction does not adversely affect infarct or expansion or cause cardiac rupture in this animal model. Therefore, there is some disagreement with regard to data in rat studies on exercise after infarction.

Musch et al.[3] studied the hemodynamic arterial blood gases and acid-base status at rest and during exercise in sedentary and trained rats with myocardial infarctions produced by coronary artery ligations, and in rats with sham operations. Their results show that the myocardial infarction rats with chronic heart failure can benefit from a program of exercise training and the beneficial effects can be clearly demonstrated during response to submaximal exercise. Therefore, the data suggest that exercise likely is beneficial in the rat model as an animal prototype for evaluation of such an intervention.

INPATIENT REHABILITATION

The application of exercise in secondary prevention has been extensively employed in the last three decades. However, until the last decade, the general consensus among physicians was that physical activity might have deleterious effects in the clinical setting of recent myocardial infarction. Treatment was rather stereotyped in that most acute coronary victims could expect 6 to 8 weeks of bed rest in the hospital before home discharge. This period of strict bed rest was based upon early studies of Levine and Brown[4] dealing with the duration of the healing process. In 1929, these authors stated that early activity post infarction could lead to mural thrombus formation, aneurysm development, or myocardial rupture. As the maximum healing process (including the formation of scar tissue) took place within 6 to 8 weeks post infarction, it seemed reasonable to markedly reduce myocardial oxygen demands and cardiac work during this time segment.

With the advent of cardiac catheterization and other refined techniques in hemodynamic assessment, it became obvious that there were certain disadvantages of maintaining a cardiac patient in a recumbent position for prolonged periods of time. Coe[5] found that cardiac work increased 29 percent when normal subjects or cardiac patients were moved from sitting to recumbent positions. The latter position resulted in an augmentation of venous return, subsequently increasing contractility through the Frank-Starling mechanism. The failing heart, or the heart with a compromised coronary circulation, could likely be unduly stressed by prolonged recumbency.

There has been controversy as to the optimal length of hospitalization post infarction and also regarding the usefulness of hospitalization itself. Because of this, a randomized study[6] was done to compare home care by the family doctor and hospital treatment. The latter involved an initial period of observation in a coronary care unit. There were 458 English general practitioners involved who allocated 343 cases at random to the two treatment groups. The groups did not differ significantly with respect to age, prior diagnosis of angina pectoris, previous myocardial infarction, or history of hypertension. The groups were also similar with respect to the prevalence of hypotension when initially examined. Of 169 hospitalized patients, the 28-day mortality rate was 14.2 percent compared to 9.8 percent for the 174 patients who were treated at home. Although the results are interesting, the study had certain definite limitations. For instance, a number of patients initially treated at home were later transferred to the hospital but were still considered to be in the home care group. Moreover, the location and severity of the infarctions were not compared in the two groups, nor was analysis made of the time lapse between the onset of symptoms and the initial call for medical help. When evaluating studies such as this, one needs to be highly critical. It is likewise important for the practitioner to utilize past experience and employ "common sense." It is certainly not difficult for most practicing physicians to recall numerous instances of life-threatening cardiac arrhythmias which were promptly recognized and treated in the coronary care unit and which probably would have resulted in the patient's demise had they occurred at home.

A more reasonable controversy centers around the question of early versus late mobilization and discharge post-myocardial infarction. Wenger et al.[7] published the results of a questionnaire as to current physician practice in managing uncomplicated myocardial infarction patients. The questionnaire was sent to 1200 general practitioners, 1200 internists, and 1200 cardiologists. The 69 percent who responded managed 70,000 patients with acute myocardial infarctions during 1970. The responses were similar for the three groups in that 95 percent of the patients were hospitalized for 21 days; most were permitted to sit in a chair on the 8th hospital day and to walk in the room on the 14th day. Rose[8] has made the following statement pertaining to old traditions and modern doubts of in-hospital care:

> Physicians have always been very cautious in their management of patients with myocardial infarction. We are less upset if our patient dies in bed than if he dies while walking in the ward or street, for in confining him to bed we feel that at least we did everything possible.

In 1952, Levine and Lown[9] published the results of armchair rather than bed rest treatment for 73 patients with myocardial infarction, indicating that there were no obvious ill effects from such therapy. They also noted the various hazards of immobilization, including rapid muscle wasting, decreased pulmonary ventilation, impaired exercise tolerance, and loss of normal postural vasomotor reflexes. The latter was clearly demonstrated by Fareeduddin and Abelmann.[10] They reported that five to ten patients treated for 9 to 24 days with strict bed rest had systemic blood pressure decreases of more than 38 mmHg during 15 minutes of passive upright tilt to 70°. This response was abolished after a period of full ambulation and was not observed in eight patients who were treated with modified bed rest. Such a significant fall in blood pressure could be catastrophic to a patient with a compromised myocardial blood supply in that it could lead to reinfarction or to extension of the initial infarction.

Saltin et al.[11] have done extensive studies on the effect of a 20-day period of bed rest on five normal subjects, ages 19 to 21. Two of the subjects were very active physically prior to the study, while the remainder had been essentially sedentary. The maximum oxygen uptake fell from a mean of 3.3 liters/minute before bed rest to 2.4 liters/minute after bed rest. Supine exercise on a bicycle ergometer at 600 kpm/minute required a rate of 180 beats/minute compared to 154 beats/minute before bed rest. An oxygen uptake that could normally be attained at a heart rate of 145 beats/minute required a rate of 180 beats/minute after bed rest. During maximal treadmill testing, the cardiac output fell 26 percent after bed rest (from 20 to 14.8 liters/minute). This was attributed to a reduction in stroke volume, since the maximal arteriovenous oxygen difference and the maximal heart rate were not altered.

Numerous recent reports have dealt with the results of early mobilization and discharge after myocardial infarction. In Northern Ireland, Adgey[12] reported 102 patients who were hospitalized for an average period of 13 days post infarction. Over a 2-week period after discharge, there was no mortality and no apparent morbidity that might have been prevented by a more prolonged hospital stay. Takkunen et al.[13] in Finland compared 146 patients who were mobilized after 3 to 7 days in the hospital and discharged between 12 to 16 days with 108 patients who were bed-ridden for 7 to 14 days and hospitalized for 21 to 28 days. There was no significant difference when the mortality rates were assessed at 7 days and again at 30 days post-discharge. This study had the limitations of not being randomized and not including long-term results. Tucker et al.[14] were more aggressive and discharged 89 percent of 289 post-infarction patients by the 10th hospital day. Of this group, 7.6 percent were readmitted during a 6-week follow-up period, and 6.7 percent of the discharged patients died. The authors seemed encouraged by this approach and noted that more importantly, 62 percent of the patients were back at work 5 months after their infarction.

Fortunately, there are reports of well-controlled studies which may serve as guidelines. Harpur et al.[15] studied 199 patients with uncomplicated myocardial infarctions. All were given 7 days of bed rest and then allocated into either Group A or Group B. In the former, patients were mobilized on day 8 and discharged on the 15th hospital day. In Group B, patients were mobilized on day 21 and discharged on the 28th hospital day. All were encouraged to return to work 1 month after discharge. The groups were well-matched with respect to previous cardiovascular history, age, sex, interval from onset of pain to admission, and site of infarction. In the first 8 months after infarction, the early and late mobilization groups did not differ significantly with respect to cardiac mortality or morbidity, congestive heart failure, serious arrhythmias, or the development of ventricular aneurysm formation. There was, however, a significant difference in the "return to work" rate 2 months after admission. In the early mobilization group, 41 percent were back to work in 2 months versus only 17 percent of the late mobilization group. This study, however, was likely not entirely free of selection bias in that patients were included in the early mobilization group only if they had been free of hypertension, congestive heart failure, or serious arrhythmias in the preceding 5 days.

Hutter et al.[16] described a prospective randomized controlled study comparing a 2-week and a 3-week hospital stay in 138 patients with uncomplicated myocardial infarction. The groups were comparable for age, sex, prior cardiovascular problems, and location of infarction. During a 6-month follow-up period, there were no group differences in terms of coronary mortality or morbidity, aneurysm formation, psychological signs and symptoms, congestive heart failure, and number returning to work. The authors concluded that there appeared to be no additional benefit from a 3-week hospital course as compared to a 2-week period for patients with uncomplicated myocardial infarction.

Bloch et al.[17] randomly assigned 154 post-infarction patients to an early mobilization group (active physical therapy beginning on day 2 or 3) and a late mobilization group (strict bed rest for at least 3 weeks). The former had a mean hospital stay of 21.3 days versus 32.8 days for the latter group. Over an average follow-up of 11.2 months, there were no significant group differences in mortality, reinfarction, arrhythmias, heart failure, angina pectoris, aneurysm formation, or exercise test results.

Unlike Bloch's study, Abraham et al.[18] considered early discharge as well as early mobilization in a prospective randomized study of 129 patients who survived for at least 5 days after a myocardial infarction. The early group was mobilized on day 6 and discharged after 12 days, while the late group was mobilized on day 13 and discharged on day 19. In a follow-up ranging from 6 to 52 weeks, cardiac complications were more prevalent in the late group than in the early group:

Complication	Early Mobilization and Discharge (64 Patients)	Late Mobilization and Discharge (65 Patients)
Myocardial ischemia	5	13
Congestive heart failure	2	15
Myocardial infarction	1	8
Pulmonary edema	1	6

With reference to the aforementioned, one must consider who is a candidate for early discharge. In an analysis of 522 consecutive patients with acute myocardial infarctions, McNeer et al.[19] found that in patients having no serious complications through day 4, the hospital mortality rate was zero and there were no serious late complications. Their definition of the "uncomplicated patient" is the individual who in the first 4 days of hospitalization has none of the following:

    1. Asystole

2. Ventricular tachycardia or fibrillation
3. High-grade heart block
4. Pulmonary edema
5. Shock
6. Extension of infarct
7. Persistent sinus tachycardia
8. Persistent hypotension
9. Supraventricular tachyarrhythmias

A study of very early discharge has been conducted in Belfast.[20] Out of 275 admissions for acute myocardial infarction, 109 (40%) who survived 6 days were *free of the following*:

1. Sustained sinus tachycardia (>1 hour) within first 2 days of hospitalization;
2. >2 mm ST segment elevation in any lead 6 days after admission;
3. The need for morphine analgesia between the 2nd and 7th days post-admission;
4. Serious rhythm and conduction disturbances between day 2 and day 7 of hospitalization.

Sixty-eight percent of those 109 patients who had none of the above complications were discharged by the 7th hospital day, and there were no deaths over a 3-month follow-up at home.

Rose[8] summarized the controversies of early versus late mobilization and has offered the following suggested policy:

1. The coronary patient free of severe pain or shock may be treated with bed or chair rest for the first 7 days of hospitalization. The legs should be exercised daily, and a bedside commode is preferred over a bedpan.
2. Beginning on the 8th hospital day, the "good risk" patient (devoid of persistent pain, congestive heart failure, and ventricular arrhythmias) can be allowed to ambulate in the ward. He can be discharged several days later and can soon return to work.
3. Patients who do not fall in the "good risk" group must be managed on a highly individualized basis. Since this is such a diverse group, fixed rules do not apply.

An ad hoc committee[21] of the American College of Cardiology felt that 9 to 14 days of hospitalization were sufficient if there was no evidence of the following: (1) continuing myocardial ischemia, (2) left ventricular failure, (3) shock, (4) important cardiac arrhythmias, (5) conduction disturbances, (6) other serious illnesses.

At most medical centers, inpatient cardiac rehabilitation teams see patients only by physician referral. The team usually consists of a physician and nurse coordinator working in conjunction with the physical therapist, dietitian, chaplain, social worker, and pharmacologist. The team follows a specific inpatient physical therapy activity regimen (Table 1 A–D) both for post-myocardial infarction post-angioplasty and post-coronary bypass surgery.

The patients perform first active assistive and then active exercise under the supervision of the physical therapist. The activities are terminated if the pulse rate is greater than 115 beats/minute or if ectopic beats occur. (At Grady Memorial Hospital, the Emory University regimen has been used on over 2,000 patients[22] with only one mishap, that being an instance of ventricular fibrillation during passive range of motion exercise that was promptly terminated by electrical defibrillation.)

Patients, in addition, are encouraged to flex and extend the feet and knees on an hourly basis. To do so on only a once or twice daily schedule is probably ineffective as suggested by the study of Browse,[23] who measured calf blood flow with venous occlusion plethysmography. The blood flow increased significantly following leg exercises but returned to the resting basal level within 1 hour of rest.

Elastic stockings, which have been known to increase the speed of venous return from ankle to groin as measured by the I-labeled Hippuran[24] injection technique, are encouraged by some. Other investigators, however, have used the tagged fibrinogen scanning technique in postoperative patients and have demonstrated counts in the lower legs indicative of venous thrombosis in 32 percent of both control and elastic stocking groups.[25] Hence, more studies involving post-coronary patients are needed before the true value of this simple form of preventive therapy can be assessed.

Multiple studies have shown that minidose subcutaneous heparin, given before surgery and continued for several doses after surgery, is effective in preventing calf vein thrombosis.[26] Handley[27] has shown that this regimen is not effective in patients with acute myocardial infarction, attributing this to the fact that the therapy in these instances is started after the event that initiated the thrombosis. Wray et al.[28] randomly allocated 92 consecutive patients with acute myocardial infarction into a control group and an anticoagulated group. The latter consisted of heparin for the initial 48 hours, followed by Coumadin. Both groups underwent active physiotherapy from the onset of admission and were mobilized to a chair within 7 days of the acute event. The groups were well-matched in the severity of cardiac illness as assessed by a coronary prognostic index. All patients were given intravenous injections of labeled fibrinogen, and the lower extremities were

---

Table 1A
Physical Therapy Inpatient Exercises
for Myocardial Infarction Patients

STEP I: ACTIVE ASSISTIVE RANGE OF MOTION EXERCISES
UPPER EXTREMITY−SUPINE
1. With the left elbow straight, lift the arm straight over the head and return back to the side. Relax and repeat. Do the same for the right side.
2. With the left elbow straight, lift the left arm away from the body and over the head and return to side. Relax and repeat. Do the same for the right side.
3. With the left elbow bent, move the left forearm over the abdomen and then out to the side of the body. Relax and repeat. Do the same for the right side.
4. With the left elbow straight, bend the elbow touching the shoulder with fingertips. Relax and repeat. Do the same for the right side.
LOWER EXTREMITY−SUPINE
1. Lift the left leg toward the chest and return to the starting position. Relax and repeat. Do the same with the right leg.
2. With the left leg straight, separate the leg out to the side of the body and return to the starting position. Relax and repeat. Do the same for the right side.
3. Roll the legs in and out simultaneously. Relax and repeat.
4. Make circular patterns with both feet. Relax and repeat.

STEP II: Do the same exercises as in Step I actively instead of actively assisted.

STEP III: Same as Step II.

STEP IV: Do the lower extremity exercises the same as in Steps II and III. Perform the upper extremity exercises the same as those in Step I in the sitting position. Exercises are to be performed *simultaneously* instead of *alternately*.

STEP V: Same as Step IV.

STEP VI: Same as Step V.
LOWER EXTREMITY−SITTING
1. Straighten and bend the knees alternately. Relax and repeat.
2. Raise the knee toward the chest alternately. Relax and repeat.

STEP VII: Perform lower extremity exercises in the sitting position the same as in Step VI.
Perform the upper extremity exercises in the standing position.

STEP VIII: Same exercises as in Step VII.

Table 1B—Flow Sheet
Physical Therapy Inpatient Activity and Exercises
For Myocardial Infarction Patients

Date of Infarction _____.

Step	Approx. Day Post MI	Date	Exercise	BP, Pulse	Remarks
1	1–2		Active assistive exercise to all extremities performed supine (5x) q.d.	Before ex After ex	
II	3–4		Active ROM (5x – 7x) q.d.	Before ex After ex	
III	5		Active ROM (8x) q.d. Do leg exercise supine, arm exercise sitting. Ambulate 30 – 60 feet.	Before ex During ex After ex Before amb During amb After amb	
IV	6		Same as III. Do exercises 9x. Walk 100 feet.	Before ex During ex After ex Before amb During amb After amb	
V	7		Same as IV. Do exercises (10x) q.d. Walk 200 feet.	Before ex During ex After ex Before amb During amb After amb	
VI	8		Same as V. Add: Standing a) arm and shoulder (5x) b) Lateral bend (5x) c) Knee raise (5x) q.d. Walk 400 feet.	Before ex During ex After ex Before amb During amb After amb	
VII	9		Same as VI. Add: a) Sitting toe touch b) Sitting trunk twist (5x) q.d. c) 1 flight stairs	Before ex During ex After ex Before amb During amb After amb	

Abbreviations: ex = exercise; MI = myocardial infarction; BP = blood pressure in mmHg; ROM = range of motion; amb = ambulation.

Table 1C
Physical Therapy Inpatient Exercises for Cardiac Surgical Patients

STEP: PREOP Instruct in diaphragmatic and nasal breathing exercises, deep coughing, splinting technique, posture, active ankle dorsiflexion exercises.

STEP I: ACTIVE ASSISTIVE RANGE OF MOTION EXERCISES
UPPER EXTREMITY–SUPINE
1. With the left elbow straight, lift the arm straight over the head and return back to the side. Relax and repeat. Do the same for the right side.
2. With the left elbow straight, lift the arm away from the body and over the head and return to the side. Relax and repeat. Do the same for the right side.
3. With the left elbow bent, move the left forearm over the abdomen and then out to the side of the body. Relax and repeat. Do the same for the right side.
4. With the left elbow straight, bend the elbow touching the shoulder with the fingertips. Relax and repeat. Do the same for the right side.
LOWER EXTREMITY–SUPINE
1. Lift the left leg toward the chest and return to the starting position. Relax and repeat. Do the same with the right leg.
2. With the left leg straight, separate the leg out to the side of the body and return to the starting position. Relax and repeat. Do the same for the right side.
3. Roll the legs in and out simultaneously. Relax and repeat.
4. Make circular patterns with both feet. Relax and repeat.

STEP II: Do same as Step I, except actively instead of active assistive.

STEP III: Same as Step II.

STEP IV: Do the same exercises as in Step I actively instead of actively assisted.

STEP V: Do the lower extremity exercises the same as those in Step IV. Perform the upper extremity exercises the same as those in Step IV in the sitting position. Exercises are to be performed *simultaneously* instead of alternately.

STEP VI: Do the upper extremity exercises the same as those in Step V. Perform standing rather than sitting.
LOWER EXTREMITY–SITTING
1. Straighten and bend the knees alternately. Relax and repeat.
2. Raise the knee toward the chest alternately. Relax and repeat.

STEP VII: Perform the lower extremity exercises in the sitting position the same as in Step VI.
ADDITIONAL–STANDING
1. Standing erect, bend trunk laterally to the left and then to the right. Relax and repeat.

STEP VIII: Same exercises as in Step VII.

Table 1D—Flow Sheet
Physical Therapy Inpatient Activity and Exercises
for Cardiac Surgical Patients

Date of Surgery _____.

Step	Approx. Day Post Surg.	Date	Exercise	BP, Pulse	Remarks
PREOP			Preoperative visits: Introduction to program. P.T. Instruction: Diaphragmatic breathing, Deep coughing, Splinting techniques, Posture, Active ankle dorsiflexion	Baseline	
SURGERY I	1		Diaphragmatic breathing, Active assist ROM (5x), Ankle dorsiflexion (10x) q.d.	Before ex After ex	
II	2		Active ROM (5x) q.d.	Before ex After ex	
III	3		Same as Step II plus walk 30 − 60 feet.	Before ex After ex Before amb After amb	
IV	4		After ROM (5x) q.d. Do upper extremity exercises sitting. Walk 100 feet.	Before ex After ex Before amb After amb	
V	5		Active exercise (5x). Do all exercises sitting. Walk 200 feet.	Before ex After ex Before amb After amb	
VI	6		Same as V. Add: Home exercise instruction. Walk 300 − 400 feet.	Before ex After ex Before amb After amb	
VII	7		Same as VI. Add: Home exercise instruction. Walk minimum 400 feet.	Before ex After ex Before amb After amb	

Abbreviations: Surg. = surgery; BP = blood pressure; P.T. = physical therapy; ROM = range of motion; ex = exercise; amb = ambulation.

scanned daily for evidence of venous thrombosis. Daily chest x-rays were done on both groups, and the last 50 patients in the study had lung scans on the 10th hospital day. The group receiving the anticoagulants had a 6.5 percent incidence of calf vein thrombosis as compared to a 22 percent incidence in the control group. The thrombosis development occurred remarkably early in the hospital course, as more than 60 percent developed within 72 hours of the clinical onset of infarction. This would suggest that the infarction itself, rather than a period of prolonged immobilization, was the precipitating factor. It is of interest that the thrombi were confined to calf veins in all instances of both control and treatment patients. Moreover, clinically important pulmonary emboli did not occur in either group. It is possible that the active physical therapy and early mobilization regimen played some role in limiting the extension of thrombosis formation.

In addition to the inpatient physical program, there are three other groups of services which are available to the patient who is referred to the cardiac rehabilitation team. *Group I* consists of *individual patient and family conferences,* and includes discussion and instruction in diet, coronary risk factors, and current cardiac problems. Religious counseling and psychological testing are done in selected instances. All phases of activities within the group are conducted in the individual patient's room. *Group II* deals with *group conferences* pertaining to the pathophysiology of coronary atherosclerosis, the psychosocial aspects of coronary disease, diet, and coronary risk factors. These conferences are held with use of various audiovisual aids and are scheduled so that a different discussion is scheduled twice monthly. The patient's spouse and family are strongly urged to attend these sessions.

Group III is the *predischarge and follow-up phase.* This includes instructions on a home walking regimen and general guidelines as to "do's" and "don'ts" during the early segment of home care (Fig. 1 [Form 1]).

The topic of sexual activity is considered as patients are often embarrassed to initiate such discussion. The energy expenditure during this activity has been studied by Hellerstein and Friedman,[29] who found that the mean pulse rate during intercourse was 117 beats per minute in post-infarction patients. This is approximately the same energy cost of climbing two flights of stairs. Patients who are stable during in-hospital stair climbing are permitted to engage in sexual activities within a week after discharge.

Form 1
Do's and Don'ts

---

1) Alternate a hard task with an easy one.
2) Spread out activities—Do some in the mornings—some in the afternoon and evening.
3) Allow plenty of time—Don't rush.
4) Rest for 20–30 minutes at least twice a day. You don't have to go to bed—just rest.
5) Stop your activity if you get tired—Rest 15–30 minutes whether you have finished the task or not.
6) Get at least 6–8 hours of sleep each night. Do not stay up late one night and try to catch up the next.
7) Don't work with arms above your head as this may be tiring. Plan many activities so that you can work with your arms at waist level.
8) Do not drink large amounts of alcohol (no more than 3 oz. per day) Limit your alcoholic intake to 1½–2 oz. per day.
9) Avoid situations or people that bring on anger or stress.
10) Do not eat large meals as this makes the heart pump harder. Eat 3–4 small meals a day instead of one large heavy one.
11) Don't eat fast.
12) Don't return to activities right after eating. Rest an hour after each meal.
13) Don't drink more than 1–2 cups of coffee, tea, and colas since they contain caffeine.
14) Avoid extremes in temperatures. It is best to perform outdoor activities mid-day in winter—late evening or early morning in summer.
15) Don't resume sexual activities until you can climb two flights of stairs without discomfort or shortness of breath. In most people, 4–6 weeks of recovery enables the heart muscle to handle the demands of sex.
16) Travel: Avoid carrying heavy suitcases.
    Avoid rushing—allow plenty of time.
    Avoid long periods of sitting—walk around at least every two hours during car or plane trips.
    Do not visit spots in high altitudes greater than 5,000 feet without consulting your physician.
17) Don't take risks.
18) Don't smoke, chew tobacco.
19) Don't eat a diet high in saturated fats.
20) Don't overeat—watch your weight.
21) Don't attempt fad diets.
22) Limit sugar and pure sweets, as they add "empty" calories.
23) Don't fry foods. Bake or broil instead.
24) Limit salt intake.
25) Don't lead a sedentary lifestyle. Follow a prescribed exercise regimen (work up gradually).
    —Don't exercise if you experience angina, fatigue or shortness of breath.
    —Stop at the first sign of angina, fatigue or shortness of breath.
    —Don't forget to use NTG if angina occurs.
    —Don't *compete* or push yourself.
    —Don't exercise after drinking alcohol, eating a heavy meal or emotional upsets.

Figure 1.

Another area of interest in the predischarge phase has been the effect of *bathing* on oxygen consumption and hemodynamic and ECG response. Reports of sudden death and ECG changes after showering have prompted new emphasis on such practices during the early phase of hospital inpatient rehabilitation. To assess this potential problem, a study was designed to obtain information on oxygen consumption and hemodynamic and ECG responses during standard in-hospital bathing practices undertaken by immediate post-myocardial infarction (PMI) patients.[30]

Twelve patients (10 male, 2 female) with uncomplicated myocardial infarction were studied. All were sequentially selected from a population of 206 patients with myocardial infarction admitted to a large metropolitan hospital between February 1978 and May 1979. All were fasting for at least 4 hours prior to testing. Immediately prior to each bath (standing shower [S], bed bath [BB], and tub bath [TB]) a resting 12-lead ECG was done with standard portable recorder, while supine blood pressure with cuff sphygmomanometer and cardiac auscultation were recorded. These measures were repeated immediately following (within 90 seconds) each bathing procedure. Every patient took one of each of three baths (S, BB, and TB) on 3 consecutive days. Patients were instructed to bathe in their usual manner, but not to wash their hair. Each bath was timed with a Wakmann stop watch. The order of the baths was determined by random numbers, and all were done during the same time period each day (near noon).

Oxygen consumption in ml/kg/min (VO_2) was determined by continuous oxygen sampling using a Max Planck respirometer technique described elsewhere (Fig. 2). Heart rate determination (taken when the patient signaled he had completed 50% of the bath) during and immediate post bathing was by palpation of radial pulse. Water temperature for all activity procedures was maintained at 96° Farenheit $\pm 2°$. All data were reduced and statistically evaluated using a noncorrelated t test.

Physiological data is recorded in Table 2. There were no significant differences in the time for each bath. VE ATPS was greater 20.83 (p < .01) for S than for TB or BB; however, none of the subjects appeared dyspneic and none hyperventilated. Shower activity demanded greater (p < .01) VO_2 than either TB or BB. Hemodynamic response peak systolic blood pressure × heart rate (PRP) was greater (p < .05) for S when compared to BB but not TB. Reduction of the shower data revealed the heart rate component of the pressure rate product was more responsible than the blood

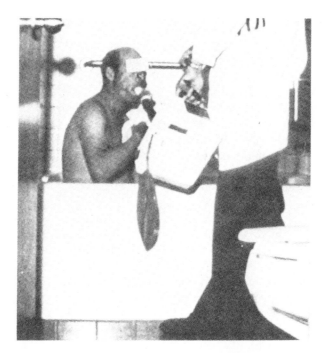

Figure 2: Patient taking tub bath during simultaneous oxygen sampling using the Max Planck Respirator. (From Johnston BL, et al. Oxygen consumption and hemodynamic and ECG responses to bathing in recent post-myocardial-infarction patients. *Heart and Lung* 1981; 10:666–671. Used with permission.)

pressure component for the changes seen in the hemodynamic data.

None of the patients complained of angina, and no arrhythmias, except for occasional premature contractions, were observed following any of the baths. However, the 12-lead ECG revealed significant ST segment displacement ($\geq$ 1 mm) after bathing in seven of the 12 (58.3%) patients (Fig. 3). Five of these seven had inferior infarctions and two had anterior infarctions. Four of the five patients with inferior infarction developed ST segment changes in their precordial leads. The other patient with inferior infarction developed T wave changes in lead II and lost the R wave in lead V_1. Of the two patients with anterior infarctions, one developed ST segment depression in the inferior leads and ST segment elevation in leads V_2 and V_3. The other anterior infarction patient developed

Table 2
Physiological Data on Twelve Patients Involved
in Postinfarction Bath Study[30]

	Shower	Bed Bath	Tub Bath
TIME	3' 07"	4' 38"	3' 34"
	SD ± 0.89	SD ± 1.2	SD ± 0.91
$\dot{V}O_2$ (ml/kg/min)	13.02*	8.94	9.01
	SD ± 3.2	SD ± 3.25	SD ± 3.22
$\dot{V}E$ ATPS (liters/min)	20.83*	13.07	14.42
	SD ± 3.41	SD ± 1.78	SD ± 2.06
METs	3.72	2.55	2.57
RQ	0.802	0.735	0.787
PRP	15070**	13189	13954
	SD ± 2009	SD ± 2494	SD ± 2592

Time, $\dot{V}O_2$, $\dot{V}E$ ATPS, and PRP are expressed in means
Abbreviations: ' = minutes; " = seconds; SD = standard deviation; $\dot{V}O_2$ = oxygen consumption; $\dot{V}E$ ATPS = total ventilation of expired air at ambient temperature pressure saturated; * = p less than .01; METs = metabolic equivalent; RQ = respiratory quotient; PRP = peak systolic blood pressure × heart rate; ** = p less than .05.

ST depression in leads V_4-V_6. This patient was taking a diuretic agent which could have influenced the ST segment displacement.

Analysis of all electrocardiograms with changes after bathing revealed that a greater number of changes occurred after S (6 of 11 − 54.4%) than after TB (4 of 12 − 33.3%) or BB (2 of 11 − 18.2%). Four of the six patients with ECG changes after S, two of the four patients with changes after TB, and both of the patients with changes after BB had inferior infarctions.

Considerations relative to showering are that more body flexion occurs in bathing lower extremities and that standing involves more use of large muscle mass. This likely results in more dynamic than static activity. The data supports this in that the heart rate was the greater component of the rate-systolic blood pressure product in the shower hemodynamic data. Although some difference in data may have been evident had the subjects taken seated showers, the standing position was chosen as this was the usual shower protocol in this hospital.

In shower activity, one must also consider adjustments for the hemodynamic response involved in changing from the supine to the upright position. The response should take place within 20 seconds. Since the patients were uncomplicated and took 20 seconds or more to go from bed to shower, it is felt that the hemo-

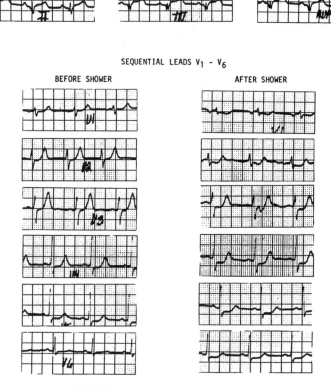

Figure 3: Precordial ECG leads (V_1 to V_6) of a patient with a recent inferior myocardial infarction. Significant ST segment changes are noted when comparing tracings before and after showering. (From Johnston BL, et al. Oxygen consumption and hemodynamic and ECG responses to bathing in recent post-myocardial infarction patients. *Heart and Lung* 1981; 10:666−671. Used with permission.)

dynamic response was related to the work of showering and not position. When considering the effect of water immersion and tub bath, this was not felt to be a factor in the hemodynamic response as 80 percent or more of the body must be immersed to obtain a water immersion effect; the patients' bodies in this study were no more than 40 percent immersed. Each of the baths required greater than 3 minutes (mean) which was felt to be adequate exposure time for the subjects to attain a physiologically stable adjustment to the bath.

In this study, the majority of additional ischemic ECG re-sponses (4 of 5) occurred in the inferior infarction patients. Find-ings of ischemia in this group caused concern about a greater degree of coronary occlusive disease involving anterior, septal, and lateral regions of myocardium. One patient had coronary arteriog-raphy which revealed left ventricular dysfunction with inferior and anterior basal hypokinesis, an ejection fraction of 35 percent, and the following coronary artery occlusions: left main, 55 percent; proximal left anterior descending, 60 percent; mid-left anterior descending, 85 percent; obtuse marginal circumflex, 75 percent; and proximal right, 100 percent. These latter findings support concern of the possible diffuse nature of disease in patients with ischemic ECG responses after bathing, especially in the shower.

Deficiencies are often inherent in clinical studies in acute care hospitals. Such is the case in this study in that matched normal controls were not included. However, with utilization of three different bathing procedures, the subjects served as their own controls, thus giving greater validity to the data.

In the absence of catheterization data, it is felt that further studies such as low level pre-discharge exercise tests may be bene-ficial in post-infarction patients, especially for inferior infarction patients. Individual discharge advice may be influenced by the exercise test. In addition, if arrhythmias are noted during hospital-ization or during the low level exercise test, a 24-hour dynamic electrocardiogram may yield significant data for use in discharge and follow-up therapy.

Other study data were analyzed on 89 post-infarction pa-tients followed for a mean of 13.5 months after hospitalization (Fig. 4).[31] Fifteen percent (14 of 89) were deceased and data were derived from the remaining 75. Fifty-six percent (42 of 75) were working, 37 full time and five part time. Four percent (3 of 75) were housewives. Forty percent (30 of 75) were retired, 15 were of retirement age, and 15 retired because of medical reasons.

All patients had been instructed in the fat-controlled diet. Sixty-six percent (49 of 75) were following the diets as instructed; 34 percent (26 of 75) changed their dietary habits from fat-controlled to regular. All were instructed in proper exercise habits and en-couraged to continue an exercise regimen at home. Seventy-seven percent (58 of 75) exercised after discharge from the hospital. Thirty-nine of these were exercising no less than two times each week; nineteen exercised once a week or less (periodic). Twenty-three percent (17 of 75 patients) did not continue an exercise regimen. Seventy-six percent (57 of 75) were overweight at the

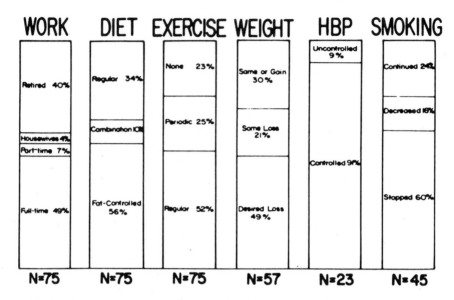

Figure 4: Bar graph showing results of inpatient cardiac rehabilitation. Lower portions of bar display desired effect in each category. (From Johnston BL, et al. Eight steps to inpatient cardiac rehabilitation: The team effort-methodology and preliminary results. *Heart and Lung* 1976; 5:97–111. Used by permission.)

time of infarction. All of these were given a goal to attain in losing the proper amount of weight. The weight goal was assessed according to recommended ideal body weight for a specific height and body frame. Forty-nine percent (28 of 57) attained this goal, 21 percent (12 of 57) partially attained their goal, and 30 percent (17 of 57) failed to attain their goal.

Thirty-one percent (23 of 75) had a history of high blood pressure prior to infarction. Ninety-one percent (21 of 23) had their blood pressure controlled and nine percent (2 of 23) were not controlled at the time of follow-up. One of these latter two patients had just begun a new antihypertensive drug regimen. Sixty percent (45 of 75) were cigarette smokers prior to infarction. Sixty percent (27 of 45) at follow-up no longer smoked cigarettes and 16 percent (7 of 45) had decreased their number of daily cigarettes to one-half their previous smoking rate. However, 24 percent (11 of 45) continued to smoke.

Recent data by Matsuda et al.[32] reflect the relationship of physical activity to angina pectoris before and during acute myocardial infarction. One hundred ninety-seven patients with a history of acute infarction were interviewed to evaluate the character of angina relative to physical activity before the infarction. In the 92 patients of the group without angina before infarction, acute infarction occurred during heavy exertion in 10 (11%), mild exertion in 43 (47%), and at rest in 28 (30%). The event occurred during sleep in 11 (12%). Therefore, this data reflect that heavy exertion and sleep seem to reflect the lesser incident of development of infarction and that infarction was likely to occur in the presence of the resting state or perhaps with mild exertion.

Other recent data by Magder[33] report the effect of potential stress of ambulatory activities in 32 patients following infarction during sitting, standing, and walking during the first 2 days. All activities were well tolerated, and the author concluded that mild ambulatory activities produced little stress for the myocardium and can be permitted in the first few days following infarction, as long as blood pressure is measured.

Pryor et al.[34] recently reported on early discharge after myocardial infarction, and reviewed existing data with reference to early discharge after infarction. They found that approximately 50 percent of patients hospitalized with acute infarction have an uncomplicated course and have an excellent prognosis. However, patients with recurring angina in the post-infarction period may be at increased risk. Early and rapidly progressive rehabilitation programs permit the safe discharge of patients with an uncomplicated course after 7 days. Functional exercise testing before or soon after early discharge may identify high-risk patients and alter their management. Therefore, more recent data continue to confirm the probable benefits of exercise in rehabilitation programs after infarction.

In summary, evidence is available to support that the uncomplicated post-myocardial infarction patient may be mobilized within the first few days of hospitalization and often can be discharged with 1 week of hospital care. The latter is enhanced with a team approach to the various facets of the post-infarction state. In small community hospitals, an interested physician and nurse, preferably with coronary care experience, will suffice to guide the patient in secondary prevention measures and to assist in handling the various psychosocial barriers that often accompany coronary disease. The hospital phase of a myocardial infarction can be a frightening experience, particularly to a person who has previously enjoyed good health. The fear of becoming a "cardiac invalid" is always present. The optimistic attitude of the rehabilitation team and the reassurance of returning to an active, productive life has done much to allay the various apprehensions and anxieties of the coronary patient.

Limited data are available on the utilization of exercise testing prior to discharge in coronary bypass surgery patients. The reason for this is that the hospital admission for this procedure is reasonably short-lived and the patients are sent home quite rapidly with hospital morbidity. One study by Eyherabide et al.[35] reviewed cardiovascular and ECG responses in 433 consecutive coronary bypass surgery patients. The test was done approximately 7 days post-operatively, using graded treadmill or cycle ergometer protocols. No complications occurred in this group of patients. However, 18 percent showed a hypertensive blood pressure response to low level exercise. Complex ventricular dysrhythmias occurred in 4 percent. The authors concluded that submaximal exercise testing is safely performed in coronary bypass surgery patients prior to discharge and that it may be useful in establishing the individual exercise prescriptions and particularly in identifying exercise-associated dysrhythmias and hypertension.

Outpatient Rehabilitation – Exercise Programs: Historic Perspectives

Outpatient exercise programs have evolved as popular activity in areas of secondary prevention. Over the past decade, numerous investigators have expounded the benefits of increased activity and regular exercise for patients with coronary artery disease. The studies dealing with the largest number of patients are the early ones of Hellerstein[36] and Gottheiner.[37] The latter reported a 5-year follow-up on 1,103 male patients with coronary disease, 548 of whom had a previous myocardial infarction (although criteria for diagnoses were not listed). The exercise program began with several months of mild strength-building activities including weight-lifting, but other specifics of this initial program are not provided. After 9 months, the men engaged in rhythmic endurance exercises such as running, hiking, swimming, cycling, rowing, and volleyball. Those who excelled in these activities and achieved a significant improvement in overall conditioning then entered competitive team games. The participants in the general exercise program basically practiced on their own on a twice-daily schedule with no medical supervision. Once a week the men met as a group for instructions and practice. The most impressive results of the study are in the mortality rate data, which was 3.6 percent for the entire group over the 5-year period in contrast to 12 percent in a comparable nonexercised group with previous myocardial infarctions. Gottheiner described other objective effects of training, such as reductions of resting heart rate and resting and exercise blood pressure levels. In addition, there was less ST segment depression on ECG taken during and immediately post exercise. Unfortunately, the complete data on these observations are not given, which makes the significance questionable.

Hellerstein[36] reported the results of physical training in 656 middle-aged males, 203 of whom had angina pectoris and/or myocardial infarctions. An additional 51 men had resting or exercise electrocardiograms compatible with silent coronary heart disease (utilizing the Minnesota code). The subjects were followed for an average of 2.7 years and participated in at least a thrice-weekly exercise program and recreational activities. The latter included swimming, basketball, volleyball, and use of a punching bag. Detailed results were presented on the first 100 cardiac patients. The average weight loss was 2.5 kg. Sixty-five percent significantly improved their level of training, as measured by bicycle ergometric testing and oxygen consumption. Sixty-three percent showed improvement in their exercise ECGs, mainly in terms of the initial slope and the junctional displacement of the ST segment. The death rate for the exercise cardiac patients was 1.9 per 100 patient-years, which was less than half the expected rate.

Rechnitzer et al.[38] reported the results of physical training in men with previous documented myocardial infarctions. There were two aspects of the study. One consisted of a comparison of the incidence of nonfatal recurrences and cardiac deaths between 77 men in the exercise group and 111 controls who were matched according to age, year of infarction, and number of infarctions. All of the controls met the criteria for entry into the exercise program but did not enter for a variety of reasons (including job conflicts and personal physician disapproval). Over a 7-year follow-up period, the results were as follows:

	No.	Nonfatal Recurrences	Cardiac Deaths
Exercise Group	77	1 (1.3)%	3 (3.9%)
Matched Control Group	111	31(28 %)	15 (11.8%)

There were several weaknesses of the aforementioned study, however, that may have influenced the results. The control groups were not "true" controls in the sense that they were randomly assigned to the inactive group. It is possible that certain members of the control group had severe angina pectoris and did not enter the exercise program for this reason. Another vulnerable aspect of the study concerns the documentation of nonfatal recurrence of myocardial infarction. In some instances, historical evidence supplied by the patient or his physician was utilized instead of more reliable criteria such as enzyme and ECG changes. Still another deficit of the study was that the exercise and control groups were not matched for important risk factors such as cigarette smoking habits, hypertension, serum cholesterol levels, and family history.

Kennedy et al.[39] reported a small study of eight men (ranging in age from 45 to 52 years) who had stable angina pectoris. None of the men developed a myocardial infarction or died during the follow-up period. This has little significance, however, since the numbers are small, the follow-up was brief (1 year), and a control group was not obtained. The study was of interest in that cardiac catheterization and coronary arteriography were performed prior to and at the completion of the 1-year exercise program. All patients had an increase in cardiac index after training (from a mean of 3.9 to 4.4 L/min/m^2). Half of the patients showed a decrease in the magnitude of ischemic changes on follow-up exercise stress testing. Surprisingly, the left ventricular end-diastolic pressure increased in seven of the eight patients (from a mean of 16 to 20 mmHg). None of the individuals showed any increase in coronary collateral circulation post training.

Perhaps the best designed study of post-infarction physical training was that of Kentala[40] who randomly assigned patients into control or exercise groups. Of those who were discharged from the hospital, 158 men met the diagnostic criteria for a documented myocardial infarction. The exercise group was comprised of 77 men, while the control group numbered 81 men. The groups were similar regarding age, smoking habits, pre-infarction physical activities, severity of infarction, serum cholesterol levels, and lung vital capacities. Over a 2-year follow-up period, there were no group differences as to coronary mortality or morbidity. However, only 10 of 77 (13%) in the training group had attended at least 70 percent of the thrice-weekly exercise sessions by the end of 1 year, while 11 of 81 controls (14%) had engaged in a regular physical training program on their own. Therefore, it is not too surprising that group differences were not detected. Those attending the exercise sessions on a regular basis showed significant weight loss, diminution of body fat, and a decrease in serum triglyceride levels. In addition, they demonstrated greater improvement in physical work capacity on exercise testing (p < .0025), had more success in giving up cigarette smoking, and had faster disappearances in Q waves on the resting ECG.

In another randomized study of post-myocardial infarction men and women (all born in 1913), 158 were allocated to an exercise group and 157 to a control group.[41] Over a 4-year follow-up period, the group differences were minimal:

	Exercise Group (# of cases)	Control Group (# of cases)
Deaths	28	35
Nonfatal myocardial infarction	25	28

As in Kentala's study, the drop-out rate was high, for after 1 year only 39 percent of the exercise group was still training at the hospital (21 percent more trained at home or at work). Of those who adhered to the exercise program for at least 1 year, the mortality rate was half as high (5 of 67, or 7%) compared to the controls (20 of 142, or 14%). The dropouts tended to be "sicker" and smoked more than the high adherence subjects.

Therefore, considerable data are available to support the benefit of physical exercise in the rehabilitation of patients in the post-infarction state. The difficulty in undertaking and completing a controlled study is apparent; however, the "trend" in available studies is quite supportive.

Recently, regarding exercise performance in men with previous infarction, more current data have been revealed regarding the influence of the location of the infarction. Wasserman et al.[42] and the National Exercise and Heart Disease Project staff reported on the 651 men evaluated in this project and found that the location and extent of a previous infarction as evaluated by the resting ECG does not significantly influence subsequent exercise tolerance. Laslett et al.[43] studied the change in myocardial oxygen consumption indices by exercise training in patients with coronary artery disease. They evaluated the experience of ten patients who had a modest-level exercise training program for 6 months. All achieved a training effect, and eight of the ten patients demonstrated an increase in heart rate at onset of ischemia. Seven of the eight had an increase in double product at onset of ischemia. Thus the rate of myocardial oxygen consumption at which ischemia developed, based on this study, was altered favorably by 6 months of moderate-level exercise training. To the contrary, Hammond et al.[44] presented clinical data in predicting improvement in exercise capacity after cardiac rehabilitation. In 59 men, after 1 year of supervised aerobic exercise, poor correlations were found between initial measurements and changes in oxygen consumption and other indices of training, therefore showing that such studies do not necessarily predict the outcome in such patients with infarction and coronary artery disease. However, in this group, a significant decrease in the amount of ischemia measured by thallium perfusion was noted after training.

With regard to patients involved in supervised exercise after coronary artery bypass surgery, Grant et al.[45] studied 25 patients who did not exercise and 27 who exercised early after surgery. They found no untoward effects of exercise in any patient, and that supervised exercise in the early post-operative period results in earlier independent activity of patients and fewer pulmonary complications, and may shorten post-operative stay. Stevens and Hanson[46] studied the comparison of supervised and unsupervised exercise training after coronary bypass surgery. They reported on 180 patients with unsupervised exercise and 24 patients with supervised exercise who were referred after bypass surgery. There were no significant differences in the maximal exercise capacity and heart rate between the groups, and they concluded that prescribed, unsupervised exercise can be performed safely and results in similar functional improvements compared with supervised exercise after uncomplicated coronary bypass surgery. This latter study further emphasizes the fact that certain subsets of coronary patients, particularly those after coronary bypass grafting with good left ventricular function, may do very well with unsupervised exercise, and this is being practiced in many clinical settings.

HOME EXERCISE PROGRAMS

In recent times, because of the limited accessibility of structured center exercise programs and difficulty at times in patient transportation to such programs, home exercise programs have become popular. Such programs have developed in various formats, and the results, applicability, and safety of these seem to be quite acceptable. Data from our program in Atlanta addressed home biking versus home walking in post-coronary bypass patients after a pre-discharge exercise test.[47] Results revealed that the home exercise with either modality was safe and effective in detecting new rate, rhythm, and blood pressure responses, and was acceptable by the patients from the standpoint of convenience and enjoyability with regards to their training. In addition, Miller et al.[48] studied 198 men after uncomplicated myocardial infarction randomly assigned to several exercise protocols. They found no significant differences in functional capacity between patients training at home and those in a group program. In addition, no training or related complications occurred. Home and group training were equally effective in increasing functional capacity of such low-risk patients after myocardial infarction.

GENERAL GUIDELINES FOR EXERCISE TRAINING

The person with known coronary heart disease, post infarction, post-coronary bypass surgery, angioplasty, and those with stable angina pectoris should be evaluated carefully before beginning a long-term conditioning program involving exercise other than walking. If such a program is limited to walking, it can be performed without medical supervision, provided a screening examination does not detect heart failure or serious cardiac rhythm disturbances. They should be taught to check their own pulse rate and should limit the intensity of walking to that producing a heart rate of less than 120 beats per minute. They should be instructed to wait 1 to 2 hours after a meal before walking, to avoid walking in extremes of weather, and to stop promptly if they experience any chest discomfort.

Post-coronary patients who wish to undergo more strenuous forms of conditioning, including jogging and swimming, should do so under the direct supervision of medical personnel and in the presence of emergency resuscitation equipment (including a defibrillator). Ten absolute contraindications to such forms of activity are as follows:

1. Moderate to severe aortic outflow obstruction (supravalvular, valvular, subvalvular);
2. Uncontrolled heart failure;

3. Acute infectious disease, including active myocarditis;
4. Unstable angina pectoris;
5. Recent myocardial infarction;
6. Aortic dissection;
7. Thrombophlebitis;
8. Poorly controlled supraventricular rhythm disorders (such as rapid atrial fibrillation) and serious ventricular rhythm disorders (such as paroxysmal tachycardia);
9. Severe systemic arterial hypertension (systolic pressure 240 mmHg, diastolic pressure 110 mmHg);
10. Cyanotic congenital heart disease.

There are, in addition, a number of relative contraindications to exercise training in which the possible benefits of exercise must be carefully weighed against the risks involved. These relative contraindications include pulmonary hypertension, ventricular aneurysm, poorly controlled metabolic diseases such as diabetes or thyroid disorders, and toxemia of pregnancy. In addition, special consideration should be given to patients with cardiac pacemakers, congenital heart disease other than the cyanotic variety, and any form of chronic disease that might make it difficult to achieve a training effect. Such diseases include chronic renal or hepatic disorders. The cardiac exercise class should not be permitted to become a "catch-all" for severe cardiac problems in which there is no other form of therapy. Patients with severe angina pectoris, three-vessel coronary disease on angiography, and an akinetic myocardium on ventriculography are usually not candidates for coronary bypass surgery or angioplasty, nor are they candidates for a progressive exercise rehabilitation program.

In the exercise program, the patient must be advised to adhere to the exercise prescription (see Chapter 3). Unless this is done, patients have a tendency to "keep up with" advanced members of the group and to see how many repetitions of one exercise can be performed without serious sequelae. The group supervisors must be alert for such instances and should report them immediately to the physician in charge. Patients should not be permitted to exercise if they have experienced any unusual type of recent chest discomfort. They are advised instead to promptly contact their personal physician.

There are several basic rules with which exercise participants must comply. They are advised against exercising within 2 hours of a large meal and to refrain from coffee, tea, cigarettes, and alcohol during the same time segment. They should warm up for 5 minutes before exercise and should cool down for the same period of time after exercise before showering. The "buddy" system is used in the dressing room. The doors on the toilets should not be locked from the inside.

Rules should be applied in an inconspicuous manner. One does not wish for the participants to look upon the exercise class as an extension of the coronary care unit but rather as a place to enjoy meaningful and pleasurable activity and social exchange. There are several ways to enhance the program and thereby to improve patient adherence. It is important for the medical staff to know the names of all class members and for the members to learn each other's names. Periodic group photographs with an accompanying name list help in this direction, as do names on the back of T-shirts. New members should be introduced to at least several of the "veterans" so that they feel more comfortable in the initial phases of the program, the period in which the drop-out rate tends to be the highest.

THE EMORY HEALTH ENHANCEMENT PROGRAM

A variety of outpatient exercise programs have been utilized by various investigators. One of the more recent programs is the Emory Health Enhancement Program developed at Emory University in the George W. Woodruff physical education facility.

The Emory Health Enhancement Program (EHEP) is a component of the Emory University School of Medicine, Department of Rehabilitation Medicine. Administered by The Emory Clinic, the EHEP staff includes a cardiologist, specially trained nurses, exercise specialists, exercise technologists, and a dietitian.

EHEP provides services to both healthy subjects and to those with heart, blood vessel, and other diseases. EHEP offers exercise testing (Figs. 5, 6) and evaluation using state-of-the-art equipment and supervised exercise programs for cardiac rehabilitation patients. Two programs are available. Phase II and Phase III. Phase II of cardiac rehabilitation complements treatment by a physician following the patient's discharge from the hospital, and helps the patient return to a productive life by developing better health habits and confidence. Intensive short-term exercise sessions are supervised by a medical team who continuously monitor

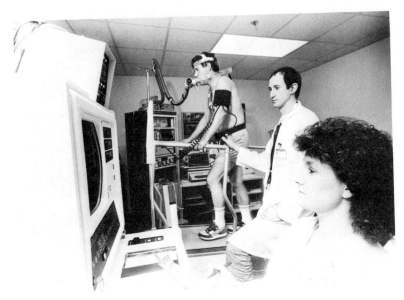

Figure 5: Exercise testing is done on a motorized treadmill with regular blood pressure recordings and constant ECG monitoring (foreground left). Continuous expired air collection for gas analysis is done as seen with subject on treadmill. Equipment in background does continuous O_2 and CO_2 measurements from expired air with intermittent (every 15 seconds) graphic display of oxygen consumption in ml/kg/min.

participants using telemetry.[49] Nonmonitored versions of Phase II and Phase III form the final phases of cardiac rehabilitation. These phases eventually place the patient in a longer-term maintenance program.

All participants should be referred by a physician, and are required to undergo evaluation before entering one of the exercise programs. Persons unable to participate in one of the exercise programs may be seen for testing and individual exercise prescriptions. Weight loss, dietary changes, stress management, and stop-smoking programs may be recommended.

All participants receive written recommendations based on their test and evaluation, and test results are forwarded to their private physician.

Testing and evaluation include:

1. Pre-exercise medical and exercise history.
2. Medically supervised graded exercise test on a treadmill

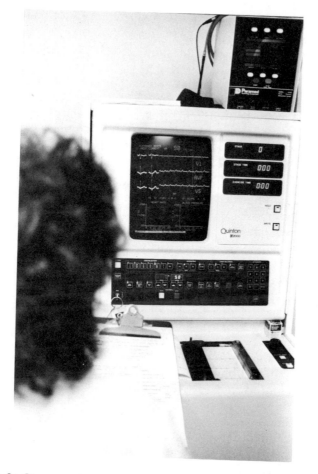

Figure 6: Close-up view at monitor-recording system for exercise testing. Screen (upper left) displays continuous two lead ECG recording for rate and rhythm. Heart rate and blood pressure (recorded and entered every 3 minutes) are displayed on lower left screen. Upper right display includes time in minutes of test duration and stage of test.

or bicycle ergometer, with continuous electrocardiographic monitoring and periodic evaluation of blood pressure and heart rate (Figs. 5, 6).

3. Measurement of oxygen consumption, metabolic functions, and pulmonary capacity and efficiency (Figure 5, 6).

4. Assessment of body composition as measured by percent

body fat, lean body weight, ideal weight, and, if necessary, projected weight loss (Figs. 7A, B).

5. Blood samples for cholesterol and HDL-cholesterol levels (Figs. 8A, B, C).
6. Assessment of flexibility and muscular strength (Figs. 9A, B).
7. Prescribed nutritional intervention for excess weight, elevated cholesterol level, and high blood pressure.
8. Evaluation of personality profile for Type A (coronary-prone behavior pattern) or Type B.

A physician, nurse, exercise specialist, and exercise technologist supervise Phase II and Phase III cardiac rehabilitation programs. A therapeutic dietitian is available for patients with need for dietary changes for total calorie, sodium, or fat control.

All cardiac classes begin with group stretching and flexibility exercises (Fig. 10). Participants then follow their individual prescription with activities that may include calisthenics, walking, jogging, bicycling, arm ergometry, rowing, and swimming (Figs. 11A-D). Modern exercise equipment is provided by EHEP. Volleyball games are also available for recreation, and 60 minutes of pool activity may be substituted for endurance activity. Exercise classes meet Monday, Wednesday, and Friday. In addition to these programs, patients may exercise at home while being monitored by means of a telephone ECG (electrocardiogram) hook-up.

Exercise retesting is performed regularly, based on each patient's condition and progress in the exercise program. EHEP regularly communicates with the patient's physician, and patients must see their physician for follow-up care on a regular basis.

Throughout the year, the staff of the Emory Health Enhancement Center and other Emory resource personnel will offer regular health-management programs with written handout materials. Topics may include nutrition, weight control, heart disease, CPR (cardiopulmonary resuscitation), exercise, preventive medicine, stress management, weight training, and smoking cessation.

Periodic screening for arrhythmias or ST segment depression during exercise is recommended. This can be done by telemetry as discussed or by using paddle electrodes on the defibrillator (Fig. 12). In one report from a large program, one of the best volleyball players was found to have significant ST segment depression by the former method. Another was found to have asymptomatic beats of ventricular tachycardia during walk/jog activity (Fig. 13).[50]

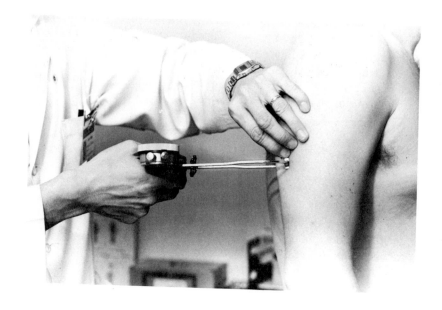

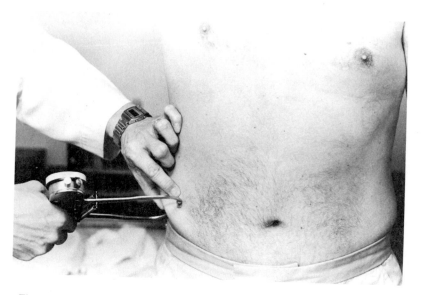

Figure 7A, B: Skin-fold measurement done by caliper technique. Measures are done at seven different sites (A—upper arm, B—abdomen shown here) to acquire data for calculation of body composition (fat) in percent.

To recapitulate, physical training is a promising new weapon in our armamentarium against coronary heart disease. The programming described herein can be modified so that it can be used in a major medical center complete with sophisticated testing devices or in a relatively small community hospital equipped with only an interested physician and patient.

RESULTS AND DATA ON OUTPATIENT
REHABILITATION PROGRAMS

A number of clinical studies from several countries emphasize the benefit of organized physical activity programs in patients with coronary heart disease and recent myocardial infarction. Although many of the known subjects with recent myocardial infarction are not incorporated into such programs, such management is becoming more popular among physicians as the feasibil-

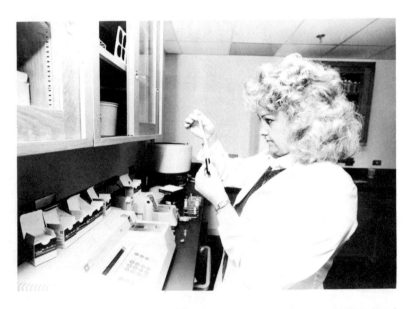

Figure 8A: View of EHEP lipid laboratory with centrifuge in background and lipid analyzer in left foreground. "Finger stick" blood sample is centrifuged and supernatant is removed as shown here. Small quantity is placed on specially prepared slide. (Slides are "prefixed" with reagent specifics for either cholesterol or high density lipoprotein [HDL] determination.) Continued.

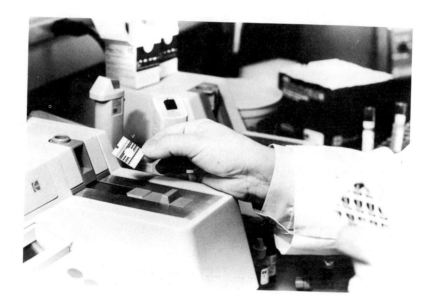

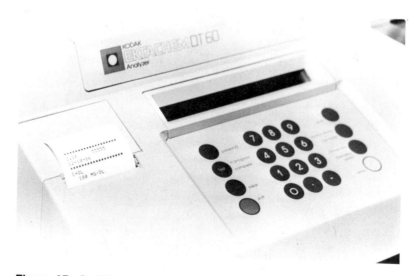

Figure 8B, C: Slide is inserted (B) into automated system and values in mgm/dl are quickly retrieved in (C) tabular format. (Cholesterol results are available in 15 minutes, HDL, 60 minutes.)

ment is becoming more popular among physicians as the feasibility and safety of these programs becomes more apparent and as more patients become motivated.

Several studies have been reported regarding the results of exercise training programs for subjects with coronary heart disease. One of the most revealing was reported by Bruce et al.[51] regarding their medically supervised program of physical training involving 30 to 60 minutes of graded levels of walk/jog and calisthenic activities three mornings per week. Of the 603 participants in this program, 230 men and 21 women remained active for 22 and 20 months, respectively; 352 (58.4%) dropped out after an average of 8.6 months for men and 5.7 months for women. Results revealed that elapsed time to morbidity tended to be longer in active persons than in dropouts. Over one-half of active men but

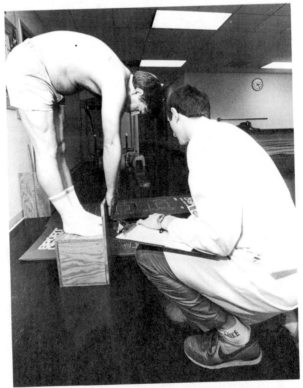

Figure 9A, B: Example of assessment of (A) flexibility by standing-flexion technique and (B) use of handgrip meter for testing strength.

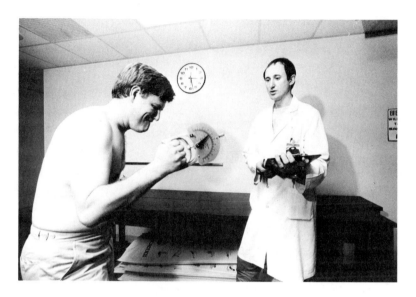

Figure 9B.

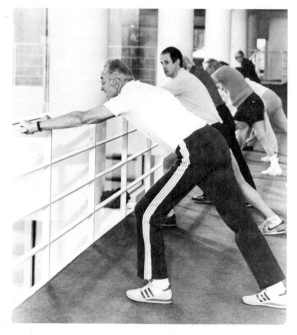

Figure 10: Technique of "stretching" prior to exercise.

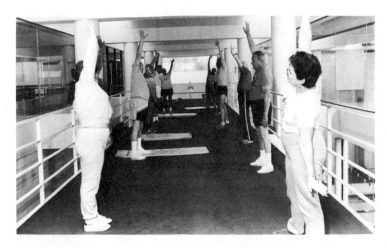

Figure 11A: Patient group doing calisthenics on balcony level of Physical Education Facility with indoor elevated track to left. Continued.

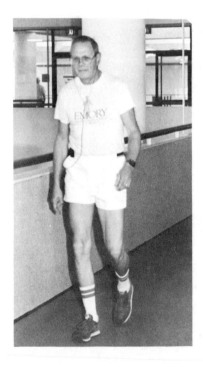

Figure 11B: Patient jogging on indoor track (eight laps on track equals 1 mile). Continued.

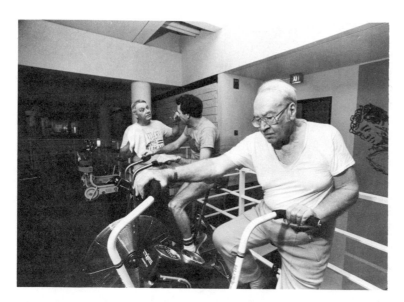

Figure 11C: Patients on stationary bicycle ergometer (arm-leg in foreground, standard leg in background). Continued.

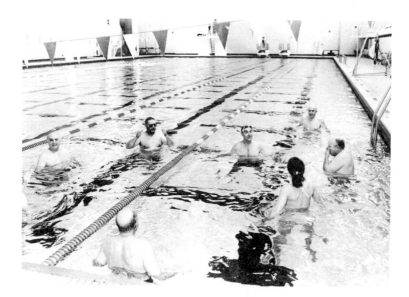

Figure 11D: Patients performing water calisthenics in four feet deep end of 50 mm indoor pool of Physical Education Facility.

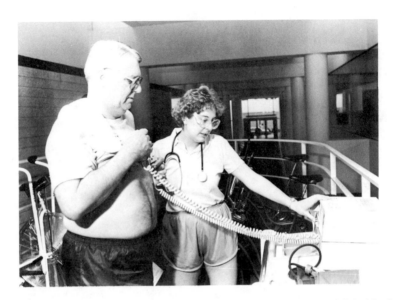

Figure 12: Technique of "instant" ECG recording. Patient to left holds defibrillator paddles for electrode leads on chest as nurse views rate and rhythm from screen and recorder of defibrillator system (lower right). Indoor track is to right.

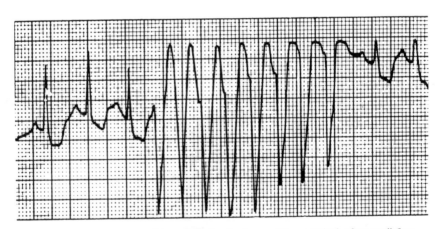

Figure 13: Asymptomatic ventricular tachycardia recorded after walk/jog activity in a post-myocardial-infarction patient participating in the medically supervised activity program. (From Cantwell JD, Fletcher GF. Instant electrocardiography—use in cardiac exercise programs. *Circulation* 1974; 50: 962–966. Used with the permission of the American Heart Association.)

only one-third of drop-outs were working. Among men, the respective total mortality rates were 2.6 and 4.9/100 person-years for active participants and drop-outs; among women, the rates were 0 and 3.8, respectively. Twenty-four episodes of cardiac arrest occurred in 13 men and three deaths outside the training program whereas in 11 instances of exertional arrests in supervised training, all defibrillations were successful (Figs. 14A, B). Therefore, the results of this follow-up study support both the benefits and the safety of medically supervised exercise training in post-infarction patients.

Data from other well-established programs have revealed various beneficial end-points.[52] Results in management of 230 patients in an Atlanta program were described in detail. Ninety-eight completed 6 months of training with an overall average of 70 percent attendance. Of these 98, 91 were male and seven were female. The ages ranged from 37 to 70 years, with a mean of 50.6

A

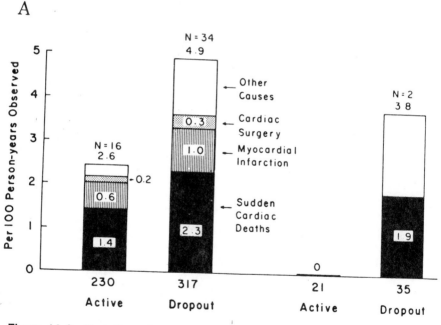

Figure 14 A: Mortality and morbidity rates among active participants and dropouts of the CAPRI cardiopulmonary rehabilitation programs. (From Bruce EH, et al. Comparison of active participants and dropouts in CAPRI cardiopulmonary rehabilitation programs. *Am J Cardiol* 1976;37:53. Used by permission.) Continued.

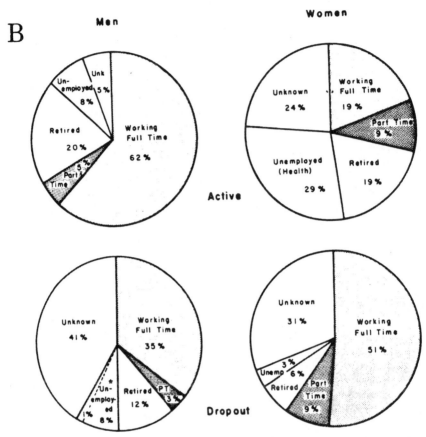

Figure 14 B: Current working status of active participants and dropouts of the programs. (From Ref. 51, with permission.)

years. Forty-one subjects had anterior myocardial infarction by ECG, 50 inferior, and seven had subendocardial infarction. Thirteen additional patients dropped out of the program prior to 3 months but cooperated in returning for follow-up studies.

Data were calculated on the 98 patients who completed 6 or more months of the training program as well as on the 13 who dropped out. All exercise testing data were recorded for the same heart rate end-point. There was an increase in mean exercise oxygen consumption in ml/kg/min from 15.6 (initial) to 18.4 at 3-month testing ($p < 0.01$) from 16.7 at 3 months to 19.5 minutes at 6-month testing ($p < 0.01$). These data are seen in Figure 15.

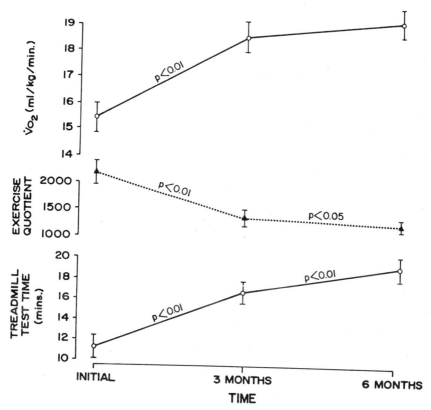

Figure 15: Graph showing changes in mean oxygen consumption, exercise quotient and treadmill test time in trained subjects from the initial to the three and six months' testing. (From Fletcher GF, Cantwell JD. Outpatient gym exercise and risk factor modification for patients with recent myocardial infarction: Methodology and results in a community program. *The Journal of the Louisiana State University Medical Society* 1975; 127:52–57. Used by permission.)

The mean resting systolic blood pressure of the study group decreased from 129.0 mmHg (initially) to 119.9 at 3 months ($p < 0.01$) but rose slightly from 119.9 at 3 months to 123.2 at 6 months. The mean peak exercise systolic blood pressure decreased from 156.9 mmHg initially to 147.9 at 3-month testing ($0 < 0.05$) and subsequently increased slightly from 147.9 (3 months) to 154.8 at 6 months. The mean diastolic blood pressure at rest decreased from 85.6 mmHg (initially) to 81.7 at 3 months ($p < 0.05$) and from that point to 81.5 at 6 months. The exercise diastolic pressure decreased from 84.4 mmHg (initially) to 79.1 at 3 months (p < 0.05) but remained the same at 6 months.

The mean resting heart rate in beats per minute decreased from 78.6 (initially) to 74.8 at 3 months (p < 0.05) and then to 74.3 at 6 months. Exercise and post-exercise testing heart rate did not change significantly during the 6-month training period.

With regard to other studies, there was essentially no change in the mean body weight, serum cholesterol, and uric acid. However, the mean serum triglycerides decreased from 214.4. mg/dl initially to 181.23 mg/dl at 3-month testing and subsequently to 169.0 mg/dl at 6 months (Fig. 16). There was a significant change in triglyceride levels from initial to 3 months (p < 0.05) and from initial to 6 months (p < 0.01). Of 81 cigarette smokers, 68 percent

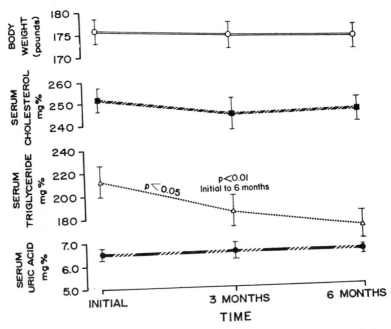

Figure 16: Graph showing changes in the mean body weight, serum cholesterol, triglycerides and uric acid in trained subjects from the initial to the three and six months testing. (From Fletcher GF, Cantwell JD. Outpatient gym exercise and risk factor modification for patients with recent myocardial infarction: Methodology and results in a community program. *Journal of the Louisiana State University Medical Society* 1975; 127:52–57. Used by permission.)

(55 of 81) stopped from initial to 6-month testing. There were no deaths and no recurrent infarctions, and 95 percent (93 of 98) of the group were gainfully employed.

Of 13 patients who dropped out of the program within the first 3 weeks, treadmill test times increased significantly on retesting 3 months after the baseline study—a mean of 11.3 minutes to 15.8 minutes ($p < 0.05$). However, the oxygen consumption did not change significantly, nor were there significant changes in triglyceride, cholesterol, and exercise pressure rate products. In addition, only 54 percent were gainfully employed. Reasons for dropping out included work conflicts in seven, unrelated medical problems in three, and lack of interest in three.

One of the most notable and significant results of this follow-up study is the gainful employment (95 percent) and improvement in oxygen consumption in the trained group. These data reflect that the most impressive training effect seems to be in the first 3 months. A similar trend is seen with the treadmill test time. These latter data show a significant change both at 3 and at 6 months, with the greatest change in mean values occurring in the first 3-month period of training. The value, perhaps, of the effectiveness of training being seen as early as 3 months is that some patients may need only this 3-month period of supervised training in order to obtain the desired level of long-term and safe exercise prescription. Therefore, earlier "graduation" from the program to an unsupervised home or community program would be both feasible and safe for selected patients. A more rapid turnover of such patients would make facilities more available for others as these programs become popular.

DIETARY INTERVENTIONS

In order to further assess the effect of multifactoral risk intervention in outpatient exercise, a subset of 60 post-infarction patients were evaluated in the early 1970s with regard to the effect of dietary control and exercise training on daily food intake and serum lipids.[53]

From a total of 60 volunteers, patients were randomized by standard random number technique into two groups. Group I (no diet control, n = 30, mean 49.2 years, mean 179.24 + 4.7 lb) underwent exercise training without dietary control; Group II (diet control, n = 30, mean 51.1 years, mean 171.21 ± 3.2 lb) combined exercise training with dietary control by individual counseling with a therapeutic dietitian.

Sources of dietary composition and related nutritional information were recorded initially and at 12 weeks by a registered dietitian from documentation of food type and source by personal interview. These data were obtained following randomization using a 3-day dietary record, recall interview, and standard reference tables. No dietary alterations were suggested in Group I. An individualized diet was prescribed for patients in Group II. The diet prescription was based on lipid phenotyping and individual caloric requirements. Six patients followed a combination fat- and caloric-controlled diet, and four patients followed a regular fat-controlled diet with no caloric restriction. Two patients had a type IIb lipid pattern indicative of elevations both in serum cholesterol and triglycerides. Eighteen patients were phenotyped as type IV. (The type IIb diet strictly limits dietary cholesterol, while in type IV diets, the cholesterol intake is only moderately restricted. Both types limit carbohydrate intake.) Caloric requirements were determined by the degree of physical activity and the patients' needs to either reduce or maintain an ideal body weight. Fasting (12-hour) blood samples were obtained prior to exercise participation initially and at the end of the study. Total cholesterol and triglycerides were determined by standard methods. None of the subjects studied were taking lipid-reducing medications. Body weight was obtained during similar conditions at the beginning and end of the experimental period. An uncorrelated t test was used to determine significant differences between group means.

Both groups showed reductions ($p \leq 0.01$) in mean total daily kilocalories consumed (2,867 ± 82 vs. 2,088 ± 77 and 2,848 ± 15 vs. 1,285 ± 68, respectively); however, no significant change occurred in total body weight. The dietary control group consumed relatively more kilocalories as protein than the group without dietary control (285 of 1,285 vs. 389 of 2,088, respectively) and less ($p \leq 0.05$) as fat (443 of 1,285 vs. 804 of 2,089, respectively). Both groups had lower ($p \leq 0.01$) mean daily dietary cholesterol after 12 weeks (811 ± 44 versus 232 ± 17 mg) versus (325 ± 18 versus 309 ± 23 mg, respectively). A reduction in serum cholesterol ($p \leq 0.05$) was seen in the dietary control group (270 ± 8 vs. 243 ± 7 mg/dl) but not in the group without dietary control (260 ± 6 vs. 261 ± 7 mg/dl). The dietary control group had a lower mean triglyceride level ($p \leq 0.05$) (229 ± 24 vs 155 ± 18 mg/dl) but no differences were seen in the group without dietary control (189 ± 15 vs. 180 ± 13 mg/dl).

It was concluded that significant reductions in caloric intake and daily dietary cholesterol complement the effects of exercise training in post-myocardial infarction patients by increasing substrate protein and fat consumption ratio and by reducing serum cholesterol and triglycerides. These effects are not seen with exercise training alone.

Recent studies of exercise training of moderate intensity in raising high density lipoprotein cholesterol has been reported by Vetrovec et al.[54] They studied low intensity exercise versus moderate intensity exercise in two groups of patients. In the moderate group, the mean high density lipoprotein cholesterol (HDLC) rose from 48.8 before training to 57.5 mg/dl after training; whereas, in the low intensity group, there was essentially no change from 47.6 to 46.7 mg/dl. They therefore concluded that HDLC increased after exercise training, provided that there is moderate intensity of exercise. Vyden et al.[55] studied physical conditioning on serum lipids in patients with type IV hyperlipoproteinemia and ischemic heart disease. Data showed that in such patients with an increase in mean exercise tolerance, there is an associated improvement with a mean decrease in serum triglycerides.

LONG-TERM AMBULATORY ECG RECORDING

Other techniques of *patient monitoring* have been utilized in the evaluation of the patients in exercise programs. In order to evaluate cardiac rate and rhythm in 20 patients, continuous ambulatory electrocardiographic recording was performed during a typical exercise training class and the subsequent 24 hours, which included activities at work and home.[56] Sixty-five percent (13) of the 20 patients had abnormal findings on recordings. Of the 20 patients studied, 40 percent (eight) had arrhythmias detected by ambulatory recording that had not been detected by resting or exercise electrocardiograms (Fig. 17). Three patients with ventricular ectopy (multiform premature ventricular beats, couplets, and bigeminy) had exercise activities temporarily curtailed and therapy with antiarrhythmic drugs begun, with subsequent resolution or improvement. Two other patients (with recorded heart rates of 160 beats per minute) were instructed to carefully monitor their heart rate in order not to exceed the target maximum. It was felt that 24-hour continuous electrocardiographic monitoring is beneficial in evaluating patients in cardiac exercise programs and

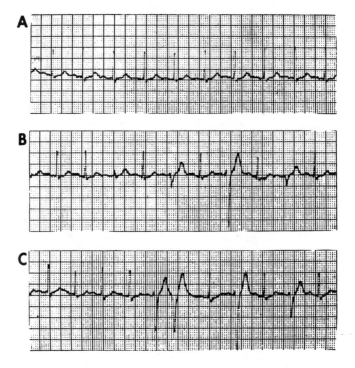

Figure 17: Home recordings (patient I). A (upper), Sinus tachycardia of 106 beats per minute just prior to coitus. B (center), Subsequent sinus tachycardia of 118 beats per minutes with period of ventricular bigeminy. C (lower), Ensuing sinus tachycardia of 118 beats per minute with ventricular bigeminy and couplets (both B and C were recorded during coitus). (From Fletcher GF, Cantwell JD. Continuous ambulatory electrocardiographic monitoring—use in cardiac exercise programs. *Chest* 1977;71:27–32. Used by permission.)

frequently influences management of such patients. Recent data in Holter recording have been presented by Plantholt et al.[57] This data was collected in evaluating patient performance in a prescribed exercise program in a coronary heart disease population. The results showed that only seven of 21 (33%) of patients accurately followed the exercise program prescription. There were complex ventricular arrhythmias in four of 21 (19%), and 14 of 21 (67%) patients required further instruction on self-monitoring after the Holter recording. It is concluded that a Holter recording obtained on patients participating in a self-monitored exercise program provided valuable evidence for guiding exercise therapy. Lillis et al.[58] evaluated ECG monitoring in cardiac rehabilitation patients on exercise training and control days. This was done by

Holter recording in 18 coronary artery disease patients. They found that ventricular ectopic activity occurred with a similar frequency during exercise training or corresponding nontraining periods. However, high risk patients had significantly greater ventricular ectopic activity during all activities and showed additional increases in ectopy during activities of daily living, such as eating and driving, on exercise days.

OXYGEN CONSUMPTION STUDIES OF VARIOUS ACTIVITIES

Current interest in exercise physiology and its application to both preventive and post-coronary rehabilitation has resulted in the use of varied exercise activities during post-coronary management. Several studies have reported activity protocols and it appears that the oxygen consumption of activities considered "low level" for the "normal" healthy subject may be significantly more physically demanding when performed by the post-myocardial infarction patients.[59] Therefore, a study was done to quantitatively assess the oxygen consumption and hemodynamic response of uncomplicated post-myocardial infarction patients during routine standardized exercise regimens used in outpatient cardiac rehabilitation.[60]

Twenty-two untrained, uncomplicated (no heart failure or refractory arrhythmias) post-myocardial infarction patients (mean age 51.3 years; mean weight 81.5 kg) were investigated. Patients had not eaten for at least 3 hours before testing, and had abstained from all physical work other than that required for their daily personal needs for 24 hours before testing. All were at least 12 weeks post-infarction. Initial baseline metabolic and hemodynamic data were obtained after the patient had rested in the supine position for 10 minutes. Resting oxygen consumption was done using the Douglas bag technique and standard equations. Immediately thereafter (within 5 seconds), with the patient still supine, blood pressure by cuff sphygmomanometer and resting heart rate were recorded. After each calisthenic activity was demonstrated, the patients completed 15 repetitions of each of 13 calisthenics (Table 3). The 15 repetitions required a mean of 25.0 seconds for the untrained and 23.53 seconds for the trained subjects (Table 4). After the 15th repetition, there was an immediate "breath-by-breath" analysis (all expired air collected for a total of

Table 3
Oxygen Consumption and Hemodynamic Response of Various Calisthenics Used to Train Patients with Recent Myocardial Infarction[60]

	$\dot{V}O_2$ (ml/kg/min)		METs (3.5 ml/O_2/kg/min)		SBP (mmHg)		DBP (mmHg)		HR (beats/min)		O_2 pulse	
	UT	T	UT	T	UT	T	UT	T	UT	T	UT	T
Toe touch	4.8	8.5	1.4	2.4	135	141	83	70	94	81	5.2	10.5
Lateral bend	5.4	6.3	1.5	1.8	142	138	84	75	91	79	5.9	8.1
Arm circling	5.6	8.6	1.6	2.5	133	134	83	74	82	75	6.8	11.5
Small jumps	11.2	13.1	3.2	3.7	133	132	79	69	91	80	12.4	16.4
Bent leg raise (ALT)	7.7	11.1	2.2	3.2	133	133	82	73	89	81	8.7	13.8
Double bent leg raise	14.8	12.5	4.2	3.6	144	142	81	74	88	84	16.8	14.8
Rocking sit-up	12.2	13.7	3.5	3.9	143	140	83	78	93	83	13.1	16.5
Leg crossover	12.9	12.1	3.7	3.4	142	145	84	82	96	73	13.4	16.5
Side leg raise	13.4	12.5	3.8	3.6	142	137	85	72	89	79	15.1	15.8
Knee push-up	12.6	14.5	3.6	4.1	146	140	85	76	95	81	13.2	17.9
Trunk twisting	7.1	14.7	2.0	4.2	145	143	85	76	100	82	7.1	17.9
Reverse push-ups	7.5	12.5	2.1	3.6	147	142	85	71	97	76	7.7	16.5
Reach and touch	6.9	11.4	1.9	3.3	144	143	85	74	96	84	7.2	13.6
Mean of means	9.3	11.7	2.7	3.3	141	139	83	79	92	80	10.2	14.6
SD	3.5	2.5	1.0	0.7	5.2	4.1	1.9	3.5	4.7	3.2	3.9	2.9
SEM	0.9	0.7	0.3	0.2	1.4	1.2	0.5	0.9	1.3	0.9	1.1	0.8

All values are means.
Abbreviations: UT = untrained; T = trained; $\dot{V}O_2$ = oxygen consumption; METs = metabolic equivalents; DBP = diastolic blood pressure; SBP = systolic blood pressure; HR = heart rate; O_2 pulse = milliliters of oxygen per heart beat; ALT = alternating.

Table 4
Comparative Data on Selected Activities Used in Training[60]

Activity	Untrained	Trained	Significance
Walk/jog (5 minutes) (mean ± SD)	36.69 ± 5.31 sec/lap*	34.3 ± 2.7 /lap	NS
Distance covered	0.454 mile	0.485 mile	
Calisthenics (time to complete each of 13 sequences) (mean ± SD)	25 ± 3.5 seconds	23.53 ± 5.4 seconds	NS
Swimming (100 feet) (mean ± SD)	85.04 ± 9.47 seconds	82.17 ± 6.84 seconds	NS
Velocity	1.17 feet/sec	1.22 feet/sec	

One lap equals 293.3 feet.
*Eighteen laps or 1 mile.

15 seconds) using a Collins two-way J valve with resistance pressure drop across valve ≤ 0.5 cm/50 L/min. The same activity was repeated on a separate day using the continuous Max Planck respirometer technique for a 5-minute collection during the activity (Fig. 18). Gas analyses were performed using Beckman automatic gas analyzers (OM-11 for oxygen and LB-2 for carbon dioxide at a constant flow rate of 3.5 ml $\times$ 100/min). Four pretrial

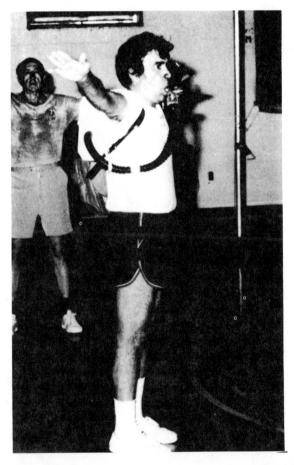

Figure 18: Patient performing calisthenic activity while wearing Max Planck respirometer. This technique allows continuous monitoring of total expired gas volume during exercise. Representative gas samples are continuously collected by means of a two-way stopcock valve system (0.6%/ Lexpired air) for analysis of oxygen and carbon dioxide contents.

calibrations were performed comparing total ventilation of expired air at ambient temperature pressure saturated (VE ATPS) by the Douglas bag technique with total VE ATPS by the Max Planck respirometer technique. The variant was ± 1.4 percent over a ventilation range of 14–70 L/min. Standard reference calibrations were done before and after each measurement using known reference gases. Blood pressures and heart rates were obtained as previously described. Patients rested (supine) for 5 to 10 minutes after each of the 13 calisthenics activities to allow for a return to baseline ± 2 percent before proceeding with the next calisthenic activity.

Patients walk/jogged 5–7 mph (mean 5.61 mph for 5 minutes), played volleyball (20-minute games), and swam (100 feet freestyle, mean time of 85 seconds in a pool heated to 30° ± 1°C) on separate days in the hospital gymnasium complex (Table 5). Exercise dance routines (Pelican, Evil Ways and Nite Owl) were introduced later in the study; consequently, those data reflect trained subjects only. With the exception of swimming, resting and exercise oxygen consumption was obtained using the identical technique previously described for calisthenics. Swimming data were derived only by the Douglas bag technique described previously. The Max Planck respirometer technique was not used to obtain oxygen consumption for the swimming for reasons of safety and technical impracticality.

At the end of 12 weeks (36 similar, medically supervised, 45-minute exercise sessions; average attendance 85 percent), the patients repeated the tests to reassess oxygen consumption and hemodynamic response after the exercise training period. A non-correlated t test was used to determine significant differences between the trained and untrained performances as well as for the two methods of oxygen consumption data collection.

The physiological data for the various activities are listed in detail in Tables 5 and 6. There were no significant differences between the two methods of determining oxygen consumption (Max Planck vs. Douglas bag technique). In all instances, oxygen consumption increased after the 12-week exercise training regimen. Oxygen consumption was highest for swimming—30.10 ml/kg/min for trained (T) vs. 22.58 ml/kg/min untrained (UT); the oxygen pulse for swimming was 16.64 ml/0_2 (T) vs. 12.05 ml/0_2 (UT), and the rate-pressure product was 21,000(T) vs. 25,991 (UT). Walk/jogging (5–7 mph) required an oxygen consumption of 23.77 ml/kg/min (T) vs. 15.83 ml/kg/min (UT); the oxygen pulse for

Table 5
Comparative Oxygen Consumption and Hemodynamic Response of Swimming, Walk/jog, Exercise Dancing, Volleyball and Calisthenics Used in Postmyocardial Infarction Exercise Training[60]

Activity	Group	Oxygen consumption (ml/kg/min)	Metabolic equivalents (3.5 ml/O_2/kg/min)	Peak oxygen pulse (ml/O_2/beat)	Rate-pressure product	Peak heart rate (beats/min)
Freestyle swimming (100 feet)	Trained	30.10 ± 2.2	8.6 ± 1.84	16.64 ± 4.84†	21,000 ± 1129†	140 ± 11.12†
	Untrained	22.58 ± 4.72	6.5 ± 1.3	12.05 ± 2.47	25,991 ± 1350	152 ± 8.37
Walk/jog (5–7 mph)	Trained	23.77 ± 6.53†	6.8 ± 1.9†	14.39 ± 3.67†	19,834 ± 1800†	134 ± 12.4†
	Untrained	15.83 ± 3.10	4.5 ± 0.8	8.8 ± 4.42	21,462 ± 990	147 ± 8.9
Exercise dancing	Trained	21.07 ± 3.40	6.02	14.07 ± 4.08	17,300 ± 187	122 ± 8.77
Volleyball (20-minute game)	Trained	12.83 ± 1.45†	3.6 ± 0.4†	11.57 ± 2.01†	11,250 ± 560†	90 ± 6.9*
	Untrained	9.87 ± 1.83	2.8 ± 0.5	8.42 ± 2.43	12,350 ± 8.10	95 ± 8.8
Sum of 13 calisthenics (mean of means)	Trained	11.70 ± 2.47	3.3 ± 0.7	14.59 ± 2.99†	11,120 ± 147†	80.0 ± 3.2†
	Untrained	9.39 ± 3.51	2.7 ± 1.0	10.2 ± 3.89	12,972 ± 240	92.0 ± 4.7

Values are mean ± SD.
*$p \leq 0.05$ (trained vs untrained).
†$p \leq 0.01$ (trained vs untrained).

Table 6
Reported Oxygen Consumption for Normals and Postmyocardial Infarction Patients[60]

Activity	Normals*				Postinfarction†			
	$\dot{V}O_2$ (ml/kg/min)		METs (3.5ml/O_2/kg/min)		$\dot{V}O_2$ (ml/kg/min)		METs (3.5ml/O_2/kg/min)	
	UT	T	UT	T	UT	T	UT	T
Swimming (100 feet freestyle)	19.95	38.0	5.7	10.8	22.58	10.10	6.4	8.2
Walk/jog (5–7 mph)	17.5	40.5	5.0	11.6	15.83	23.77	4.5	6.8
Volleyball (20 minute game)	8.0	14.0	2.3	4.0	9.87	12.83	2.8	3.6
Sum of means of 13 calisthenics	7.3	13.5	2.1	3.8	9.39	11.70	2.7	3.3
Exercise dancing						21.07		6.0

*Comparative data were compiled from proceedings of the International Symposium of Physical Activity and Cardiovascular Health: *Can Med Assoc J* 96: 910, 1967; *Energy, Work and Leisure*, London, Heineman, 1970; *JR Army Med Corp* 61, July 1933; *Textbook of Work Physiology*, New York, McGraw-Hill, 1970.

†Oxygen consumption variability when compared with normals may be due to differences in intensity of performance.

Abbreviations: UT = untrained; T = trained; METs = metabolic equivalents.

walk/jog was 14.39 ml/O_2 (T) vs. 8.8 ml/O_2 (UT), with a rate-pressure product of 19,834 (T) vs. 21462 (UT). Exercise dancing (trained only) required an oxygen consumption of 21.07 ± 3.4 ml/kg/min; the oxygen pulse was 14.07 ml/O_2 and the rate-pressure product was 17,300 ± 187. Volleyball required an oxygen consumption of 12.83 ml/kg/min (T) vs. 9.87 ml/kg/min (UT); the oxygen pulse for volleyball was 11.57 ml/O_2 (T) vs. 8.42 ml/O_2 (UT), and the rate-pressure product was 11,250 (T) vs. 12,350 (UT). The mean oxygen consumption for all 13 calisthenics was 11.7 ml/kg/min (T) vs. 9.39 ml/kg/min (UT); the oxygen pulse for these activities was 10.2 ml/O_2 (T) vs. 14.59 ml/O_2 (UT) and the rate-pressure product was 11,120 (T) vs. 12,972 (UT).

Total body weight decreased from 81.5 ± 1.14 kg to 78.82 ± 1.8 kg with training, but not significantly. The amount of work performed by the patients before and after training was essentially the same. No symptom other than fatigue and no clinically apparent dysrhythmias were noted in any patients during the oxygen consumption studies.

The oxygen consumption of the various activities for exercising cardiac patients varies—swimming required the highest and volleyball the lowest. The calisthenics (Table 3) showed considerable variability—oxygen consumption was greatest during trunk twisting and least during lateral bending. In most instances, the trained group had the highest mean oxygen consumption, while the mean rate-pressure products were less. Although the sample of patients is relatively small, it was sufficient to obtain a reliable index of oxygen consumption for the individual activities because of both the extensive number of tests and methods used. The increased oxygen consumption with associated decrease in mean rate-pressure products reflects greater oxygen delivery and extraction at the cellular level. As this change occurred at submaximal work levels in these subjects, it was felt that aerobic pathways of metabolism are being used more extensively, thus delaying the significant dominance of anaerobic pathways that is characteristic of maximum work loads.

In all instances, oxygen consumption varied considerably for the same calisthenics when performed by the same patients after the 12-week conditioning program. This was expected, for the individual effort during low-level calisthenics undoubtedly varies, regardless of exercise training effect. Patients were instructed to perform the activities at similar levels of intensity and skill, and by general assessment appeared to do so (Table 4). The higher oxygen-pulse values in the trained subjects, along with the other hemodynamic responses (Table 5), support the view that exercise training effects are favorable when performing the activities.

The greater oxygen consumption and hemodynamic response attributed to swimming versus walk/jogging confirms that swimming can be an integral part of a cardiac conditioning program. However, because of the high energy demands it places on the cardiopulmonary system, swimming should be carefully prescribed and monitored in cardiac patients who do not swim routinely. Similar observations of training specificity have been noted comparing peak attained oxygen consumption and heart rates in patients performing leg versus arm ergometry.[61] Few of the post-infarction patients preferred swimming to walk/jogging; consequently, training specificity may have influenced the higher oxygen values observed. Other studies have shown that compared with walk/jogging, swimming in either the prone or supine position can result in initial differences in heart rate, blood pressure, and stroke volume that are further complicated by the effects of immersion.[62] Immersion in warm water (35−37°C) causes an increased heart rate and subsequent increased and extensive vasodilation, while a decrease in heart rate has been associated with immersion in water of an average swimming pool (temperatures 27−32°C). Furthermore, with the physiologic response to immersion in cold water (15−20°C) or warm water (35−37°C), careful observation of pool temperatures is necessary. A water temperature of 30° ± 1°C is satisfactory for post-infarction swimming based on experience herein described. Although few well-controlled studies on swimming have been undertaken with post-coronary subjects, the literature on the physiology of swimming in normal patients is extensive.[63,64] Although not comparable to data from our cardiac patients, data in normals indicate that maximum oxygen consumption in swimming is approximately 15 percent lower than that in cycling, jogging, and skiing (Table 6); however, swimming velocity, stroke, and speed were not reported. These data are in contrast to reports for normal subjects, as our subjects had a notably greater oxygen consumption for swimming than for walk/jogging. Of 22 subjects studied in the pool, 19 chose breast stroke, one side stroke, and two the crawl. Swimming speeds ≤ 2 feet/sec may be considered vigorous, but not competitive.[64] Breast stroke at speeds ≤ 2 feet/sec is generally considered less demanding and, therefore, more appropriate for the post-coronary patient. Using time as the criterion for estimating the speed of the swimmers for 100 feet—mean time 85.04 seconds or 1.17 feet/sec (UT) vs. mean time 82.17 seconds or 1.22 feet/sec (T)—

swimming at these speeds was considered less strenuous and, therefore, acceptable as a conditioning exercise for the post-coronary patient, if carefully monitored.

The calisthenics data are generally in agreement with the classic work of Kennedy, which showed less oxygen consumption during calisthenics than during other activities. The low oxygen consumption and hemodynamic response attributed to volleyball and certain "low level" calisthenics, in both normals and post-infarction patients, poses the question of including those activities in an outpatient exercise program. However, based on previous work supporting the thesis that 20–30 minutes of walk/jogging two to three times weekly can maintain a training effect in patients, it is felt that higher work loads are not necessary for these latter activities, providing the walk/jog/swimming prescription is maintained. The calisthenics routine emphasizes stretching and flexibility, which may help reduce musculoskeletal complications of the walk/jog sequence. Most of the patients enjoy the camaraderie of volleyball, and it is felt this helps to maintain compliance ($\geq$ 75%) over a long-term period.

To vary exercise training programs, the study investigated exercise dancing. The patients appeared to enjoy exercise dancing, which requires a considerable degree of coordination. The oxygen demands of exercise dancing are not too severe for patients without heart failure or refractory arrhythmias. Exercise dancing was slightly less demanding than walk/jogging.

This study documents oxygen consumption by post-infarction patients during exercise in actual gymnasium conditions and confirms the variability in oxygen consumption and heart rate–blood pressure response to various activities in such training programs. In addition, the training effect (12 weeks) of increased oxygen consumption and lower heart rate–blood pressure product (T vs. UT) is apparent in all activities. The data further substantiate the probably beneficial effect of volleyball, calisthenics, and especially walk/jogging, exercise dancing, and swimming in increasing oxygen consumption and decreasing heart rate–systolic blood pressure product in post-myocardial infarction patients.

EVALUATION OF SEXUAL ACTIVITIES

In order to evaluate the effects of exercise training on sexual habits in the post-myocardial infarction and post-revascularization state, questionnaires were mailed to 130 patients enrolled in an outpatient exercise program. Of 87 (67%) responding, 68 were post-myocardial infarction and 19 had undergone myocardial revascularization. The post-infarction group significantly decreased their coital frequency after infarction by 28 percent; the revascularization group, however, decreased by only 10 percent. The myocardial infarction group waited 9.4 weeks after infarction to resume sexual intercourse, while the revascularization group waited only a mean of 5.7 weeks. These data suggest that physically trained post-myocardial infarction patients decrease frequency of coitus significantly more than physically trained patients with myocardial revascularization. The overall decrease, however, is notably less than reported in nontrained post-myocardial infarction patients and therefore supports the possible "bedroom benefit" of medically supervised exercise both in post-infarction and in post-revascularization patients.[65]

The aforementioned study has been one of a number relating to this area. Various authors[29,56,66-68] have related pertinent data regarding sexual activity in the cardiac patient; however, overall information and clinical research leading to definitive conclusions remains limited. The classification of coitus as benign in the cardiac patient has recently been questioned as a result of ambulatory monitoring in a physically conditioned post-myocardial infarction patient. This particular subject was active in a medically supervised exercise program. He had ventricular ectopy identified during coitus on a 24-hour dynamic electrocardiographic recording and subsequently experienced reversible ventricular fibrillation while participating in the medically supervised program.[56] To extend the data collection in both post-myocardial infarction and post-myocardial revascularization patients, a study on sexual activity was done with dynamic ECG recordings (Holter).[69] The group of subjects involved were not in a regular exercise training program but had been involved in an inpatient rehabilitation program post event.

They were requested to return to the hospital for follow-up evaluation approximately 2 weeks after hospital discharge. All patients were asked if they were currently engaging in sexual activity. Those responding positively were submitted to a 24-hour dynamic electrocardiographic recording and were asked to participate in sexual activity during the 24-hour period of recording. The recorder was returned to the hospital on the following day. The tape was scanned utilizing an Avionics 660A Dynamic Electrocardioscanner and was referred to two cardiologists for final interpretation. In addition, 40 consecutive minutes of "real time" were recorded to include equal periods of time before and after sexual activity. This 40-minute strip was then analyzed for heart rate and dysrhythmias. The heart rate was calculated every minute utilizing a "heart rate ruler" for consistent accuracy.

The patient population was composed of nine post-myocardial infarction and 15 post-myocardial revascularization patients. Although these are not comparable groups, the data are considered together since both have the same underlying disease process, i.e., coronary atherosclerosis. The nine post-myocardial infarction patients were all males with an age range of 37 to 66 ($\bar{x}$ 50.8) years. The infarction localization included five inferior, three anterior, and one subendocardial. The myocardial revascularization patients consisted of 12 males and three females with an age range of 39 to 57 ($\bar{x}$ 48.4) years. In all cases the indication for surgery was angina pectoris which could not be well-controlled by medical therapy. The number of aortocoronary grafts per patient ranged from one to five, with a mean of 3.2. Six of the myocardial revascularization group had previous myocardial infarctions and four of these occurred within 3 months prior to surgery. The operative course in all cases was uneventful and the postoperative recovery was uncomplicated. The time lapse from cardiac event to date of recording ranged from 21 to 38 days ($\bar{x}$ 30.1) in the post-myocardial infarction group and 20 to 38 days ($\bar{x}$ 31.5) in the myocardial revascularization group. This was the first sexual activity since cardiac event for 10 of the total 24 patients. None of the patients had associated diseases. Medications and other clinical data are itemized in Table 7.

Three of the nine post-myocardial infarction patients and nine of the 15 post-myocardial revascularization patients had dysrhythmias during sexual activity (12 of the total 24). Of the three myocardial infarction patients, one had occasional premature ventricular contractions (PVCs) ($\leq$ six isolated PVCs/minute) with sexual activity as well as throughout the 24-hour period. The second had rather constant ventricular bigeminy and ventricular coupling noted only during the 10-minute period of coitus (Fig. 19) and the third patient had an occasional premature atrial contraction (PAC) noted during coitus.

Of the nine myocardial revascularization patients having abnormalities recorded during sexual activity, five had occasional PVCs which were also noted at other times during the 24 hours. One of these five experienced sexual activity twice during the

24-hour period and with a different partner for each episode. The noon coitus was with his girlfriend, and a heart rate range of 96 to 150 BPM with PVCs was noted. During the evening coitus with his wife, normal sinus rhythm with a rate range of 72 to 92 BPM was recorded. Occasional PVCs were inscribed at other times during the recording. The remaining four of the nine myocardial revascularization patients with sexual activity abnormalities had these recorded either with sexual activity only, or more frequently with sexual activity (none of these four had infarction within 3 months prior to surgery). One had occasional PVCs, pairs of PVCs, and an episode of chaotic atrial tachycardia at a rate of 135 BPM during sexual activity. The PVCs, PACs, and paired ventricular extrasystoles were recorded at other times on the recording, but chaotic atrial tachycardia was recorded only with sexual activity. The other two myocardial revascularization patients had sexual activity twice within the 24-hour period. One of them demonstrated frequent PVCs in addition to two consecutive ventricular beats (probably reentry) during his evening coitus but no arrhythmias during his morning coitus. Only occasional PVCs were recorded during the remaining portion of the 24 hours. The other patient demonstrated an almost constant Wolff-Parkinson-White (WPW) pattern throughout sexual stimulation in both the morning and evening episodes, with only intermittent WPW during the other portion of the record (Fig. 20). This patient (a widow) utilized a mechanical vibrator for stimulation.

Of the total of 12 patients (50 percent) experiencing abnormalities during sexual activity (nine post-myocardial revascularization and three post-myocardial infarction), five (one myocardial infarction and four myocardial revascularization, a total of 20 percent) were considered to have more serious changes than the other seven myocardial revascularization and myocardial infarction patients demonstrating occasional PVCs or PACs. These more serious changes were defined as frequent PVCs (five PVCs in a 15-second period), paired PVCs, ventricular bigeminy, and a constant WPW pattern.

The data support, in part, those previously documented by Hellerstein and Friedman.[29] In the analysis of coitus in 14 post-coronary patients, they found a mean heart rate of 117.4 bpm with an average duration of intercourse of 16.3 minutes. This time interval was calculated between retiring to bed and attainment of maximal heart rate associated with coitus. Three of 14 subjects developed ectopic beats. Two of these had ventricular ectopy and

Table 7

Clinical Data on 24 Patients Having Dynamic Electrocardiographic Recording with Sexual Activity Either Post-Infarction or Post-Revascularization[69]

Pa-tient	Age (years)	Sex	Race	Infarction location	Drugs	Days MI to DER	HR with S.A. Rest	HR with S.A. Peak	Dysrhy. With S.A.	Sysrhy. at other times
Infarction Group										
1	46	M	W	Anterio	Glyceryl trinitrate	28	62	100	1 PVC	Same
2	49	M	W	Subendocardial	Procainamide, Propranolol	38	93	116	None	None
3	46	M	W	Infero-posterior	isosorbide dinitrate	34	84	90	None	Occ. PVC's
4	51	M	W	Inferior	Glyceryl trinitrate	36	86	150	None	Occ. PVC's PAC's
5	65	M	W	Antero-lateral	Glyceryl trinitrate, Warfarin sodium, Isosorbide dinitrate, Diazepam	30	68	90	None	Occ. PVC's
6	37	M	W	Infero-posterior	Chlordiazepoxide, Procainamide	21	58	86	None	Same
7	49	M	W	Infero-posterior	None	34	56	136	Vent. bigeminy, Vent. coupling, Frequent PVC's	Occ. PVC's
8	54	M	W	Inferior	Procainamide	24	82	102	Occ. PAC's	None
9	38	M	W	Antero-lateral	Insulin, Propranolol, Isosorbide dinitrate	26	72	100	None	None
Revascularization Group										
1	53	M	W	5	Aspirin	36	106	144	None	Occ. PVC's
2	46	M	W	3	Aspirin	31	100	120	One fusion beat	Occ. PVC's
3	43	M	W	4	Procainamide	31	82	122	Occ. PVC, PAC	Occ. PVC

No.	Age	Sex	Race	Episode	Medication				DER findings	
4	51	M	W	1	Aspirin, Lanoxin, hydrochlorothiazide	32	72	96	None	Occ. PVC's Vent. coup,
5	53	M	W	5		35	100	120	Occ. PVC's Chaotic atrial Tach. (135/min), Vent. couplet	Occ. PVC's
6	44	M	W	3	Percodan (Oxycodone)	29	(1)86 / (2)82	116 / 106	(1) Freq. PVC's Vent. couplet (2) None	Occ. PVC's
7	39	M	W	1	Aspirin	21	80	156	None	None
8	51	F	W	1	Flurazepam, Acetaminophen	31	78	92	None	None
9	53	F	W	1	Glyceryl trinitrate, Acetaminophen	32	(1)104 / (2)102	116 / 130	(1) WPW with vibrator (2) WPW with vibrator	Intermittent WPW
10	46	M	B	5(3/23/77) 3(9/22/77)	Aspirin	28	(G)96	150	(G) Occ. PVC's	Occ. PVC's
11	49	M	W	3	None	38	(W)72 / 95	92 / 140	(W) None Occ. PVC's	Occ. PVC's
12	50	M	W	5	Percodan (Oxycodone)	20	98	116	Occ. PVC's	Occ. PVC's
13	57	M	W	2	Aspirin, Lanoxin	36	100	100	None	Occ. PVC's
14	43	M	W	3	Quindine gluconate, Triampterene, hydrochlorothiazide	34	74	94	None	None
15	53	F	W	3	Acetaminophen, hydrochlorothiazide	38	96	110	Frequent PVC's	Occ. PVC's

Abbreviations: M = male; F = female; DER = dynamic electrocardiographic recording; HR = heart rate in beats per minute; PVC = premature ventricular contraction; Vent. = ventricular; PAC = premature atrial contraction; Occ. = occasional; Tach. = tachycardia; (G) = girlfriend; (W) = wife; WPW = Wolff-Parkinson-White pattern; (1) and (2) in patient No. 6 and 9 data = first (1) and second (2) sexual act of the 24-hour period; Dysrhy. = dysrhythmias; MI = myocardial infarction; S.A. = sexual activity; coup = couplet; Freq = frequent.

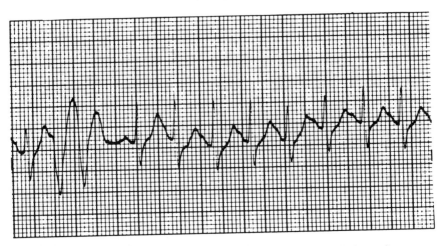

Figure 19: Example of paired ventricular ectopy occurring during coitus.

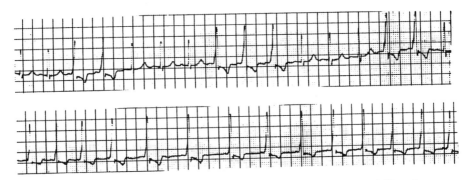

Figure 20: Comparison of dynamic ECG recording during daily activities of a patient while walking (top) with only intermittent Wolff-Parkinson-White pattern compared to a constant Wolff-Parkinson-White pattern (bottom) during sexual stimulation.

one had both atrial and ventricular ectopy. When comparing ECG response during coitus to other times during the day, they concluded that the cardiovascular response was similar during coitus and usual occupational activities. In comparison, the data reported herein described an average peak heart rate of 107.8 for myocardial infarction patients and 117.8 for myocardial revascularization patients, with a duration of sexual activity of 18.6 minutes (myocardial infarction) and 18.8 minutes (myocardial revascularization). In contrast to three of 14 subjects experiencing dysrhythmias with sexual activity in previous reports,[29] the data herein reveal that 12 of 24 patients developed abnormalities (three of nine myocardial infarction patients, and nine of 15 myocardial revascularization patients). When eliminating occasional PVCs and PACs, five of 24 patients (one myocardial infarction and four myocardial revascularization) had abnormalities either with sexual activity only or more frequently with sexual activity. These changes were not seen during other portions of the 24-hour recording when daily activities included such chores as bathing, shaving, dressing, cooking, putting groceries in the pantry, and other light housework or when exercise activities included one or two flights of "stair climbing" or walking less than one-half mile at a leisurely pace.

When considering the difference in yield of abnormalities with sexual activity between the data presented here and that reported elsewhere, one must consider the time of data collection in relation to the cardiac event. Hellerstein and Friedman's patients[29] were post-coronary patients already participating in an outpatient exercise program. The patients herein described, in contrast, were studied earlier, a mean time of 30.1 days post-myocardial infarction and 31.5 days post-myocardial revascularization.

Stein[70] has shown an increase in aerobic capacity and a reduction in peak coital heart rate from 127 bpm to 120 bpm in trained post-myocardial infarction patients. These patients had experienced a 16-week bicycle ergometer training program at 12 to 15 weeks following their first myocardial infarction. The author did not, however, discuss dysrhythmias.

The data herein presented relate a notable degree of cardiac electrical instability recorded with sexual activity in 12 of 24 patients (50 percent). Of the total of 12, five had abnormalities only with or notably more with sexual activity as compared to other times on the 24-hour record. More myocardial revascularization patients had abnormalities than myocardial infarction patients (0 of 15 vs. 3 of 9), and there was also a slightly higher peak heart rate in this group compared to the myocardial infarction group. Considering the number of higher grade dysrhythmias, there were no early fatalities in this group of 24 patients. However, there may be some cause for concern regarding the ultimate long-term prognosis, as data[74] suggest a higher incidence of sudden death associated with such degrees of ventricular ectopy.

Based on the data in this group of subjects, it is therefore felt that sexual activity in recent post-myocardial infarction and post-myocardial revascularization patients may be a stimulus for cardiac electrical instability. In accord with this, appropriate concern should be expressed in patient management and counseling, and consideration should be given to the use of antidysrhythmic drugs.

THE NATIONAL EXERCISE AND HEART DISEASE PROJECT

Regardless of the apparent benefit and safety of exercise programs for post-myocardial infarction patients, there is still a lack of controlled data to support this. In order to study all aspects of the question, the National Exercise and Heart Disease Project (NEHDP)[72] was initiated in 1972 as a multicenter study involving Emory University School of Medicine, Case Western Reserve University, University of Alabama, George Washington University, and Lankenaw Hospital. After a pre-randomization period of exercise, 651 post myocardial infarction patients were randomized into either an organized medically supervised exercise class (323) or to free activities at home (328).

Characteristics of the study population revealed that the patients were predominately married, white, middle class, educated, with good incomes, and average age of 52 years. More than half entered the study within one year of experiencing the myocardial infarction. Most patients (83 percent) had only one myocardial infarction, the qualifying one. The exercise test taken at the end of the pre-randomization exercise period as the final evaluation before entry to the study revealed that the candidates could perform quite well.

More than 81 percent were already back at work; therefore, only 103 were available to study the rehabilitation effects of the exercise program with respect to return to work. The percent already working did not seem to depend upon the "months elapsed" since the myocardial infarction. The initial psychological evaluations indicated that a fair proportion of the patients had scores above the upper limits of normality, indicating potential for improvement from the exercise program or other influences.

Changes observed during the pre-randomization exercise period (PREP) were clearly noticeable; measurement of systolic blood pressure and heart rate suggest that the PREP had some conditioning effect. Changes were also noted in various psychological scores. Most of these were of questionable clinical significance even though "statistically significant" at the customary .05 level.

No serious events occurred during the PREP sessions—no deaths and no recurrent myocardial infarctions. There were two deaths after the first evaluation before scheduled entry into the study. One of these died of unknown cause before entering the PREP. The other died of a myocardial infarction 2 weeks after successfully completing PREP. He had not come in for the second evaluation but was continuing PREP-like exercising at the clinic. He died at the race track one day after his last (nontraining) exercise session. One nonfatal myocardial infarction occurred during the trial period. This patient had completed the PREP; he had been through the second evaluation and was awaiting the randomization step. He had been continuing in PREP-like sessions and experienced the myocardial infarction on a nonexercising day. He did not complain of pain in the previous exercise session and withdrew from candidacy for the study.

The final phase of the study has recently been reported. There was no difference in morbidity between the two groups; however, the nonexercise control group had a higher (not significant) mortality than the exercise group: 7.3 versus 4.6 percent. It was concluded that this study supports the value of supervised exercise in decreasing mortality in male survivors of myocardial infarction. Figure 21 displays the data graphically. Table 8 summarizes results from the NEHDP along with other publicated trials (some recent) of exercise training and rehabilitation.

STANDARDS FOR EXERCISE PROGRAMS

The American Heart Association in 1979–1980 published two sets of carefully prepared and properly reviewed and approved *Standards*.[73,74] These were written by ad hoc committees under the auspices of the Rehabilitation and Exercise Committee of the American Heart Association. Because of the impact of these standards in the area of cardiovascular exercise *treatment* and *maintenance*, certain sections of these standards are included here either verbatim or paraphrased. The exercise prescription discussed is omitted and the reader is referred to Chapter 3.

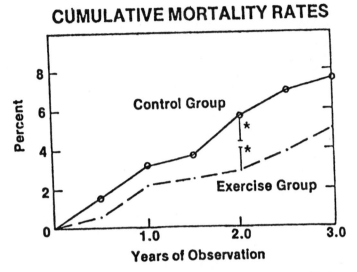

Figure 21: Display of percent difference in mortality of patients in the control versus the exercise group studied in the National Exercise Heart Disease Project (From Shaw LW, for the Project Staff. Effects of a prescribed, supervised, exercise program on mortality and cardiovascular morbidity in patients after a myocardial infarction. The national exercise and heart disease project. *Am J Cardiol* 1981;48:39−46. Used with permission.)

CARDIOVASCULAR EXERCISE TREATMENT PROGRAM

The goals of any cardiovascular exercise treatment program should be:

1. To help the individual return to activities important to the quality of his life prior to the onset of illness;
2. To prepare the individual and his family for healthy alternatives in life-style that might reduce the risk of occurrence (primary prevention) of coronary heart disease;
3. To prepare the individual and his family for healthy alternatives in life-style that might reduce the recurrence (secondary prevention) of coronary heart disease;
4. To return the individual to optimal physiological function;
5. To reduce costs of health care through shortened treatment time and prevention of disability; and
6. To reduce occupational losses caused by cardiovascular disease.

Table 8
Summary of Published Trials of Exercise Training in Subsets of Coronary Artery Disease

Study	Disease Subset	No. of Patients		Duration (Mo.)	Death (%)		Nonfatal MI (%)		Return to Work (%)		Overall Mortality (%)		Comments
		EX	C		EX	C	EX	C	EX	C	EX	C	
Bruce[51]	Angina, MI, CABS	230	352	22	0.6	2.3	0.6	1.0	62	35	2.7	4.7	Controls are dropouts. Significant increase in return to work in exercisers vs. dropouts.
Kallio[96]	Post-MI FC I, II	183	187	32	5.8	14.4	18.1	11.2			21.8	29.9	Significant decreases in sudden deaths, exercisers vs. controls.
Kentala[40]	Post-MI	74	74	20	1.3	4.1	8.1	5.4			14.9	14.9	No significant differences exercisers vs. controls.
NEHDP[72]	Post-MI	328	328	36	2.4	1.8	4.6	3.3			4.7	7.3	37% reduction in deaths, exercisers vs. controls.
Waites[80]	Post CABS	11	11	6	0	0	0	0	82	36	0	0	82% return to work in exercisers, 36% in controls.
Rechnitzer[97]	Post-MI	66	127	84			3	27.9			7.6	11.8	Significant decrease in nonfatal infarction in exercisers vs. controls.
Wilhelmsen[41]	Post-MI	158	157	48	3.8	1.9	15.7	17.9			18	22	31% reduction in deaths in exercisers vs controls.
Vermeulen[98]	Post-MI	47	51	2	0	0	9	18			5	10	Death rate significantly lower in exercisers vs. controls.
Kellerman[99]	Post CABS	51	45	58					58.8	20			Exercise group significantly greater % return to work.

Abbreviations: **Data in per 100/person year observed; C = Control; CABS = coronary artery bypass surgery; ETT = exercise treadmill test; EX = exercise; F.C. = New York Heart Association functional classification; MI = myocardial infarction; mo = month; NEHDP = National Exercise Heart Disease Project.

Candidates for Exercise Treatment Programs

Candidates for the cardiovascular exercise treatment programs include those with proven heart disease and those highly vulnerable to its development. Individuals with proven cardiovascular disease are those with either documented myocardial infarction or stable angina pectoris or who are postoperative cardiovascular surgical or angioplasty patients. Other candidates for the program include patients who are vulnerable to premature coronary heart disease due to significant coronary risk factors.

A patient should enter the program through a proper referral from the physician responsible for his continuing care. The physician responsible for the medical component of the rehabilitation program should report to the referring physician on status changes of significance and status on discharge with recommendations for maintenance programs.

Informed Consent

The physician responsible for the cardiovascular exercise treatment program must explain the exercise procedure carefully and thoroughly to the patient. The patient must understand why the exercises are being done, how they will be conducted, and the potential risks involved. The physician should emphasize that the patient must report immediately to a staff member any unexpected symptoms such as chest discomfort, shortness of breath, weakness, or dizziness. In addition to a notation in the patient's record concerning the substance of their conversation about the exercise program, the physician should obtain from the patient a signed consent form. (A sample is provided in Fig. 22 [Form 2]).

After an evaluation of personal history (emphasizing risk factors), a physical examination, laboratory assessment, and an exercise tolerance test, the patient may be accepted into the program.

Candidates with Known Cardiovascular Disease

Generally, myocardial infarction patients may be admitted to an exercise treatment program as early as 3 weeks following a myocardial infarction, at the discretion of the physician. Patients

---

Form 2
Informed Consent for Exercise Treatment

(It is recommended that this form be submitted to local counsel for review and modification to insure that it conforms with the appropriate state and local laws governing consent.)

I desire to engage voluntarily in the _____ exercise program in order to attempt to improve my cardiovascular function. This program has been recommended to me by my physician, Doctor _____ . Before I enter this exercise program I will have a clinical evaluation. This evaluation will include medical history and physical examination consisting of, but not limited to, measurements of heart rate and blood pressure, EKG at rest and with effort. The purpose of this evaluation is to attempt to detect any condition which would indicate that I should not engage in this exercise program.

The program will follow an exercise prescription prepared by Doctor _____ _____ . I understand that activities are designed to place a gradually increasing work load on the circulation and to thereby attempt to improve its function. The reaction of the cardiovascular system to such activities cannot be predicted with complete accuracy. There is the risk of certain changes occurring during or following the exercise. These changes include abnormalities of blood pressure or heart rate, or ineffective "heart function," and possibly, in some instances, "heart attacks" or "cardiac arrest."

I realize that it is necessary for me to promptly report to the supervisor of exercises any signs or symptoms indicating any abnormality or distress. I consent to the administration of any immediate resuscitation measures deemed advisable by the supervisor of exercise.

I have read the foregoing and I understand it. Any questions which have arisen or occurred to me have been answered to my satisfaction.

Date _____

Patient Signature _____

Physician Signature _____

Witness _____

Figure 22.

with stable angina pectoris may also be admitted. Postoperative cardiovascular surgical patients are admitted approximately 4 to 8 weeks following surgery or at the discrection of the physician. These patients include those having myocardial revascularization, peripheral arterial obstructive surgery, and, on occasion, valve replacement and repair of congenital heart defects.

Candidates at High Risk of Developing Cardiovascular Disease

Persons who have a *high risk* of developing cardiovascular disease may be admitted to the program. These include: (1) patients who are vulnerable to developing coronary heart disease because of risk factors such as diabetes, obesity, hyperlipidemia, and smoking; (2) asymptomatic patients with an abnormal exercise test; (3) patients with or without other clinical evidence of coronary artery disease with dysrhythmias induced or aggravated by activity; and (4) patients with significant hypertension and a low functional capacity may be candidates for the program. (The hypertensive patient with normal functional capacity usually does not require a therapeutic program but may benefit from a nonsupervised prescribed exercise program.) The program provides an opportunity for simultaneous counseling for behavioral factors shown to influence coronary heart disease such as smoking, diet, and stress management.

Special Precautions for Exercise Program Candidates

The following conditions usually require special precautions before engaging in an exercise treatment program:

- Uncontrolled congestive heart failure (Class III or IV)
- Myocarditis or cardiomyopathy within the past year
- Uncontrolled hypertension
- Dysrhythmias
  - Second- and third-degree atrioventricular block
  - Uncontrolled atrial fibrillation
  - Excessive or complex PVCs
- Significant cardiac enlargement
- Valvular disease (moderate to severe)
- Outflow tract obstructive disease (IHSS)
- Recent pulmonary embolism
- Anemia with a hemoglobin below 10 gm/100 ml
- Uncontrolled metabolic disease (diabetes mellitus, thyrotoxicosis, myxedema)
- Transient illness that includes acute febrile illnesses
- Certain orthopedic disabilities
- Inappropriate blood pressure response to exercise testing

Personnel

Requirements for staff members conducting an exercise treatment program vary according to program, location, and characteristics of the patient group. All personnel must share a common background in the art and science of medicine with an emphasis on cardiovascular disease. Health professionals who work in such a program must be directed by the physician, whose judgment is a key factor. Personnel may be nurses, social workers, rehabilitation counselors, clinical psychologists, exercise physiologists, physical therapists, occupational therapists, dietitians, recreational leaders, and physical educators. Certified exercise technologists, exercise specialists, and program directors can provide depth to the program. All staff members should be certified in cardiopulmonary resuscitation and supervisors should be trained and certified in advanced life support. In addition, patients and their families should be taught cardiopulmonary resuscitation.

Training requirements vary for staff members. Subgroups of interested, informed, and active persons are found in many broader disciplines. Since certification within a larger professional body does not guarantee quality performance in this field, special requirements should be met because of the multidisciplinary nature of this program.

The physician should have both the personal interest and the multiple skills needed to supervise the program. He should have a broad medical background with a fundamental understanding of cardiovascular disease and its treatment, exercise physiology, educational techniques in behavior modification, concepts of prevention, and administrative experience. A registered nurse with coronary care unit experience is important for monitoring physiological and electrocardiographic response to exercise and for emergency resuscitation.

The exercise physiologist may be trained in medicine, nursing, physical therapy, or physical education. He must be trained properly within one professional discipline and acceptable to the associated disciplines within the program. This implies some quality control by the peer group. A physical therapist hired for a cardiovascular exercise treatment program should be qualified for cardiovascular physiology. Occupational therapists and recreational directors should possess at least a bachelor's degree. Dietitians, social workers, clinical psychologists and vocational rehabilitation counselors also add specialization to the program.

Program directors should be considered authoritative in the field of exercise cardiology and/or physiology and should be administratively competent. The exercise specialist's primary responsibility is to the exercise program. They often are well qualified to conduct adult fitness programs and programs for the maintenance of cardiovascular fitness under proper conditions. Exercise technologists should understand the dynamics and technology of exercise and are of particular value in the diagnostic section.

Training in Resuscitation and Safety

All personnel, patients, and patients' families should complete basic life support courses in cardiopulmonary resuscitation. Key personnel should have completed the advanced life support course and be at the instructor level in basic life support. Personnel, patients, and their families should be recertified periodically according to American Heart Association standards.

Any exercise program involving patients with cardiovascular disease or subjects at risk, such as adult fitness programs, maintenance programs, and inpatient and outpatient therapeutic programs, should have the proper equipment and drugs for evaluating and correcting life-threatening cardiac dysrhythmias. There also should be a written plan for dealing with emergencies. Appropriate emergency equipment, including a portable defibrillator and drugs, should be available immediately. The portable defibrillator should be tested daily for its ability to deliver an adequate charge. Personnel should inventory drugs every 3 months as well as after each entry to the sealed container. Nitroglycerin should be available outside the sealed container for immediate use. In addition, a stretcher or other patient-carrying device should be available.

Personnel must instruct patients about significant symptoms they might experience as a result of exercising and teach them how to recognize those symptoms. If special discomfort or distress is sensed, the patient should be told to report it immediately and reduce the intensity of effort or discontinue the exercise.

Exercise activities using swimming pools require special attention so that electrical shock hazards for both patient and personnel are eliminated.

The Exercise Treatment Program

The rehabilitation process is structured into divisions based primarily on site, equipment, and personnel needs. These divisions should be viewed as links in a continuous chain of return to function. The divisions include: (1) the exercise testing laboratory, (2) the inpatient program, (3) the outpatient therapeutic exercise and cardiac rehabilitation program, and (4) the maintenance program. Placement of the subject in a proper program depends on the preliminary evaluation.

The Exercise Testing Laboratory

The laboratory can be a useful component for teaching exercise terminology and precautions determined by individual performance levels. It is desirable for the physician responsible for the therapeutic program to be present during the testing procedure. In addition to providing the hard data base for the exercise prescription, this can be a valuable teaching experience for both patient and staff. The measurement of physiologic findings associated with exercise can be taught to the patient at this time and related to the onset of symptoms when present.

The Inpatient Program

For hospitalized patients, the therapeutic program starts early in the hospital phase and is followed by a therapeutic outpatient phase. The hospital inpatient component is important for early ambulation, increased activity to prevent deconditioning, and for beginning education and psychological acceptance of the outpatient program. Components in the inpatient program are: (1) medical treatment, (2) risk factor education (including psychological support and family counseling), and (3) education for physical activity.

Medical treatment is under the direction of the physician. The physician is responsible for providing the proper psychological climate that influences the mood for the rehabilitative program and for initiating the sequence that leads to functional return to optimal performance. Risk factors are discovered during the hospital phase by taking the patient's history regarding nutrition, smoking, occupational demands, family medical problems, and exercise and sports, as well as the traditional physical examination and laboratory assessment of lipids, glucose, and renal function.

The educational program identifies and introduces the elements of patient education that will be included in the outpatient program. Emphasis is on risk factor modification and principles of exercise and physical performance. The coronary care unit nurse instructs the patient on his daily care in the hospital. Psychosocial support for the family and patient is started as soon after admission as possible by appropriately trained rehabilitation team members.

Education for physical activity is an important part of the in-hospital phase. Exercise terminology and the concept of energy cost of activity, using MET units, is introduced. The groundwork for understanding physiologic response to effort and emotions also is introduced. The outpatient program should be discussed with the patient prior to discharge.

The Outpatient Therapeutic Program

Following progressive low level activity in the hospital and the basic educational and psychosocial support programs given there, patients with heart disease may enter a prescribed, medically supervised exercise program. For those whose cardiac problems have been discovered by exercise testing, an educational session covering in-hospital topics must be given.

The treatment program consists of at least three sessions per week for purposes of delivering the desired goals of individually prescribed behavioral counseling, vocational counseling, and physical conditioning. The program is structured in 3-month units, but may be shortened (see *Exit Criteria from the Therapeutic Program*) or extended with justification.

The Exercise Maintenance Program

The physician may determine the patient's need for continued physical conditioning and maintenance of the status achieved after he has reached criteria for release from the therapeutic program. The maintenance program is preventive (secondary prevention) and, if very stringent criteria are met, may function with primary prevention programs supervised by a physician or health professional trained in therapeutic exercise programs.

COMPONENTS OF THE REHABILITATION PROGRAM

The components of the outpatient cardiac rehabilitation program are medical, educational, and physical.

The Medical Component

In the medical component, the physician in charge of the program is responsible for the patient and the training area. He evaluates the patient at entry and supervises progress, making appropriate recommendations to the personal physician for therapy and safety. Evaluation by the physician in charge takes place at the beginning of the program, at scheduled intervals, whenever significant changes occur in the status of the patient, and at the conclusion of the program. The physician should be present during therapeutic exercise sessions in order to:
- Observe the patient's performance during exercise;
- Evaluate symptoms;
- Evaluate drug effects and recommend changes when appropriate;
- Assess progress of the disease;
- Determine when catheterization, myocardial imaging, or repeat exercise testing should be done;
- Counsel the patient and give psychological support;
- Maintain patient discipline;
- Maintain discipline among health professionals;
- Assist in emergencies and cardiopulmonary resuscitation.

The Educational Component

Educational elements of the program are directed toward modifying risk factors and changing the patient's attitude toward health and occupational status. Formal classes are scheduled for teaching the physical aspects of daily living including energy cost of activity defined in METs (metabolic equivalent) and the principles of physiologic response to activity and environmental influences. The groundwork for these outpatient classes is formulated in the in-hospital phase.

Emphasis on the risk factors includes: (1) dietary counseling, (2) psychosocial counseling regarding stress management, smoking, and weight control utilizing group education and participation techniques where appropriate, (3) referral for further occupational and psychological counseling when necessary, and (4) education regarding physical activity.

The Exercise Component

The exercise format may consist of circuit training exercise sessions and a less rigid gymnasium program. The decision regarding the type of program is determined by characteristics of the individual entering the program. In exercise sessions using individually prescribed circuit training, the patient spends the prescribed amount of time at one exercise station and then moves to the next one until the entire prescription is completed. Circuit training allows for close monitoring of the patient and is recommended for the individual shortly after entry into the program or for the individual whose condition is less stable and requires closer supervision. Exercise sessions are scheduled on three nonconsecutive days per week for at least one-half hour and are supplemented by individual and group counseling. The exercises are prescribed individually. In addition to the physiological value of the exercise, the exercise session is used to teach the patient his personal limits of performance and the prescription of physiological work loads.

The exercises may include as many as eight stations, some isotonic and some resistive, such as:

Warm-up	Walking steps
Treadmill walking	Dumbbells
Arm crank ergometer	Rowing machine
Barbells	Bicycle ergometer

The less rigid gymnasium programs add flexibility to the exercise sessions. A gymnasium program requires a competent exercise leader who can judge performance demands and response. When available, water exercises in a swimming pool are valuable.

The therapeutic section of the cardiac exercise program should take place in a facility that is either: (1) physically within the hospital, (2) in a hospital-allied facility, or (3) a facility remote from the hospital that is subject to peer review.

Most hospital-based programs provide only fixed-position exercise stations including treadmill, bicycle, and step stations with dumbbells, barbells, and arm crank ergometers. Hospital-allied and outside facilities usually have the additional advantage of swimming pools, gymnasia, and walking trails. Physical training away from the hospital helps develop a sense of independence from the hospital and a feeling of personal progress.

Physical Features

Space requirements should be adequate to meet the needs of the individual program. Ideally, the exercise testing facility should be close to the therapeutic section so that there can be a sharing of responsibility between the personnel. The temperature should be regulated between 20° and 23°C (68° and 75°F) with humidity between 40 percent and 60 percent. When the temperature is unusually warm, the exercise intensity should be reduced proportionally to keep the target heart rate constant.

Easy access to the facility is important for patients and for emergency equipment in the event of cardiorespiratory crisis. Signs indicating exits, emergency equipment, and procedures in the event of an emergency should be clearly visible.

The program involving early post-hospital treatment (usually 3 to 12 weeks) requires the availability of electronic monitoring of patients. Frequency of monitoring depends upon the electrical stability of the patient, elapsed time since the acute event, and the stage of rehabilitation. Monitoring one of every three sessions is reasonable in a short-term therapeutic program, decreasing in frequency after the first few weeks. Monitoring may be by hardwire or telemetry. Telemetry, although expensive, is more versatile and psychologically more appealing than hard-wire monitoring.

As the patient moves into a less controlled environment, the gymnasium activities use simple exercise equipment and include noncontact sports, such as volleyball, under close supervision. Swimming pools should have shallow water, 1.3 meters (4 feet) or less, for walking exercises. Water temperature should be between 25° and 30°C (77° and 84°F).

Personal activity programs to be followed at home add to the rehabilitation effort. As appropriate exit criteria are met, the patient may be promoted into an organized maintenance program.

EXIT CRITERIA FROM THE THERAPEUTIC PROGRAM

At the discretion of the rehabilitation program staff, a patient may be discharged from the program after having met the following criteria:

Functional Capacity: A functional level adequate for the occupation of the individual and an activity level appropriate for the individual's life-style after consultation with the physician, staff, and social and/or vocational counselor. A peak functional capacity of about 8 METs is more than adequate for most occupations.

Time: It is the consensus of exercise treatment program professionals that the time necessary for therapeutic physical reconditioning of most patients with cardiovascular disease may be 1 to 3 months. The need for supervision is more demanding during the therapeutic phase of the rehabilitation process to which these standards are directed. After the initial program, extensions may be provided in the highly structured program when medically justified by individual evaluation.

Medical Status: Discharge from the program depends on the judgment of the cardiac rehabilitation team's physicians, based on the (1) resting ECG, (2) exercise ECG, (3) blood pressure response, and (4) symptoms.

Education: Patients should understand the basic pathophysiology of their cardiovascular disease process. They should be taught the signs and symptoms associated with this disease process and, in particular, the signals that might indicate a changing situation and the appropriate response to such signals. They also should understand reasons for the intervention methods used in cardiac rehabilitation, including benefits of physical activity ir improving functional capacity, the importance of safe heart rate range and limiting symptoms during physical activity, the benefits of optimal nutrition in weight control and blood lipid control, and the importance of identifying and modifying personal stress and tension. The evaluation of the success of the educational process for each patient should be determined by the staff, either by personal evaluation of the patient or by objective testing.

The Decision to Discharge a Patient: A final decision for early discharge of patients should be made by the cardiac rehabilitation staff. It also is necessary to decide on a maintenance program at that time. In addition, the vocational counselor, with the help of other rehabilitation staff members, should make a recommendation concerning the patient's employment.

QUALITY CONTROL

Maintaining standards of personnel, program, and facilities is the responsibility of the medical director and is possible through several mechanisms, but the fundamental principle is peer acceptance.

Hospital-Based Program: A hospital accredited by the Joint Commission on Accreditation of Hospitals (JCAH) is assured of certain physician and operational standards. The quality of the program is acceptable since peer review by staff is implied.

Hospital-Allied Program: Since a hospital accredited by JCAH meets standards of operations, reliance by hospital staff on the hospital-allied program, either on a contractual or on an agreement basis, implies peer review.

Independent or Free-Standing Program: Standards for peer review may be established by the local society or by national medical organizations, such as American Heart Association, American College of Physicians, American College of Cardiology, American Medical Association, American College of Chest Physicians, and American College of Sports Medicine, in cooperation with local peer groups.

Cardiovascular Exercise Maintenance Programs[74]

Candidates for cardiovascular maintenance programs as described in these *Standards* are:

1. Those persons with cardiovascular disease who meet the exit criteria from a therapeutic exercise program;
2. Those who are at risk for developing ischemic heart disease;
3. Those who are markedly deconditioned;
4. The well individual who is interested in improving and maintaining cardiovascular health and wants to participate in a formal comprehensive program.

The maintenance program represents the interface between medical care and personal responsibility for health. It may be: (1) coordinated personally by the individual, or (2) structured and supervised. In either circumstance, efforts are directed toward acquiring independent and personal responsibility for health. Whichever pathway the individual chooses, the goals are the same. For patients with known heart disease, participation in a supervised exercise maintenance program is desirable.

Principles for maintaining cardiovascular health also apply to primary prevention, secondary prevention, and rehabilitation. Since these principles are largely behavioral, responsibility for maintaining personal health belongs primarily to the individual. On the other hand, it is the responsibility of health professionals acting in concert with other available resources to provide guidelines and access to information and to teach the skills that lead to healthy cardiovascular habits.

Goals

The primary goal for cardiovascular exercise maintenance programs is to maintain life with vitality and to reduce morbidity and mortality from cardiovascular disease. In an effort to accomplish this, the program should attempt to help the individual:

1. Understand the principles for maintenance of cardiovascular health through risk factor intervention;
2. Maintain activities and attitudes important to quality of life in keeping with cardiovascular health;

3. Maintain optimal physiologic function;
4. Learn to deal with psychological stresses;
5. Enhance occupational performance;
6. Reduce the cost of health care through primary and secondary prevention.

Components of the Program

Program components include: (1) medical, (2) educational, and (3) exercise. Various combinations of available resources may be used with these components. The program should be flexible and tailored to the individual and to the community in which it operates.

Whether the program is coordinated by the participant (personal program) or directly supervised by health professionals (structured program), the same principles and components apply.

Medical Component

Participants should have a medical assessment prior to beginning a maintenance program. The assessment includes evaluation of previous medical history, present physical status, identification of risk factors, and current exercise performance level. Individuals with known or suspected heart disease should have a medically supervised exercise test. The features of a personal program are developed during this assessment. Recommendations for emphasis on various educational, environmental, and medical aspects of the program are also initiated during this phase.

Educational Component

The cardiovascular maintenance program should provide educational materials of the best scientific quality for cardiovascular health enhancement. Resources in the format of films, lectures, group conferences, printed material, etc., are available from the American Heart Association. The educational strategies included in the maintenance program are designed to promote health education for people of all ages.

Exercise Component

Physical activity is the focal point around which the maintenance program functions. Evidence indicates that moderate and vigorous occupational or leisure-time physical activity may protect against coronary heart disease and improve the likelihood of survival from a heart attack. Exercise training can increase cardiovascular functional capacity and decrease myocardial oxygen demand for any given level of physical activity in normal persons as well as in selected cardiac patients. Regular physical activity is required to sustain the effects of training and may serve as an adjunct to reducing the risk factors of coronary heart disease such as cigarette smoking, hypertension, lipid abnormalities, obesity, and emotional stress. The potential risk of vigorous physical activity can be reduced by appropriate medical clearance, education, and guidance.

RISK FACTOR INTERVENTIONS

Risk factors include those related to: (1) host susceptibility (family history, age, sex), (2) atherogenic personal attributes (altered blood lipids, arterial hypertension, hyperglycemia), and (3) living habits (diet, physical activity, obesity, cigarette smoking, oral contraceptives, and psychosocial factors) which predispose the individual to disease.

Many communities have developed structured and supervised programs for maintenance of cardiovascular health. These programs have the advantage of group participation and peer reinforcement. A satisfactory alternative is a properly developed, personally coordinated program. Specific interventions include the following.

Regular Physical Activity

Physical activity is an integral part of life. Regular exercise can improve exercise tolerance and can favorably modify certain risk factors such as hypertension, body weight, and HDL cholesterol.

Nutrition Counseling

Nutrition counseling may help reduce risk of recurrence of coronary heart disease through control of blood lipid abnormalities, obesity, and carbohydrate intolerance. The program should present: (1) principles of food purchase, labeling, and interpretation of the label as it applies to food components (fat, salt, etc.); (2) diet formulation; (3) principles of food preparation for nutritious but tasty and inviting meals; (4) good nutrition counseling to enable the participant to adopt a suitable dietary pattern. Information on diet formulation is available through the American Heart Association.

Elimination of Cigarette Smoking

Elimination of cigarette smoking is of critical importance in cardiovascular disease prevention. Smoking also affects exercise performance. Adverse effects on lung function are compounded by a decreased oxygen carrying capacity of arterial blood due to carbon monoxide from smoke inhalation. No single technique for stopping is uniformly successful, but group programs with peer support appear to help. For this reason, maintenance programs should continue to remind participants of the health hazards inherent in smoking and insist on its elimination.

Stress Management

There are implications that emotional factors play a role in the development of cardiovascular disease. Many techniques of stress management have been advocated. Their value in cardiovascular disease management is not established.

COMPLIANCE AND REPORTING

Program compliance depends upon individual commitment. Group activities help provide support and motivation to continue. For those individuals with cardiovascular disease, a good doctor/

patient relationship is an important element in sustaining compliance. Documentation of initial individual status and interventions is an important tool in measuring results. It is useful both to patient and to physician.

PERSONNEL

Program development and administration may be provided by persons of various backgrounds. Qualified personnel should be available to provide: (1) participants' safety, (2) initial evaluation, (3) education, (4) exercise prescription, (5) exercise program, and (6) documentation and reporting of interventions and results. Some model programs may serve as a resource for interested industries and organizations.

Minimal personnel for the maintenance program are the participant and the physician. The program may also include other appropriate specialists, such as nurses, exercise physiologists, physical therapists, dietitians, occupational therapists, physician's assistants, clinical psychologists, physical educators, health educators, recreational therapists, social workers, and vocational rehabilitation counselors.

SITE AND EQUIPMENT

A gymnasium, swimming pool, classrooms, outdoor exercise areas, and space for circuit training and games are desirable. Cool-down facilities and dressing rooms are desirable so that participants are refreshed and comfortable as they leave the site.

The gymnasium should be environmentally controlled. Pleasant lighting, sound baffles, temperature control—20–24°C (68–75°F), and humidity control (less than 60 percent) are recommended. A swimming pool should have shallow water, 1.3 meters (4 feet), for walking exercises. The water temperature should be maintained between 25–30°C (77–84°F); 28°C (82°F) is ideal.

Accessibility, space, weather, safety, and cost factors must be considered in the design of a personal program. Heat injuries during activity can be avoided if principles of exercise physiology as related to heat, humidity, and fluid ingestion are followed. This is especially important in high performance activity if the energy cost is greater than 50 percent of the individual's maximum energy level or when the temperature is greater than 32°C (90°F) with humidity greater than 60 percent.

Requirements for site and equipment may be met by a number of public or private facilities such as school or community gymnasia, pools, "Y's," or community centers. Recognizing the value of "adult physical fitness," many businesses and industries have built facilities or contracted locally for adult exercise programs. In these circumstances, the maintenance program should serve as a specialized component of the overall health program emphasizing cardiovascular risk factor modification.

SAFETY

It is important that access to the community emergency care system be clearly identified. The participants should be instructed to recognize and deal with symptoms or signs of cardiovascular distress.

It is felt that these standards will serve as general guidelines for those interested in these cases of cardiovascular treatment. There are no intentions to "referee" or certify programs. However, peer and patient "pressure" will likely promote adherence to these realistic guidelines in setting up and maintaining this type of treatment.

STUDIES IN EVALUATING CARDIAC REHABILITATION

Current data in the early 1980s reflect methodology to evaluate and data to support the effectiveness of cardiac rehabilitation. Jensen et al.[75] reported results of radionuclear ventriculography in 19 consecutive patients before and after 6 months of exercise training. They found that, after training, a higher maximal mean systolic pressure, heart rate, and work load were achieved. In addition, at equivalent subnormal work loads after training, similar levels of mean heart rate and systolic blood pressure were achieved but a significantly greater mean ejection fraction. These results suggest that exercise training may improve cardiac function in selected patients with coronary artery disease.

Rehabilitation programs for coronary patients continue to be under close scrutiny with regard to benefits and safety. Jackson et al.[76] evaluated 2,644 patients in 69 centers by questionnaires. Fifty percent of the patients continued to be active in the programs. They concluded that cardiac rehabilitation can be done with a high degree of safety (no deaths in 3 years in the active treatment group) and that a mortality rate of less than 1 percent in 3 years suggests a decreased mortality in post-myocardial infarction patients active in chronic cardiac rehabilitation.

Superko et al.[77] studied the benefits of cardiac rehabilitation training in patients with fixed heart rates (with pacemakers). They found that even with no heart rate response, these subjects had improved oxygen consumption (VO_2) after training and decreased systolic blood pressure (after training) with fixed work load and fixed VO_2. Ritter et al.[78] evaluated angina pectoris status in cardiac rehabilitation patients. They found that in 59 patients undergoing cardiac rehabilitation, there was a 50 percent increase in maximal exercise capacity in contrast to only 10 percent in 22 subjects not in cardiac rehabilitation.

Hertanu et al.[79] have recently reported results of an outcome assessment of a 3-month rehabilitation exercise program in 38 patients with coronary artery disease. All patients improved in exercise performance and 57 percent of the group complied with a post-discharge exercise routine. Of the total, 16 remained employed and seven of 12 patients not employed initially returned to work during the time of the rehabilitation program.

Over and above the results of cardiac rehabilitation programs in post-myocardial infarction patients, one must consider the value of such therapy in patients after coronary artery bypass surgery. Insufficient data are available to support that surgical intervention coupled with a rehabilitation program is of greater benefit than surgery alone, nor has the value of a structured versus nonstructured rehabilitation program been examined. For the post-bypass patient, does a structured, supervised cardiac rehabilitation program improve cardiopulmonary function more than an individualized, nonsupervised program? Are there other benefits of compliance in a rehabilitation program?

These questions were precisely studied in a long-standing cardiac rehab program by comparing two groups of post-bypass patients. One group was enrolled in an organized rehabilitation program[80] which consisted of medically supervised and individually prescribed walk/jog, calisthenic and recreational activities. The subjects participated in these activities three times weekly for approximately 1 hour each session (20–25 minutes of walk/jog activity) with an average of 75 percent attendance. Education in coronary risk factor modification was an integral part of the program with both individual and group teaching. The other group had begun the same program but had voluntarily dropped out. To recruit the dropouts, 18 post-coronary bypass patients were identified in the Atlanta area who had previously been regular participants (now dropouts) of the outpatient cardiac rehabilitation program. In follow-up phone calls to solicit enrollment, 11 patients agreed to participate. Of those who refused, one cited medical reasons (recent prostate surgery). The other six declined for non-medical reasons (either travel distance or job conflict). None of these were involved in an exercise program elsewhere. A comparable control group of 11 post-bypass patients who were active in the rehabilitation program was chosen for study. All active patients were at least 9 months post bypass and had been enrolled in the rehabilitation program for at least 6 months with ≥ 75 percent attendance.

Presurgical catheterization data and angiograms of all patients were reviewed. Particular note was made of coronary artery anatomy, left ventricular end diastolic pressure, regional wall dynamics, and ejection fraction. There was, however, no data on the presurgical exercise capacity (baseline peak oxygen consumption) of the two groups. Post-surgical exercise tests performed at least 3 months postoperatively for entry into the rehabilitation program were reviewed and compared.

All subjects were then scheduled for treadmill exercise testing to be done with both physiologic and hemodynamic studies. The testing procedure was explained and use of the modified Douglas bag technique was demonstrated. Precisely at the peak of exercise, a single breath sample of expired air was collected for calculation of peak oxygen consumption. Exercise testing results were interpreted independently by two physicians. Rate-pressure product was calculated from peak heart rate in beats per minute (bpm) and peak systolic blood pressure in millimeters of mercury (mmHg). Standard equations were used to calculate peak oxygen consumption from the expired air sample. Gas was analyzed by Beckman automatic gas analyzer (OM-11 for oxygen and LB-2 for carbon dioxide). Standard reference calibrations were performed before and after each measurement using known reference gases. Data were analyzed by paired and nonpaired t testing using two-way tables (one degree of freedom) and standard chi-square equations.

Clinical features and physiologic and functional data are seen in Tables 9–11.

There was no difference in age between the active and the dropout groups: active $\bar{x} = 53.45$ years, dropout $\bar{x} = 55.81$ years. However, the age of patient no. 9 in the actives (71 years) may have influenced that data to a degree especially with the small group numbers. Body weights and heights were comparable: active $\bar{x} = 80.95$ kg, dropout $\bar{x} = 80.57$ kg, and active $\bar{x} = 27.46$ cm, dropout $\bar{x} = 27.43$ cm, respectively. All active patients were male while three of the drop-outs were female. Peak oxygen consumption in ml/kg/min was significantly different between the two groups: active $\bar{x} = 29.78$, dropout $\bar{x} = 23.73$ ($p < 0.005$). Total treadmill time was also significantly different: active $\bar{x} = 11$ minutes, 3 seconds; inactive $\bar{x} = 8$ minutes, 8 seconds ($p < 0.001$). Peak rate-pressure products, however, were not signficantly different between the groups.

Nine of 11 (82%) actives had returned to full working status compared to only four of 11 (36%) dropouts ($p < 0.01$). Only one active patient had been hospitalized (on two different occasions); however, five of 11 dropouts had been rehospitalized for a total number of seven rehospitalizations. All of the rehospitalizations were because of patient symptoms or circumstances and none were solely by request of the medical-surgical team. None of the actives but four of 11 dropouts continued to smoke. The period of time for follow-up from start of the program was comparable between groups.

Peak oxygen consumption correlates well with cardiovascular conditioning and is an index of maximal cardiovascular and pulmonary function. An increase in the habitual level of physical activity will increase peak oxygen consumption and revascularization resulting from bypass surgery will also increase peak oxygen consumption. It has not previously been shown that bypass surgery plus an organized program of exercise improves results over bypass surgery alone; however, in this study the active patients attained a higher mean peak oxygen consumption than those in the dropout group.

Symptom-limited end-point time on an exercise test is an indirect measurement of myocardial oxygen consumption and is an indication of myocardial blood flow. Successful coronary bypass

Table 9A
Clinical Features of Dropout Patients[80]

Patient	Years Age	Sex	Extent of Coronary Disease*	Ventricular Function	Drugs	Cigarette Smoking
1	48	M	Double	Normal	Aspirin	No
2	64	M	Triple	Inferior hypokinesis LVEDP = 12	Propranolol Furosemide	No
3	61	F	Double	Normal	Hydrochlorothiazide Propranolol Diazepam	Yes
4	47	M	Double	Normal	None	Yes
5	63	M	Triple	Inferior akinesis LVEDP = 30	Digoxin Propranolol Hydrochlorothiazide	No
6	53	F	Single	Normal	Nitroglycerin Aspirin Propranolol	Yes
7	51	F	Triple	Normal LVEDP = 13	Propranolol	Yes
8	55	M	Triple	Akinetic apex LVEDP = 14	Digoxin	No
9	59	M	Left main and triple	Aneurysm	None	No
10	58	M	Single	Anteroapical hypokinesis	None	No
11	55	M	Single	Normal	Propranolol Digoxin Sulfinpyrazone	No

*Number of major vessels with ≥75 percent cross-sectional luminal narrowing.
LVEDP = left ventricular end-diastolic pressure in mmHg (No comment implies<12)

Table 9B
Clinical Features of Active Patients[80]

Patient	Years Age	Sex	Extent of Coronary Disease*	Ventricular Function	Drugs	Cigarette Smoking
1	52	M	Double	Normal	Aspirin	No
2	52	M	Triple	Akinesis of postero-inferior wall LVEDP = 18	None	No
3	61	M	Triple with left main	Hypokinetic infero-posterior wall	Aspirin	No
4	46	M	Triple with left main	Normal LVEDP = 18	Hydrochlorothiazide	No
5	53	M	Single	Normal	Propranolol	No
6	62	M	Single	Inferior hypokinesis LVEDP = 14	Aspirin	No
7	54	M	Triple	Anterolateral hypokinesis LVEDP = 12	None	No
8	41	M	Double	Inferior hypokinesis apical akinesis LVEDP = 18	Propranolol	No
9	71	M	Triple	Normal	Sulfinpyrazone Digoxin	No
10	48	M	Double	Normal	Propranolol Aspirin Cholestyramine Clofibrate	No
11	58	M	Double	Infero-apical hypokinesis	Aspirin	No

*Number of major vessels with ≥75% cross-sectional luminal narrowing.
LVEDP = left ventricular end-diastolic pressure in mmHg (No comment implies<12)

Table 10A
Exercise Testing Data in Dropout Patients[80]

Patient	V̇O₂	METs	Time on Treadmill (minutes)	Peak Heart Rate (beats/min)	Peak Blood Pressure (mmHg)	Rate Pressure Product	Treadmill Results in ST Displacement	Weight (kilograms)	Height (centimeters)
1	35.07	10.02	14.0	180	160/60	28800	None	85.91	190.5
2	17.85	5.1	7.1	120	160/70	19200	.2 mv	97.27	180.0
3	17.73	5.1	6.3	135	160/90	21600	None	69.09	161.3
4	23.47	6.7	6.5	155	180/40	27900	None	88.18	180.32
5	21.90	6.3	7.0	100	180/70	18000	None	86.36	177.42
6	22.47	6.4	8.0	108	180/90	19440	None	83.18	181.55
7	19.47	5.6	9.0	125	170/70	21250	None	63.64	166.32
8	26.09	7.5	9.0	155	180/90	27900	None	87.73	180.32
9	29.04	8.3	10.0	160	140/80	22400	None	76.36	174.84
10	20.17	5.9	6.9	150	200/80	30000	.2 mv	69.54	176.77
11	27.83	7.9	9.8	154	220/70	33880	Indeterminant	79.09	177.42
Mean values	23.74	6.8	8.5	140	175/74	24579		80.57	176.96

V̇O₂ = peak oxygen consumption in ml/kg/min
MET = metabolic equivalent (one MET = 3.5 ml/kg/min of oxygen consumption)
mv = millivolts in horizontal negative displacement

Table 10B
Exercise Testing Data in Active Patients[80]

Patient	$\dot{V}O_2$	METs	Time on Treadmill (minutes)	Peak Heart Rate (beats/min)	Peak Blood Pressure (mmHg)	Rate Pressure Product	Treadmill Results in ST Displacement	Weight (kilograms)	Height (centimeters)
1	25.74	7.3	9.0	145	145/50	21025	None	87.27	182.9
2	27.77	7.9	10.0	155	136/72	21080	None	86.36	179.9
3	30.33	8.6	9.0	150	190/74	28500	None	86.36	172.25
4	28.36	8.1	12.3	160	185/80	29600	None	80.91	177.8
5	40.80	11.6	13.5	130	160/75	20800	None	78.64	179.9
6	35.30	10.1	13.0	150	172/74	25800	None	60.91	167.6
7	29.05	8.3	12.0	165	160/40	26400	None	84.9	176.77
8	28.56	8.3	12.0	140	158/60	22120	None	85.0	180.32
9	30.20	8.6	5.0	145	180/90	26100	None	88.18	179.35
10	36.33	10.4	12.4	160	160/70	25600	Indeterminant	78.18	180.32
11	22.77	6.5	8.0	118	150/74	11700	None	74.54	171.62
Mean values	30.5	8.7	10.6	147	163/69	23520		80.95	177.16

$\dot{V}O_2$ = peak oxygen consumption in ml/kg/min
MET = metabolic equivalent (one MET = 3.5 ml/kg/min of oxygen consumption)
ST displacement in millivolts

Table 11
Functional Features of Patient Population[80]

Patients	Work Status	Hospital Admissions Since Surgery
Dropouts		
1	Full time work	None
2	Not working	1-for recath-patent grafts
3	Not working	2-1 for recath-patent grafts
4	Not working	2-1 for recath-patent grafts
5	Not working	1-for recath-patent grafts
6	Not working	None
7	Not working	1-for recath-patent grafts
8	Full time work	None
9	Not working	None
10	Full time work	None
11	Full time work	None
Actives		
1	Full time work	None
2	Full time work	None
3	Full time work	None
4	Full time work	None
5	Full time work	2-for recath-patent grafts
6	Full time work	None
7	Full time work	None
8	Full time work	None
9	Not working (Retired before "heart trouble")	None
10	Full time work	None
11	Not working	None

Recath = repeat coronary arteriography

surgery improves myocardial blood flow and thus increases exercise test duration. Previous data have shown that bypass patients further improve their time on treadmill testing after participation in an exercise program. These data also revealed improvement in treadmill duration time for bypass patients who were not regularly exercising. In this study, the active post-bypass patients were capable of a greater duration on the treadmill test than the dropouts.

There was no significant difference in peak rate-pressure product between the two groups. This contradicts the oxygen consumption data but there are two possible explanations. First, the difference in oxygen consumption between groups likely reflects a "total body" training effect over and above the effect on the rate-pressure product. Secondly, three active and six drop-out patients were on propranolol. When the work load is the same, exercise with propranolol results in lower heart rate, blood pressure, and myocardial oxygen consumption than exercise without proprano-lol. This greater number of patients on propranolol in the dropout group (six) versus the active (three) may have accounted for some differences between groups.

General state of well-being is difficult to assess. However, based on personal interview, it seems that the actives "felt better" than the drop-outs because they were enjoying the program and the "comradeship" with other patients and staff. Of note, four of the 11 drop-outs (patients no. 2, 4, 6, and 8) (Table 9A) later rejoined the exercise program. Two of these four (patients no. 4 and 6) (Table 9A) were smokers. None of the actives smoked cigarettes, whereas eight of them had previously. Four of the 11 dropouts continued to smoke. Peer pressure is likely a factor in this differ-ence and the motivation to remain in a triweekly rehabilitation program probably also motivates them to stop cigarettes.

Nine of the 11 actives are still working. One received disabil-ity retirement prior to surgery; the other (age 71 years) retired at age 65. Only four of 11 dropouts are working. Two had physical disability retirement prior to surgery. The other five listed various health reasons (prostatism in two, low back pain in two, and peripheral vascular disease in one); however, none in either group listed angina pectoris as a reason for not working. As noted, only one of the active versus five of the inactive were rehospitalized. All hospitalizations for the dropouts occurred 6 or more months after withdrawing from the program. In each instance, the reason for rehospitalization was for repeat coronary arteriograms because of symptoms to evaluate status of the bypass grafts. Results of stud-ies revealed patient grafts in all subjects (Table 11).

The actives, therefore, seemed to benefit from the rehabilita-tion program; however, was compliance with the program a signif-icant factor? It is concluded that it likely was based on certain available baseline data: The two groups were matched by presurgi-cal data. The groups had comparable numbers of significantly diseased coronary arteries, left ventricular wall contraction and end-diastolic pressure. According to operative notes, revascular-ization was considered complete in all cases. In addition, we evalu-ated post-surgical pre-exercise data by comparing entry treadmill tests for the rehabilitation program. These post-surgical treadmill test results were comparable in that there was no difference between the groups on treadmill testing with respect to duration time, ECG changes, arrhythmias, systolic blood pressure increase, or attained heart rate. Therefore, it was felt that the groups were comparable in degree of underlying cardiovascular disease.

All patients were medically stable and motivated to begin the rehabilitation program. Though it is possible that the reason for dropping out was due to physical or medical inability to continue, none of the drop-outs stated such as reasons. Although most had conflicts of time or distance given as reasons for dropping out, the true reasons are not clear and are likely multifactoral.

Based on these results, coronary bypass patients in a medically supervised program have greater oxygen consumption and exercise test duration, are more often at full working status, have less hospital readmissions, and are less likely to smoke. These data support benefits of coronary bypass patient compliance in an organized cardiac rehabilitation exercise program.

From another perspective, the Council on Scientific Affairs of the American Medical Associations has published a statement on physician-supervised exercise programs in rehabilitation of patients with coronary heart disease.[81] Conclusions stated are (quoted or paraphrased):

1. Exercise training can improve the objective and subjective rehabilitation of some patients with coronary heart disease and result in increased functional capacity.
2. Physician direction and supervision of exercise programs are critical to the proper assimilation of these services into the heart care system.
3. Exercise testing is important for prescribing and monitoring exercise rehabilitation programs in such patients and may provide prognostic information. Serial testing may help to individualize the length of the exercise program.
4. While rehabilitation programs appear to provide many subjective benefits to the cardiac patient, they have not yet been shown to improve survival.
5. Cardiac rehabilitation should be considered one of the treatments for coronary heart disease in addition to drug therapy or surgery.
6. Further studies that examine the long-term benefit of the different types of exercise programs are indicated.

Special Considerations in Rehabilitation

Arm and Weight Training

With the increasing use of various modalities in exercise training for both healthy subjects and cardiac patients, various interventions are now being used in cardiac patients that were not popular in previous times. Arm training has been more often used for coronary artery disease patients as done by Savin et al.[82] Their data were reported in ten coronary artery disease patients who were trained with arm training on a modified bicycle ergometer three times weekly for 15 minutes a day for 15 weeks. No complications occurred during the arm testing or arm training. They concluded arm training may be safely prescribed in coronary patients and that dynamic arm training increases capacity for dynamic arm effort but not for static arm effort. Increased capacity for dynamic arm effort caused ischemia in some patients probably because of an increased myocardial work load. Balady et al.[83] studied physiological differences between upper and lower extremity exercise testing in patients with coronary disease. They concluded that the differing physiological response to upper extremity and lower extremity exercise is likely due to size and conditioning of the exercising muscle groups. Myocardial oxygen demand appears to be greater during leg than upper extremity exercise despite similar rate pressure product. Schram et al.[88] used weighted walking as part of an exercise prescription for cardiac rehabilitation patients. This intervention was done in 13 patients with increases in oxygen consumption and heart rate with added weight load which were not related to initial body weight. The authors concluded that weight load walking may be used as an alternative mode of exercise training in most patients with low exercise capacity. Kelemen et al.[85] evaluated circuit weight training in 20 cardiac patients compared to 20 controls. The circuit weight training utilized a series of weight-lifting exercises with moderate load with frequent repetitions. The patients participated in a supervised cardiac rehabilitation program for a minimum of 3 months before the study. No sustained arrhythmias or cardiovascular problems occurred in the patients. The experimental group significantly increased treadmill time from 619 to 694 seconds, while the time of the control group did not change. Strength in the experimental group increased by an average of 24 percent with no change in the control patients. They concluded that circuit weight training appears to be safe and results in significant increases in aerobic endurance and musculoskeletal strength compared with traditional exercise used in cardiac rehabilitation programs.

It is therefore felt that various types of exercise (arm versus leg, weight walking, and circuit weight training) may be effectively used as adjuncts to exercise prescriptions in cardiac patients. The limited aforementioned studies reflect that this type of training is safe and perhaps beneficial. Experiences in our own programs are in accord with this, and this type of exercise training is utilized in addition to (and oftentimes in place of) the standard, dynamic training that has been traditionally employed.

Influence of Chronic Adrenergic Beta Blockade

Because of the widespread use of beta adrenergic blocking drugs in patients with cardiovascular disease, the question has been posed as to whether or not exercise training effects can be attained in such patients. A number of studies have been done to assess this and, in general, the results have been positive that patients can obtain the training effect with beta blockade.

Dressendorfer et al.[86] studied 88 coronary patients (71 on propranolol and 17 on no drugs). They found that the mean maximal oxygen consumption (VO_2 max) before and after training and changes in VO_2 max were similar between the groups. Laslett et al.[90] studied 37 coronary disease patients (16 on propranolol and 21 on no drugs). They found that all patients significantly increased their functional capacity in METs with training. Vanhees et al.[88] studied 29 subjects with ischemic heart disease (15 on beta blockers and 14 on no beta blockers). They found that all patients significantly increased their oxygen uptake with exercise training.

To determine whether a variety of cardioselective and nonselective beta-blocking agents impair exercise training effects in patients with cardiovascular disease, 50 subjects were evaluated in the Emory University program.[89] All were in a three times weekly medically supervised outpatient program for 3 months or longer. Treadmill exercise tests were done initially and at 3-month intervals. Eight patients were receiving atenolol, 23 propranolol, three timolol, six metoprolol, and eight nadolol. One patient receiving timolol changed to atenolol and one receiving nadolol changed to propranolol during their training period. Treadmill test duration increased significantly ($p < 0.05$), from 7.5 ± 2.5 to 9.9 ± 2.3 minutes, with exercise training. In 35 of the 50 subjects heart rate at rest decreased significantly ($p < 0.05$) from 67.5 ± 11.7 to 60.4 ± 10.5 beats/min. The other 15 subjects were excluded from heart rate analysis because beta blockade was begun 1 to 2 weeks after the initial exercise test. It was concluded that exercise training effects (increase in exercise test duration and decrease in resting heart rate) can be achieved in patients with cardiovascular disease in the presence of both cardioselective and nonselective beta-blocking agents.

In summary, patients with cardiovascular disease can most likely become "trained" on beta blockade. Sometimes there are problems with mental depression or cardiovascular limitation on very high doses of beta blockade. These circumstances, however, are relatively unusual and in most clinical instances beta-blocking drugs may be utilized in exercise training programs without problems.

Exercise Training in Left Ventricular Dysfunction

With the evolution of the use of exercise in the prevention and management of cardiovascular disease, programs have begun to incorporate a number of types of patients. In accord with this, the more liberal utilization of exercise in subjects with coronary disease has permitted referral of patients with left ventricular dysfunction. In the past, there has been considerable concern about this type of patient and potential problems that may be precipitated by exercise. However, there are recent data to suggest (and experience of our own) that patients with some degree of left ventricular dysfunction may be "exercise trained" without difficulty.

One study of endurance training in rats with chronic heart failure clearly supports the positive effect of exercise in heart failure. In this study, Musch et al.[90] sham-operated 20 rats (11 sedentary, nine exercise trained) and induced myocardial infarction with resultant heart failure in 22 rats (11 sedentary and 11 exercise trained). After the training period of 10 to 12 weeks, of treadmill running at a 10 percent grade, at 20 m/min. for 60 min/day for 5 days/week, they found the following:

	Mean VO$_2$max (ml/kg^{-1}/min^{-1})
Sham-Operated Rats	
Sedentary (n = 11)	57 ± 1
Trained (n = 9)	67 ± 1 (p < 0.05)
Myocardial Infarction Rats	
Sedentary (n = 11)	52 ± 1
Trained (n = 11)	59 ± 1 (p < 0.05)

Therefore, in this animal study, experimental infarction with associated heart failure does not impair the training capability of the animal as evidenced by the improvement in mean VO$_2$max. One shortcoming of the study, however, is the lack of clarity with regard to the exact degree of left ventricular dysfunction that resulted from the experimental infarction.

In humans, Litchfield et al.[91] have reported on the preservation of exercise capacity despite severe left ventricular dysfunction. These authors found that 32 percent of patients with severe left ventricular dysfunction have normal exercise capacity. Paumer et al.[92] reported the benefits of exercise training in relation to left ventricular function in 28 patients with coronary artery disease. Several of these patients had left ventricular ejection fractions of less than 40 percent. However, even these patients showed benefits in exercise testing, thus suggesting that training programs can afford beneficial effects in functional capacity and submaximal heart rate even in patients with depressed left ventricular function. Lickoff[93] reported on patients with chronic congestive heart failure and potential benefits from a physical conditioning program. They found that in all their groups, the magnitude of change in exercise testing duration greatly exceeded the change in VO$_2$max after the training program. They concluded that patients with chronic heart failure can benefit from physical conditioning through several possible mechanisms. These changes may occur by increase in muscle recruitment, use of increased numbers of muscle motor units, enhanced joint flexibility, and factors other than the role of the left ventricle per se. A recent study by Ehsani et al.[94] is encouraging, though not conclusive, regarding improvement of left ventricular contractile function by exercise training in patients with coronary artery disease. In this study, 25 patients completed a 12-month endurance exercise training program and were compared to 14 who did not exercise. Maximal attainable VO$_2$ increased by 37% (p < 0.001). Of ten patients with effort angina, eight had less or no angina. Ejection fraction increased with maximal exercise from 52 to 58 ± 3% (p < 0.01) after training. The results, therefore, revealed that exercise training can cause an improvement in left ventricular function independent of cardiac loading conditions in some patients with coronary disease. The authors feel that this improvement is likely due to improved oxygenation of some underperfused region of the myocardium.

Therefore it is felt that the presence of an abnormal left ventricle does not necessarily prohibit the improvement of physical conditioning in patients with coronary disease. This probably reflects the fact that physical conditioning is actually more of a peripheral alteration through improvement of pulmonary capacity, skeletal muscle capacity, improved arteriovenous oxygen difference and that the myocardial alterations per se are only a small part of the conditioning process.

THE PEDIATRIC PATIENT

Data in cardiac rehabilitation in this population is limited and primarily confined to that in subjects after correction of congenital heart disease defects. Bradley et al.[98] did monitored aerobic training in 11 patients who had undergone repair of transposition of the great arteries or tetralogy of Fallot. Their results were similar to others and revealed no change in heart rate or ventilation after training but subjects did improve systolic blood pressure, treadmill time, and oxygen consumption. They felt that such programs can improve aerobic conditioning of young children even in the presence of moderate hemodynamic and electrophysiologic residual disturbance from their intrinsic cardiac problem. Therefore cardiac rehabilitation is feasible in the pediatric population though data is limited at this time.

Therefore, rehabilitative exercise activities are becoming more widespread in use in our population and, in addition, address many subjects of coronary artery disease. As emphasized previously, proper exercise with appropriate integral medical supervision testing is of utmost importance in assuring safety and proper follow-up of all subjects involved in such activities.

REFERENCES

1. Kloner RA, Kloner JA: The effect of early exercise on myocardial infarct scar formation. *Am Heart J* 1983; 106:1009–1013.
2. Hochman JS, Healy B: Effect of exercise on acute myocardial infarction in rats. *JACC* 1986; 7:126–132.
3. Musch TI, Moore RL, Zelis R: Beneficial effects of exercise training in the rat model of chronic heart failure. *Circulation* (Abstr) 1985; 3:(Suppl) 72:III–256.
4. Levine SA, Brown DL: Coronary thrombosis: Its various clinical features. *Medicine* 1929; 8:245–418.
5. Coe WS: Cardiac work and the chair treatment of acute coronary thrombosis. *Ann Intern Med* 1954; 40:42–48.
6. Mather HG, Pearson NG, Read KL, et al: Acute myocardial infarction: home and hospital treatment. *Br Med J* 1971; 3:334–338.
7. Wenger NK, Hellerstein HK, Blackburn H, et al: Uncomplicated myocardial infarction, current physician practice in patient management. *JAMA* 1973; 224:511–514.
8. Rose G: Early mobilization and discharge after myocardial infarction. *Mod Concepts Cardiovasc Dis* 1972; 41:59–63.
9. Levine SA, Lown B: Armchair treatment of acute coronary thrombosis. *JAMA* 1952; 148:1365–1369.
10. Fareeduddin K, Abelmann WH: Impaired orthostatic tolerance after bed rest in patients with myocardial infarction. *N Engl J Med* 1969; 280:345–350.
11. Saltin B, Blomqvist G, Mitchell JH, et al: Response to exercise after bed rest and after training. *Circulation* 1968; 38(Suppl) 7:1–78.
12. Adgey AAJ: Prognosis after early discharge from hospital of patients with acute myocardial infarction. *Br Heart J* 1969; 31:750–752.
13. Takkunen J, Huhti E, Oilinki O, et al: Early ambulation in myocardial infarction. *Acta Med Scand* 1970; 188:103–106.
14. Tucker HH, Carson PHM, Bass NM, et al: Results of early mobilization and discharge after myocardial infarction. *Br Med J* 1973; 1:10–13.
15. Harpur JE, Conner WT, Hamilton M, et al: Controlled trial of early mobilization and discharge from hospital in uncomplicated myocardial infarction. *Lancet* 1971; 2:1331–1334.
16. Hutter AM, Sidel VW, Shine KI, et al: Early hospital discharge after myocardial infarction. *N Engl J Med* 1973; 288:1141–1144.
17. Bloch A, Maeder JP, Haissly JC, et al: Early mobilization after myocardial infarction. *Am J Cardiol* 1974; 34:152–157.
18. Abraham AS, Sever Y, Weinstein M, et al: Value of early ambulation in patients with and without complications after acute myocardial infarction. *N Engl J Med* 1975; 292:719–722.
19. McNeer JF, Wallace AG, Wagner GS, et al: The course of acute myocardial infarction, feasibility of early discharge of the uncomplicated patient. *Circulation* 1975; 51:410–413.

20. Chaturvedi NC, Walsh MJ, Evans A, et al: Selection of patients for early discharge after acute myocardial infarction. *Br Heart J* 1974; 36:533–535.
21. Swann HJC, Blackburn HW, De Sanctis R, et al: Duration of hospitalization in "uncomplicated completed acute myocardial infarction." *Am J Cardiol* 1976; 37:413–419.
22. Wenger NK: Physical activity, exercise testing, and exercise training programs for patients with myocardial infarction: The state of our knowledge. *Acta Cardiol* 1973; 28:33–37.
23. Browse NL: Effect of bed rest on resting calf blood flow of healthy adult males. *Br Med J* 1962; 1:1721–1723.
24. Makin GS, Mayes FB, Holroyd AM: Studies on the effect of "Tubigrip" on flow in the deep veins of the calf. *Br J Surg* 1969; 56:369–372.
25. Rosengarten DS, Laird J, Jeyasingh K, et al: The failure of compression stockings (Tubigrip) to prevent deep venous thrombosis after operation. *Br J Surg* 1970; 57:296–299.
26. Kakkar VV, Corrigan T, Spindler J, et al: Efficacy of low doses of heparin in prevention of deep vein thrombosis after major surgery: double-blind, randomized trial. *Lancet* 1972; 2:101–106.
27. Handley AJ: Low-dose heparin after myocardial infarction. *Lancet* 1972; 2:623–624.
28. Wray R, Maurer B, Shillingford J: Prophylactic anticoagulant therapy in the prevention of calf-vein thrombosis after myocardial infarction. *N Engl J Med* 1973; 288:815–817.
29. Hellerstein HK, Friedman EH: Sexual activity and the post-coronary patient. *Arch Intern Med* 1970; 125:987–999.
30. Johnston BL, Watt EW, Fletcher GF: Oxygen consumption and hemodynamic and electrocardiographic responses to bathing in recent post myocardial infarction patients. *Heart and Lung* 1981; 10:666–671.
31. Johnston BL, Cantwell JD, Fletcher GF: Eight steps to patient cardiac rehabilitation: The team effort methodology and preliminary results. *Heart and Lung* 1976; 5:97–111.
32. Matsuda M, Matsuda Y, Ogawa H, Moritani K, Kusukawa R: Angina pectoris before and during acute myocardial infarction: Relation to degree of physical activity. *Am J Cardiol* 1985; 55: 1255–1258.
33. Magder S: Assessment of myocardial stress from early ambulatory activities following myocardial infarction. *Chest* 1985; 87:442–447.
34. Pryor DB, Hindman MC, Wagner GS, Calif RM, Rhoads MK, Rosati RA: Early discharge after acute myocardial infarction. *Ann Intern Med* 1983; 99:528–538.
35. Eyherabide A, Bruskewitz E, Stevens R, Hanson P: Predischarge monitored exercise following coronary surgery. *Circulation* (Abstr) 1983; 68:III–123.
36. Hellerstein HK: The effects of physical activity: patients and normal coronary-prone subjects. *Minn Med* 1969; 52:1335–1341.
37. Gottheiner V: Long-range strenuous sports training for cardiac reconditioning and rehabilitation. *Am J Cardiol* 1968; 22:426–435.

38. Rechnitzer PA, Pickard HA, Paivio AU, et al: Long-term follow-up study of survival and recurrence rates following myocardial infarction in exercising and control subjects. *Circulation* 1972; 45:853–857.
39. Kennedy CC, Spiekerman RE, Lindsey MI, et al: Evaluation of a one-year graduated exercise program for men with angina pectoris by physiologic studies and coronary arteriography. *Am J Cardiol* (Abstr) 1973; 31:141.
40. Kentala E: Physical fitness and feasibility of physical rehabilitation after myocardial infarction in men of working age. *Ann Clin Res* 1972; 4:(Suppl) 9:1–84.
41. Wilhelmsen L, Sanne H, Elmfeldt D, et al: A controlled trial of physical training after myocardial infarction: effects on risk factors, non-fatal reinfarction, and death. *Prevent Med* 1975; 4:491–508.
42. Wasserman AG, Gorman PA, Leiboff R, Ross AM, Rios JC: Characteristics of exercise performance in men with previous myocardial infarction: (Non) influence of infarct location. *Am J Cardiol* (Abstr) 1980; 45:391.
43. Laslett LJ, Paumer L, Amsterdam EA: Increase in myocardial oxygen consumption indexes by exercise training at onset of ischemia in patients with coronary artery disease. *Circulation* 1985; 71: 958–962.
44. Hammond HK, Kelly TL, Froelicher VF, Pewen W: Use of clinical data in predicting improvement in exercise capacity after cardiac rehabilitation. *J Am Coll Cardiol* 1985; 6:19–26.
45. Grant VSP, Wilkinson W, Czekaj LM, Katz RI, Weintraub WS, Helfant RH: Benefits of supervised exercise early after myocardial revascularization. *Chest* (Abstr) 1983; 83:362.
46. Stevens R, Hanson P: Comparison of supervised and unsupervised exercise training after coronary bypass surgery. *Am J Cardiol* 1984; 53:1524–1528.
47. Fletcher GF, Chiaramida AJ, LeMay MR, Johnston BL, Thiel JE, Spratlin MC: Telephonically-monitored home exercise early after coronary artery bypass surgery. *Chest* 1984; 86:198–202.
48. Miller NH, Haskell WL, Berra K, DeBusk RF: Home versus group exercise training for increasing functional capacity after myocardial infarction. *Circulation* 1984; 70:645–649.
49. Fletcher BJ, Thiel J, Fletcher GF: Phase II intensive monitored cardiac rehabilitation for coronary artery disease and coronary risk factors—a six-session protocol. *Am J Cardiol* 1986; 57:751–756.
50. Cantwell JD, Fletcher GF: Instant electrocardiography, use in cardiac exercise programs. *Circulation* 1974; 50:962–966.
51. Bruce EH, Frederick R, Bruce RA, et al: Comparison of active participants and dropouts in CAPRI cardiopulmonary rehabilitation programs. *Am J Cardiol* 1976; 37:53–60.
52. Fletcher GF, Cantwell JD: Outpatient gym exercise and risk factor modification for patients with recent myocardial infarction: Methodology and results in a community program. *J Louisiana State Med Soc* 1975; 127:52–57.
53. Watt EW, Wiley J, Fletcher GF: Effect of dietary control and exer-

cise training on daily food intake and serum lipids in postmyocardial infarction patients. *Am J Clin Nutr* 1976; 29:900−904.

54. Vetrovec GW, Parker G: Exercise training of moderate intensity raising high density lipoprotein cholesterol in cardiac patients. *Clin Res* (Abstr) 1981; 29:247A.

55. Vyden JK, O'Connor L, Kanazawa M, Rose HB: Effect of physical conditioning on serum lipids in patients with type IV hyperlipoproteinemia and ischemic heart disease. *Clin Res* (Abstr) 1981; 29:248A.

56. Fletcher GF, Cantwell JD: Continuous ambulatory electrocardiographic monitoring: use in cardiac exercise programs. *Chest* 1977; 71:27−32.

57. Plantholt S, Gillilan R, Kennedy H, Kalaria D, Ruffier J: Usefulness of Holter recording in evaluating patient performance in a prescription exercise program. *Clin Res* (Abstr) 1981; 29:231A.

58. Lillis D, Hanson P: Ambulatory ECG monitoring in cardiac rehabilitation patients on exercise training days and control days. *Circulation* (Abstr) 1985; 3:(Suppl) 72:III−342.

59. Kitamura K, Jorgensen CR, Gogel FL, Taylor HL, Wang Y: Hemodynamic correlates of myocardial oxygen consumption during upright exercise. *J Appl Physiol* 1972; 32:516−522.

60. Fletcher GF, Cantwell JD, Watt EW: Oxygen consumption and hemodynamic response of exercises used in training of patients with recent myocardial infarction. *Circulation* 1979; 60:140−144.

61. Kennedy TF: Report on an investigation of energy expended on the exercises of the physical training tables for recruits of all arms. *J R Army Med Corps* 1933; 3:1.

62. Keatinge WR, Evans M: The respiratory and cardiovascular response to immersion in cold and warm water. *Q J Exp Physiol* 1961; 46:83−94.

63. Faulkner JA: Physiology of swimming. *Res Quart Amer Assoc Health Phys Educ* 1966; 37:41−54.

64. Andersen KL: Energy cost of swimming. *Acta Clin Scand* 1960; 253:169.

65. Johnston BL, Cantwell JD, Fletcher GF: Sexual activity in exercising patients after myocardial infarction and revascularization. *Heart and Lung* 1978; 7:1026−1031.

66. Green AW: Sexual activity and the post-myocardial infarction patient. *Am Heart J* 1975; 89:246−252.

67. Tuttle WB, Cook L, Fitcher E: Sexual behavior in post-myocardial infarction patients. *Am J Cardiol* 1964; 13:64.

68. Block A, Maedor JP, Haissley JC: Sexual problems after myocardial infarction. *Am Heart J* 1975; 90:536−537.

69. Johnston BL, Fletcher GF: Dynamic electrocardiographic recording during sexual activity in recent post-myocardial infarction and revascularization patients. *Am Heart J* 1979; 98:736−741.

70. Stein RA: The effect of exercise training on heart rate during coitus in the post-myocardial infarction patient. *Circulation* 1977; 55:738−740.

71. Coronary Drug Project Research Group. Prognostic importance of

premature beats following myocardial infarction. *JAMA* 1973; 223:1116–1124.

72. Shaw LW: Effects of prescribed supervised exercise program on mortality and cardiovascular morbidity in patients after a myocardial infarction. The national exercise and heart disease project. *Am J Cardiol* 1981; 48:39–46.

73. Erb BD, Fletcher GF, Sheffield LT: Standards for cardiovascular exercise treatment programs. *Circulation* 1979; 59:1084A–1089A.

74. Erb BD, Fletcher GF, Sheffield LT: Standards for supervised cardiovascular exercise maintenance programs. *Circulation* 1980; 62:669A–673A.

75. Jensen D, Atwood JE, Froelicher V, McKirnan MD, et al: Improvement in ventricular function during exercise studied with radionuclide ventriculography after cardiac rehabilitation. *Am J Cardiol* 1980; 46:770–777.

76. Jackson F, Hensel P, Morganroth J: Cardiac rehabilitation: natural history and physiologic cardiac changes. *Clin Res* (Abstr) 1979; 27:176A.

77. Superko HR: Effects of cardiac rehabilitation in permanently paced patients with third degree heart block. *J Cardiol Rehabilitation* 1983; 3:561–568.

78. Ritter WS, Neuner GM, Fiore JP: Sustained cardiac conditioning and improvement in angina following cardiac rehabilitation. *Clin Res* (Abstr) 1980; 28:813A.

79. Hertanu JS, Davis L, Focseneanu M, Lahman L: Cardiac rehabilitation exercise program: outcome assessment. *Arch Phys Med Rehabil* 1986; 67:431–435.

80. Waites TF, Watt EW, Fletcher GF: Comparative functional and physiologic status of active and dropout coronary bypass patients of a rehabilitation program. *Am J Cardiol* 1983; 51:1087–1091.

81. Council on Scientific Affairs. Physician-supervised exercise programs in rehabilitation of patients with coronary heart disease. *JAMA* 1981; 245:1465–1466.

82. Savin W, Berra K, Houston N, Doucette J, DeBusk R, Haskell W: Effects of arm training in coronary artery disease patients. *Circulation* (Abstr) 1981; 64:IV–83.

83. Balady GJ, Weiner DA, McCabe CH, Cutler SS, Dagostino G, Ryan TJ: Physiological differences between upper and lower extremity exercise testing in patients with coronary disease. *Clin Res* (Abstr) 1984; 32:149A.

84. Schram VG, Hanson P: Exercise prescription for cardiac rehabilitation patients using weighted walking. *Circulation* (Abstr) 1985; 72:III–39.

85. Kelemen MH, Stewart KJ, Gillilan RE, Ewart CK, Valenti SA, Manley JD, Kelemen MD: Circuit weight training in cardiac patients. *J Am Coll Cardiol* 1986; 7:38–42.

86. Dressendorfer R, Smith J, Gordon S, Timmis G: Improved maximal oxygen uptake during phase 2 cardiac rehabilitation is independent of beta-blockade therapy. *JACC* (Abstr) 1984; 3:500.

87. Laslett L, Paumer L, Baier P, Amsterdam E, Foerster J: Exercise

training efficacy is not affected by propranolol administration in coronary patients. *Am J Cardiol* (Abstr) 1982; 50:1000.

88. Vanhees L, Fagard R, Amery A: Influence of beta-adrenergic blockade on the hemodynamic effects of physical training in patients with ischemic heart disease. *Am Heart J* 1984; 108:270–275.

89 Fletcher GF: Exercise training during chronic beta blockade in cardiovascular disease. *Am J Cardiol* 1985; 55:110D–113D.

90. Musch TI, Moore RL, Leathers DJ, et al: Endurance training in rats with chronic heart failure induced by myocardial infarction. *Circulation* 1986; 74:431–441.

91. Litchfield RL, Kerber RE, Benge JW, et al: Normal exercise capacity in patients with severe left ventricular dysfunction: compensatory mechanisms. *Circulation* 1982; 66:129–134.

92. Paumer L, Laslett LJ, Amsterdam EA: Benefits of exercise training in relation to left ventricular function. *Circulation* (Abstr) 1985; 72:III–267.

93. Likoff MJ, Hare T, Gumbardo D, Chadwick B: An assessment of the response in oxygen uptake and exercise duration in patients with chronic cardiac failure. *Heart Failure* 1986; August/September: 164–175.

94. Ehsani AA, Biello DR, Schultz J, et al: Improvement of left ventricular contractile function by exercise training in patients with coronary artery disease. *Circulation* 1986; 74:350–358.

95. Bradley LM, Galioto FM, Jr., Vaccaro P, Hansen DA, Vaccaro J: Effect of intense aerobic training on exercise performance in children after surgical repair of tetralogy of Fallot or complete transposition of the great arteries. *Am J Cardiol* 1985; 56:816–818.

96. Kallio V, Hamalainen H, Hakkila J, Luurila O, et al: Reduction in sudden deaths by a multifactorial intervention program after acute myocardial infarction. *Lancet* 1979; 2:1091–1094.

97. Rechnitzer PA, et al: The effects of training: reinfarction and death: An interim report. *Med Sci Sports Exercise* 1979; 2:381.

98. Vermeulen, Lie KI, Durrer D: et al: Effects of cardiac rehabilitation after myocardial infarction: changes in coronary risk factors and long-term prognosis. *Am Heart J* 1983; 105(5):798.

99. Kellerman JJ, Ben-Ari E, Fisman EZ, Pines A, Peled B, Drory Y: Benefits of long-term physical training in patients after coronary artery bypass grafting—58-month follow-up and comparison with a nontrained group. *J Cardiopulmonary Rehabil* 1986; 6:165–170.

6

Exercise in Pulmonary Disease

Jonne B. Walter, M.D.

INTRODUCTION

Although this section will review pulmonary response to exercise in health and several common diseases, it should be kept in mind that exercise involves the integration of complex neurologic, psychiatric, circulatory, respiratory, and muscular mechanisms (Fig. 1). Pulmonary responses cannot be viewed in isolation in a patient with exertional dyspnea. Therefore, the first part of this chapter will consider primarily normal cardiopulmonary response to exercise. Excellent reviews and textbooks are available which cover physiologic and metabolic effects of conditioning and exercise in detail.[1-12]

Since cardiovascular exercise response is discussed in depth elsewhere, only a superficial review important to understanding cardiopulmonary interactions will be presented in the section on oxygen delivery. Pulmonary ventilation, gas exchange and drive will be discussed under pulmonary responses. The second part will review pulmonary exercise testing strategies, measurements, and a few of the settings in which this kind of data is clinically useful.

From: Fletcher GF: *Exercise in the Practice of Medicine,* 2nd Revised Edition. Mount Kisco, NY, Futura Publishing Co., Inc., © 1988.

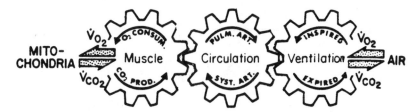

Figure 1: Schematic representation of the essential elements in gas exchange between the cell mitochondria and the external environment. During exercise, the oxygen consumption ($\dot{V}O_2$) and CO_2 production ($\dot{V}CO_2$) depend on the metabolic rate of the muscles. The interconnecting gears denote the precise coupling of circulatory and ventilatory mechanisms to muscle metabolism. (From Wasserman K: Breathing during exercise. *N Engl J Med* 1978; 298:780. Used by permission.)

CARDIOVASCULAR RESPONSE

Oxygen Delivery

The chief energy source for exercise is oxidation of dietary substrate in mitochondria of the exercising muscles. The added oxygen demand is met by increased O_2 transport and increased O_2 extraction by the muscles. The increased O_2 transport is achieved by elevation of the cardiac output and *minute ventilation* proportional to the work intensity. Cardiac output is determined by the product of stroke volume and heart rate, and since stroke volume increases only modestly, the increase in heart rate accounts for most of the augmented cardiac output. A recognized linear relationship exists between heart rate and cardiac output, oxygen consumption ($\dot{V}O_2$), and work load[4,13] (Fig. 2). A useful index of stroke volume easily obtained from a gas exchange study is the oxygen pulse defined as the ratio of heart rate observed to $\dot{V}O_2$. This relationship is derived from the Fick equation:

The oxygen pulse

$$Qt = SV \times fc = \frac{\dot{V}O_2}{CaO_2 - C\dot{V}O_2} \text{ (Fick's principle)}$$

Rearranging: "O_2 pulse" $= \dfrac{\dot{V}O_2}{fc} = SV (CaO_2 - C\dot{V}O_2)$

Qt = total or cardiac output, SV = stroke volume,

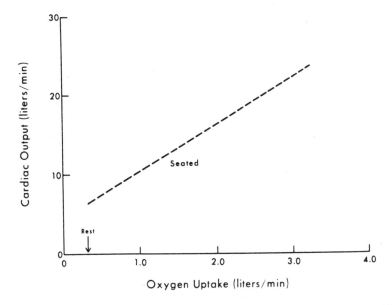

Figure 2: The relationship of oxygen consumption to cardiac output with exercise.

fc = heart rate, CaO_2 = arterial O_2 content, $C\dot{V}O_2$ = mixed venous O_2 content.
A low stroke volume is usually associated with a low oxygen pulse. Deconditioning may result in low stroke volume and oxygen pulse values which overlap those seen in heart disease[14] and a rapid heart rate will result.

Patients whose exercise is limited by pulmonary ventilation, unless markedly deconditioned, will have a normal O_2 pulse—a useful diagnostic measure when considered with all the exercise data. Chronic exercise training improves stroke volume, capillary and mitochondria density in muscle, leading to increased oxygen consumption and work capacity at lower cardiac output and heart rate.[7,15] Exercise cardiac output and maximal heart rate decrease with age, accounting for the reduced exercise capacity with age.[16]

Exercise is said to be at "steady state" when O_2 delivery and ventilation precisely match O_2 demand and CO_2 production ($\dot{V}CO_2$). Steady state exercise below 50 or 60 percent of maximal O_2

consumption can be continued for long periods. When O_2 delivery lags behind metabolic demand, anaerobic metabolism can sustain work only briefly. Anaerobic metabolism occurs during the first minute or two of moderate work, until the circulatory and ventilatory adjustments have time to balance O_2 need, and also at heavy work loads beyond about 60 percent of maximal O_2 uptake when O_2 transport is inadequate to meet the metabolic demand. As lactate is the product of anaerobic metabolism, its accumulation causes metabolic acidosis during exercise and "points" to the onset of anaerobic metabolism. The level of work or oxygen consumption ($\dot{V}O_2$) at which this "anaerobic threshold"[17] appears is a function of the oxygen delivery system and therefore is influenced by training and degree of heart disease. Elevation of the blood lactate level is known to occur at lower work rates in patients with heart disease and sedentary habits—two conditions associated with a lower cardiac output than in trained subjects[1,18,19] (Fig. 3). Elevated lactate leads to greatly increased minute ventilation

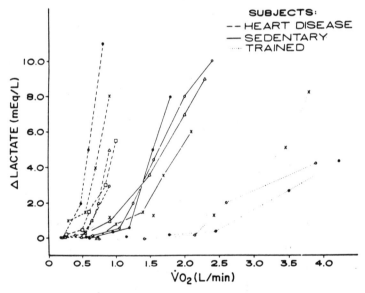

Figure 3: Change in lactate concentration during graded exercise in patients with cardiac disease (primarily mitral valve disease), sedentary subjects, and trained normal subject. (From Wasserman K, Whipp BJ: Exercise physiology in health and disease. *Am Rev Resp Dis* 1975; 112:219–249. Used by permission.)

($\dot{V}E$) and $\dot{V}CO_2$ which is easy to recognize on a plot of $\dot{V}E$, $\dot{V}CO_2$, $\dot{V}O_2$ (Fig. 4).

In normal individuals, the major limitation to oxygen delivery

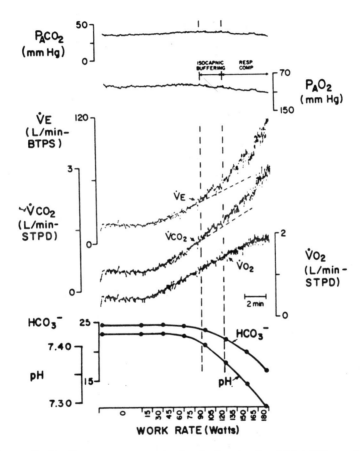

Figure 4: Continuous measurements of alveolar (end-tidal CO_2 and O_2 tension [$PaCO_2$ and PaO_2]), minute ventilation $\dot{V}E$), CO_2 production ($\dot{V}CO_2$), O_2 consumption ($\dot{V}O_2$), arterial bicarbonate (HCO_3) and pH for a one-minute incremental work test on a cycle ergometer in a 43-year-old male subject. "Isocapnic buffering" refers to the period when $\dot{V}E$ and $\dot{V}CO_2$ increase curvilinearly at the same rate, thus reflecting a constant $PaCO_2$. After the period of isocapnic buffering, $PaCO_2$ decreases, reflecting respiratory compensation for the metabolic acidosis of exercise. (From Wasserman K, Whipp BJ: Exercise physiology in health and disease. *Am Rev Resp Dis* 1975; 112:219–249. Used by permission.)

and aerobic work is not pulmonary ventilation but cardiac output, peripheral distribution of blood flow, and mitochondrial density in working muscles.

PULMONARY RESPONSES

Pattern of Breathing

At low or moderate work rates, increased ventilation is due mainly to an increased tidal volume, the respiratory rate increasing to a lesser extent. Tidal volume increases to about 60 percent of the vital capacity at heavy work, beyond which minute ventilation is augmented by an increased breathing frequency. Respiratory rate in normal people varies with age and lung size, is higher in children than in adults, and higher in untrained than in fit subjects. Young adults have a maximum respiratory rate of about 40−45 per minute. Respiratory rate is affected by many other factors including physiological dead space, central and chemoreceptor drive, pain, and other central factors such as anxiety. During bicycle ergometry, it has been noted that breathing frequency may adopt a pattern related to pedaling frequency, increasing stepwise almost as if in a rhythm. The accessory muscles of ventilation are recruited when $\dot{V}E$ exceeds about 30 l/min or when tidal volume is large, thereby increasing the energy expenditure or "oxygen cost" of breathing. At heavy work the oxygen cost of breathing may increase from a resting level of 2 to 10−15 percent of total $\dot{V}O_2$.[20] Milic-Emili demonstrated in 1960 that normal subjects will adopt a breathing pattern that accomplishes the greatest alveolar ventilation for the least energy expense.[21] Respiratory muscle fatigue may contribute to dyspnea at high work loads.[22] Recent evidence has shown that respiratory muscles, like skeletal muscles, can be trained in normal individuals[23−25] and in patients with chronic obstructive lung disease,[16,26,27] quadriplegia,[28] and cystic fibrosis.[29] These findings have renewed interest in training as a form of therapy in these conditions, and stimulated much new thinking about the physiology of the respiratory muscles[25] and their contribution to respiratory failure. It is likely that "fitness" of the respiratory as well as skeletal muscles contributes to the lower breathing frequency in trained subjects. Slow, deep breathing minimizes dead space ventilation, enhances alveolar ventilation, and has a beneficial effect on gas exchange as seen in the example below:

	$\dot{V}E$	Rate	VT	$\dot{V}D/VT$	$\dot{V}D$	$\dot{V}A$
(1)	10 l/min	40	250	0.6	6.01	4.01
(2)	10 l/min	20	500	0.3	3.01	6.01
(3)	10 l/min	10	1000	0.15	1.51	8.51

Breathing pattern can alter alveolar ventilation ($\dot{V}A$) and therefore gas exchange. Rapid shallow breathing increases $\dot{V}D/VT$, reduces alveolar ventilation and CO_2 elimination, resulting in a higher arterial CO_2 tension. If CO_2 production were the same in each of the examples, arterial pCO_2 would be highest in (1) and lowest in (3) by the alveolar ventilation equation:

$$\dot{V}A = \frac{\dot{V}CO_2}{PaCO_2}$$

$\dot{V}E$ = minute ventilation, VT = tidal volume
$\dot{V}D$ = physiological dead space

Exercise minute ventilation ($\dot{V}E$) and alveolar ventilation ($\dot{V}A$) increase proportionally to $\dot{V}O_2$ and $\dot{V}CO_2$ up to about four times the resting level of 60 percent of the maximal oxygen intake ($\dot{V}O_2$ max), (Fig. 4). When anaerobic metabolism further stimulates ventilation out of proportion to $\dot{V}O_2$, the buffering of lactate to CO_2 increases $\dot{V}CO_2$ and appears to stimulate drive centrally by metabolic acidosis. Animal studies suggest the possibility that CO_2 receptors in right heart, pulmonary vessels, or alveolar tissue may contribute to respiratory drive.[30]

Normal values for minute ventilation in the linear portion of the curve relating $\dot{V}E$ to $\dot{V}O_2$ (Figs. 5A, B) have been expressed by Jones et al.,[31] but the variation is wide and the age and activity level of the subjects not defined. According to Jones,[31] the ventilatory volumes in the linear portion of the $\dot{V}E/\dot{V}O_2$ or $\dot{V}CO_2$ curve are expressed by $\dot{V}E$ = 4.54 + 0.0221 $\dot{V}CO_2$ (SD 2.5). $\dot{V}E$ is expressed in l/min BTPS* and $\dot{V}CO_2$ in ml/min STPD†. The wide normal variation is probably related to the difference in individual ventilatory responsiveness to CO_2.[32] Physiologic dead space is small in normal subjects, adding little to anatomic dead space (about 1 cc/l lb) and is included in Jones' formula above, since

---

* = Body temperature press standard.
† = Standard temperature, pressure dry.

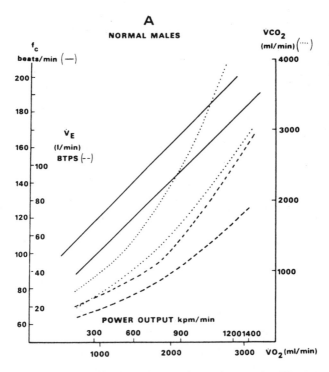

Figure 5: Normal values for Jones' stage I exercise test for (A) adult males, and (B) adult females. The boundaries represent ± standard deviation from the mean values at each power output. (From Jones NJ, et al: *Clinical Exercise Testing*. WB Saunders 1975. Used by permission.)

minute ventilation equals the sum of physiologic dead space ventilation and alveolar ventilation.

The maximum voluntary ventilation ($MV\dot{V}$) at rest is also used to predict maximum exercise ventilation. $MV\dot{V}$ is best measured directly for 12 to 15 seconds with a spirometer, but has been estimated from the product of the $FE\dot{V}_1 \times 35$.[33] In normal people, the end point of exercise is reached at 70 percent of the $MV\dot{V}$, again reflecting that ventilation does not limit exercise in normal individuals.[34]

Any ventilatory stimulus such as hypoxemia, metabolic acidosis, or idiopathic hyperventilation may elevate $\dot{V}E$ out of proportion to that needed for CO_2 elimination. Conversely, $\dot{V}E$ may be lower than expected in some disease states because chemoreceptors lose sensitivity to arterial CO_2 tension, or pulmonary me-

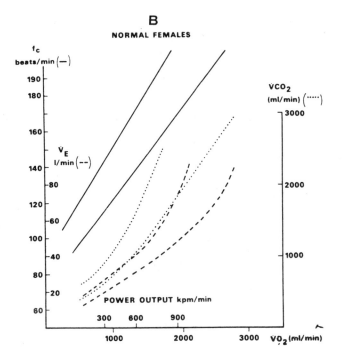

Figure 5B.

chanics are so impaired as to be incapable of response appropriate to the stimulus resulting in hypercapnea. These responses to alteration in respiratory drive cannot be estimated from studies at rest, but may become important factors limiting exercise potential.

Carbon Dioxide Clearance (R, Alveolar Ventilation, Physiological Dead Space)

Carbon dioxide production by the exercising muscle is related to oxygen consumption by the respiratory exchange ratio, R.

R equals the ratio of CO_2 produced to O_2 consumed ($R = \dfrac{\dot{V}CO_2}{\dot{V}O_2}$)

Its value depends on the mixture of fat or carbohydrate fuel substrate being metabolized. An average American diet results in an R of 0.8 to 0.9 both at rest and exercise below anaerobic threshold.

Hughson and Kowalchuk[35] showed that a low carbohydrate diet lowered exercise metabolism, indicating a higher contribution of fat relative to carbohydrate metabolism at exercise in their subjects. The high carbohydrate in central hyperalimentation formulae can increase R to 1.0 or above, thereby also increasing the CO_2 burden for pulmonary ventilation and occasionally leading to frank respiratory failure in ill patients. At heavy work the lactate buffering increases CO_2 production beyond that anticipated from substrate utilization as discussed above and the R rises, often exceeding 1.0. Hyperventilation also increases R by "blowing off" CO_2 at a rate exceeding metabolic production, resulting in respiratory alkalosis and an R of 1.0 or more.

The amount of ventilation required for CO_2 elimination depends on CO_2 production and the resulting concentration of CO_2 in alveolar gas, the proportion of "wasted" or dead space ventilation to alveolar ventilation ($\dot{V}D/\dot{V}T$ ratio), and the arterial pCO_2 to which the respiratory control mechanisms adjust ventilation.[32,36]

$\dot{V}CO_2$ increases proportionally to alveolar ventilation and work load below anaerobic threshold as the product of oxidative metabolism, and increases greatly during anaerobic metabolism apparently as lactate is buffered to CO_2 by the bicarbonate buffer system.

The alveolar ventilation is that volume of inspirate which reaches perfused terminal alveolar units and takes part in gas exchange. About one-third of each tidal volume inspired remains in the conducting airways (anatomic dead space) or is distributed to alveoli such as those at the pulmonary apex which are ventilated but not perfused (alveolar dead space). Together the anatomic plus alveolar dead space are termed *physiologic dead space* ($\dot{V}D$). In a normal resting adult breathing 16 times per minute (500 ml per breath), 150 cc fills the dead space × 16 breaths so 2400 ml is "wasted" ($\dot{V}D$) and the alveolar ventilation ($\dot{V}A$) involved with gas exchange is 5600 ml. The expired minute ventilation is the sum of alveolar ventilation and physiologic dead space ($\dot{V}E = \dot{V}A + \dot{V}D$). Because alveolar gas cannot be measured directly without contamination from the conducting airways, arterial pCO_2 is taken as the best estimate of the mean alveolar CO_2 tension and used to calculate the proportion of each tidal volume "wasted" in the dead space (the $\dot{V}D/\dot{V}T$) by the Bohr equation (modification):

$$\dot{V}D/\dot{V}T = \frac{PaCO_2 - PEO_2}{PaCO_2}$$

The Bohr Equation expressing the dead space ($\dot{V}D$) to tidal volume $\dot{V}T$ ratio. $PaCO_2$ = arterial CO_2 tension, $PECO_2$ = CO_2 tension in mixed expired air.

Alveolar ventilation is inversely related to arterial pCO_2, as shown below:

$$PACO_2 = PaCO_2 = \frac{\dot{V}CO_2 \times 0.863}{\dot{V}A}$$

This equation expresses the relationship between CO_2 tension in alveolar gas and arterial blood. In the ideal lung these are identical. $\dot{V}A$ = alveolar ventilation. $\dot{V}CO_2$ = CO_2 production and 0.863 is a constant. The equation shows that if CO_2 production is constant, a reduction in alveolar ventilation will increase arterial CO_2 tension.

With exercise, as tidal volume increases, more blood enters the lung, capillary recruitment occurs, and gas exchange is improved towards ideal decreasing the $\dot{V}D/\dot{V}T$ from the normal resting value of 0.3 to .15−.20.[4,6] An elevated physiological dead space as in pulmonary vascular or parenchymal lung disease increases the total minute ventilation required to achieve an alveolar ventilation appropriate to any work load, and in disease states may be a major obstacle to exercise, due to increased ventilatory work and inefficient gas exchange (Figs. 6, 7). Exercise-induced hypoxemia may occur in patients with low ventilation:perfusion ratios due to lung disease confounding oxygen delivery. Since arterial CO_2 tension is known to remain constant at moderate work levels, the alveolar ventilation must increase proportionally to metabolic production of CO_2 (Fig. 6).

Diffusing Capacity

The increased cardiac output to the lung seen with exercise recruits capillaries not open at rest and increases flow to others. Ventilation and perfusion become better matched and gas exchange improves, and the increased pulmonary blood volume correlates with an increased membrane diffusion capacity. Failure of

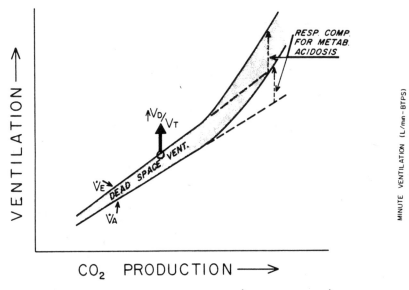

Figure 6: Factors that determine alveolar ($\dot{V}A$) and minute ($\dot{V}E$) ventilation during exercise. (From Wasserman K: Breathing during exercise. *New Engl J Med* 1978; 298:780. Used by permission.)

the diffusion capacity (DLCO) to nearly double suggests restriction of filling of the pulmonary vascular bed.[37]

Alveolar-Arterial O$_2$ Difference

Improved ventilation-perfusion matching in the lung with exercise reduces the alveolar-arterial O$_2$ gradient (A-aO$_2$D) at all but extreme work.[6]

Ventilatory Drive

Ventilatory regulation with exercise has been extensively studied but remains poorly understood. Respiratory drive increases with exercise in a manner that so precisely links alveolar ventilation to oxygen consumption that alveolar and arterial gas tensions change very little. A review by Dejours[38] and other recent papers[3,39] are of interest.

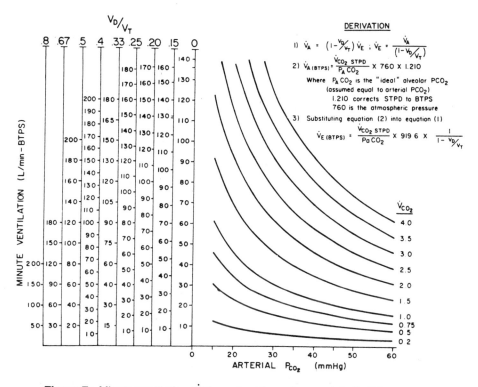

Figure 7: Minute ventilation ($\dot{V}_E$) required for various metabolic CO_2 production rates as modified by the level of $PaCO_2$ and the V_D/V_T ratio. (From Wasserman K, Whipp BJ: Exercise physiology in health and disease. *Am Rev Resp Dis* 1975; 112:219–249. Used by permission.)

EXERCISE STRATEGIES

Choosing a Device

Testing should be performed on a bicycle ergometer or treadmill which can be calibrated and allows work load to be progressively increased and quantitated in watts, kilogram meters/min, or speed and grade. Bicycle ergometry makes calculation of load simpler (patient's tendency to lean on the treadmill arm supports makes work load calculations inaccurate), but is more difficult for patients with unconditioned legs. Maximal $\dot{V}_{O_2}$ may be higher on the treadmill than on the ergometer,[40] but this is unimportant for submaximal clinical studies. Collection of expired gas, heart rate, and blood pressure readings, ear oximetry, and physical examinations are generally easier with the patient on an ergometer than on most treadmills, and ergometers take less space.

Incremental work load tests are more discriminating than single-level tests which might miss the point at which symptoms develop, or be so far above a given patient's tolerable exercise as to yield no information. Many protocols have been published[14,31,36,41] employing from 1- to 4-minute increments in work load, some with intermittent rest periods. The equipment and resources of the laboratory will obviously determine protocol to an extent, but steady state tests changing load no more than every 4 minutes are vastly more informative and easier to interpret.

Noninvasive Measurements with Exercise

The noninvasive measurement of ECG and expired air volume or flow are essential to any protocol and will permit calculation of tidal volume ($\dot{V}T$), $\dot{V}E$ and respiratory rate. Expired air can be collected into a Tissot spirometer, Douglas bag, or passed through a pneumotachygraph for electronic derivations of these variables. Most laboratories find a modified lead V_5 ECG provides acceptable tracings, sensitive to ST segment changes. Heart rate can be read from the written tracing which is also analyzed for ischemic changes and arrhythmias. A tracing should be taken during voluntary hyperventilation as abnormalities in the ST segment may be seen during this maneuver. Analysis of the exercise ECG is discussed elsewhere.

Ear oximetry is easy to perform and helpful in calibrating home O_2 doses and in detecting worsening of hypoxia in some individuals (those whose O_2 saturations fall at exercise into the steep portion of the oxyhemoglobin saturation curve). Elevation of patient carboxyhemoglobin levels lead to falsely high ear oximetry readings. Measurement of CO_2 and O_2 in mixed expired air allows calculation of $\dot{V}O_2$, $\dot{V}CO_2$, R, O_2 pulse, and the ventilatory equivalents for O_2 and CO_2 ($\dot{V}E/\dot{V}O_2$ or $\dot{V}CO_2$).[34] Prediction of $\dot{V}O_2$ and $\dot{V}CO_2$ from heart rate is inaccurate in pulmonary patients who often have increased $\dot{V}D/\dot{V}T$ and heart rates either higher or lower than expected. Quantitation of exercise by oxygen consumption makes the errors in calibration of the treadmill or ergometer less important, since heart rate, blood pressure, and derived variables are all interacting and interpreted together. The international use of $\dot{V}O_2$ makes communication between laboratories and compared data more meaningful. $\dot{V}O_2$ can be divided by weight in kg ($\dot{V}O_2$/kg) expressed in cc/kg, or divided by basal $\dot{V}O_2$ (one MET) and expressed as METs. A CO_2 rebreathing method for noninvasive estimation of cardiac output is used by Jones.[31]

Invasive Measurements with Exercise

Cannulation of the radial artery permits exercise analysis of lactates, physiologic dead space, arterial oxygenation, alveolar-arterial O_2 gradient, and venous admixture and is sometimes necessary in patients with normal resting lung function and gas exchange. Occasionally, passing a Swan-Ganz catheter into the pulmonary artery may be indicated if accurate cardiac output measurement is needed and pulmonary hemodynamic monitoring is warranted. The rise in steady state DLCO from rest to exercise is helpful in evaluating possible vascular disease, but requires an arterial puncture for pCO_2 measurement (Filley technique) since the end-tidal gas sampling device is not likely to be accurate during moderate exercise. A normal rise in DLCO of 1.5 ml/mmHg/min per 100 cc in $\dot{V}O_2$ has been reported.[9,42]

Terminating the Test

Ideally, exercise tests should reproduce the patient's specific symptoms and continue through several work loads. Baseline measurements of $\dot{V}E$, $\dot{V}O_2$, $\dot{V}CO_2$, blood pressure, and heart rate should be taken at rest and while riding "free-wheel" on the ergometer. The patient should be questioned about symptoms such as leg fatigue, dyspnea, chest pain, and leg cramps. Accepted indications for stopping the test are the same as for a cardiac exercise examination. The patient should be coached to continue to his subjective maximum work load.

Indications for Testing

Not every patient with dyspnea on exertion needs an exercise test. However, when this is needed to explain exercise symptoms, the information gained should be helpful to the patient's clinician in diagnosis and in constructing a treatment scheme.

Resting cardiopulmonary function studies may be normal while the normally vast reserves in either system may be sufficiently reduced to evoke symptoms on exertion. The larger the reserves in cardiopulmonary function, the less sensitive are studies at rest in detecting abnormality of corroborating a patient's history of exertional symptoms. Breathlessness is a nonspecific symptom potentially related to any number of cardiac and pulmonary problems, common psychiatric affective disorders, acute or chronic hyperventilation and, at times, anemia and neuromuscular dysfunction. A thorough history and physical examination may elucidate the problem without further search. Often the history reveals a symptom of chest pain, weakness, fatigue, wheezing, or dyspnea while the physical examination, resting ECG and ventilatory studies either fail to reveal its source, or show only subtle changes. The exercise test properly conducted then becomes an extension of the physical examination. The complexity of the test performed and measurements made should be dictated by the clinical presentation and differential diagnosis, and there should be a specific question to answer. Because exercise involves a complex integration of respiratory, circulatory, metabolic, and neurologic mechanisms, the exercise test should be designed to explore as many of these entities as possible. This need not be complicated and usually a noninvasive test can describe the patient's capacity to exert, the factors causing limits to exercise, the reasons for specific exertional symptoms, and sometimes establish a diagnosis.

The most common indications for exercise testing in pulmonary medicine are listed below. Referral patterns vary with the community and capability of the laboratory:

1. Unexplained dyspnea: Diagnoses ultimately established in patients with normal resting ventilation studies and physical examinations often include hyperventilation syndrome (where the normal study is often therapeutic as well as diagnostic), exercise-induced asthma, angina pectoris, cardiomyopathy, mitral stenosis, and rarely in our experience, pulmonary hypertension.
2. Pulmonary rehabilitation.
3. Interstitial lung disease: Staging, following therapy or calibrating oxygen dose.
4. Disability assessment.

Interpreting the Pulmonary Response to Exercise

Patterns of response to exercise may be common to more than one condition. For example, a rapid shallow breathing pattern may be seen with exercise in patients with pulmonary venous hypertension, diffuse pulmonary fibrosis, and severe pulmonary hypertension. Interpretation of the exercise response is made in lieu of the clinical history and physical exam and adds depth to the patient's overall evaluation. In such instances the diagnosis is usually known, and the exercise study is required for functional assessment or follow-up.

Chronic obstructive pulmonary disease is a common cause of exertional dyspnea, often coexisting with cardiac disease. Frequently the clinical problem is to discern whether a patient's dyspnea is related to cardiac or to ventilatory limitation.

PULMONARY EXERCISE RESPONSE IN CHRONIC OBSTRUCTIVE PULMONARY DISEASE (COPD)

Exertional dyspnea is not an early symptom in patients with chronic lung disease, and static pulmonary function studies will show some flow rate reduction, often with air trapping and vital capacity reduction. The correlation between exercise performance and resting blood gases or pulmonary function tests is poor, perhaps because these static tests cannot predict ventilation perfusion balance with exercise or the patient's ability or willingness to tolerate discomfort.[43-46]

BREATHING PATTERN

The minute ventilation ($\dot{V}E$) is usually increased for a given work load. The relationship between $\dot{V}E$ l/min per 100 cc $\dot{V}CO_2$ is called the ventilatory equivalent for CO_2 (or O_2) and is high in COPD patients. The physiological dead space ($\dot{V}D/\dot{V}T$) is increased by uneven $\dot{V}/Q$ matching. $\dot{V}D/\dot{V}T$ often increases at exercise because the final volume does not increase normally, probably for mechanical reasons related to airflow obstruction but possibly also influenced by vagal reflexes from the chest wall. A high $\dot{V}D/\dot{V}T$ increases the ventilatory requirement to maintain alveolar ventilation for gas exchange. Normal subjects and cardiac patients reach exhaustion and stop exercise at a $\dot{V}E$ below 50 or 60 percent of their maximum voluntary ventilation. The $\dot{V}E$ max/MV$\dot{V}$ ratio is called the *dyspnea index*,[34,43] normal under 60 percent. The high values of 70 percent and greater found in COPD patients at the point of exercise exhaustion reflect their greater use of ventilatory reserves at exercise and implies a ventilatory rather than a cardiovascular limit to exercise. Although COPD patients at exercise more closely approach their resting MV$\dot{V}$ values, the reported variation is wide, ranging from 30 to 130 percent. Since ventilation in COPD requires increased respiratory muscle work, the high $\dot{V}E$/MV$\dot{V}$ in COPD patients suggests the possibility that respiratory muscle fatigue may be a factor limiting exercise in these patients. The MV$\dot{V}$ is measured for only 12 seconds, and probably represents a work load exceeding what the respiratory muscles of normal subjects can sustain even for a few minutes.[47] Smidt[48] detected diaphragm fatigue by EMG at 40 percent of MV$\dot{V}$.

Freedman[47] found normal subjects could sustain only 72 percent of MV$\dot{V}$ for 4 minutes and estimated that only 50 percent of the static MV$\dot{V}$ could be sustained indefinitely. Flow-volume loops in COPD patients are abnormal at rest and despite the high expiratory pleural pressures and respiratory work done the flow limitation seems not to be overcome at exercise,[44,48,49] and may even worsen. Physical examination often detects wheezing not present at rest.

GAS EXCHANGE

Ventilation-perfusion mismatch may change with exercise to result in worsening of hypoxemia and widening of the alveolar-arterial O_2 tension difference (A_aO_2). This effect appears to be more common in patients with predominant emphysema, whereas patients with bronchitis in predominance often show improved arterial oxygen tension (PaO_2) during exercise.[44,50-52] Hypoxemia may act further as a potent stimulus to increase ventilation via the carotid chemoreceptors.[53-55] The resting PaO_2 shows no correlation with degree of airway obstruction and does not predict changes in PaO_2 which may occur with exercise.[56,57] Significant hypoxemia may improve with exercise, or develop only during exercise. Hypoxemia does not appear to limit exercise in COPD. Hypercapnia may occur during heavy work usually in bronchitic patients with such severe airway obstruction that alveolar ventilation cannot increase appropriately, or in those whose chemoreceptor responsiveness seems blunted.[51,58]

Cardiovascular performance in COPD patients is usually normal unless inactivity and detraining are pronounced. These patients usually have slow pulse rates and achieve low maximal oxygen consumptions because their reduced ventilatory capacities do not allow them to continue exercise long enough to stress the cardiovascular system. The O_2 pulse is normal for the work level in normal subjects. The O_2 pulse is three or four at rest and rises progressively with exercise and $\dot{V}O_2$ in COPD patients. Exercise may need to be terminated before cardiac output and $\dot{V}O_2$ have increased greatly enough to develop the O_2 pulse to its maximum. For the same reason, anaerobic threshold is not often seen in these patients whose ventilatory limits are reached before the cardiovascular limit. The ECG rarely shows abnormalities, although patients with cor pulmonale may develop supraventricular premature beats. Physical examination of the heart may occasionally reveal an exercise-induced right ventricular gallop rhythm.

Ventilatory response to exercise in patients with heart disease has not been extensively studied except in mitral stenosis, where anaerobic threshold appeared at extremely low work loads, inducing anaerobic metabolism and hyperventilation.[19] One could expect the lungs to become stiffer if left ventricular end-diastolic pressure were elevated during exercise, and this has been documented in mitral stenosis.[59] Peripheral airway function can change, apparently due to engorgement of peribronchial blood vessels compromising the airway lumen.[31] Airway conductance falls during angina pectoris induced by atrial pacing, concomitant with a rise in left ventricular end-diastolic pressure in one study.[60] Decreased conductance or compliance, or stimulation of vagal receptors within alveolar walls could initiate a rapid shallow breathing pattern. More information is needed on breathing patterns and its correlation with hemodynamic data in patients with various forms of heart disease. A patient who develops rapid shallow breathing at a low $\dot{V}O_2$ may have a low cardiac output. There is overlap in the response of patients with heart disease and poor conditioning which becomes very important in older patients with sedentary habits, and makes noninvasive exercise studies less specific. A low $\dot{V}O_2$ max with hyperventilation at low work loads in a sedentary patient may not discriminate between heart and pulmonary disease in some situations. The more debilitated the patient, the less useful is the exercise test[14] for separating cardiac and pulmonary work limits.

CASE EXAMPLE: NONINVASIVE TEST

The patient is a 51-year-old male with a sixth grade education, chronic obstructive pulmonary disease, osteoporosis, and dumping syndrome following subtotal gastrectomy for ulcer disease. He worked until a year ago as a commercial refrigeration technician, carrying 40 pounds of tools and equipment over long distances from parking lots into large buildings. He is applying for disability related to dyspnea. Physical examination revealed normal breath sounds without wheezing at rest, 1¾ inch chest expansion, and normal cardiac examination. His height is 67 inches and his weight is 140 pounds.

FVC = 3.01 FEV_1 = 1.81 $MV\dot{V}$ = 631 $FE\dot{V}_1/FVC$ = 60%
predicted max heart rate 184, predicted $\dot{V}O_2$ max 2.56 l/min

Interpretation of Case Example (Table 1)

Pulmonary Response

Airflow at rest was moderately limited. Tidal volume increased normally to 58 percent of vital capacity, and respiratory rate remains slow until onset of anaerobic metabolism at the last two loads. The ventilatory equivalent for O_2 was high throughout, and his $\dot{V}E$ max/$MV\dot{V}$ was 109 percent, indicating ventilatory limit to exercise at this point. He hyperventilated at rest and "free wheeling" (R > 1), but was at steady state at 150 and 350 kpm/min (R < 1). Ear oximetry revealed no hypoxemia during exercise.

Cardiovascular Response

The R of 1.1 at 450 kpm/min suggests onset of anaerobic metabolism at a low $\dot{V}O_2$ of 1261 cc/min. The O_2 pulse at the higher loads was at the lowest limit of normal,[61] suggesting a low stroke volume. The increase in blood pressure and heart rate were appropriate and he reached 95 percent of his age-predicted heart rate.

Summary

These data show poor O_2 delivery and reduced cardiovascular performance, but do not distinguish between poor conditioning

Table 1
Ergometer Load

	Rest	Freewheeling	150 kpm/min	300 kpm/min	450 kpm/min	600 kpm/min
Resp. rate	17.9	21.7	14.5	23.7	30	41.7
$\dot{V}_E$/min	18.5	31.1	28.6	39.1	52.4	68.9
Vtidal	1036	1438	1977	1653	1748	1652
$\dot{V}_{O_2}$ cc/min	353	463	758	976	1150	1348
$\dot{V}_{CO_2}$	352	582	664	925	1261	1533
R	1.0	1.26	.88	.95	1.1	1.14
Ear Oximetry % O_2 saturation	95	97	97	96	96	96
Dyspnea Index ($\dot{V}_E$ max/MVV)				62%	83%	109%
Heart rate	100	112	124	136	144	176
Blood Pressure mmHg	135/82	142/82	150/90	160/90	280/100	180/95
$\dot{V}_E/\dot{V}_{O_2}$ (100 cc)	5.2	6.7	3.7	4	4.52	5.1
O_2 pulse $\dfrac{\dot{V}_{O_2}}{\text{heart rate}}$	3.53	4.12	6	7.2	8	7.6
Predicted $\dot{V}_E$ (Jones) $4.54 + (.0221 \times \dot{V}_{CO_2})$	12.1	17.1	19.1	25.1		

and heart disease. The patient's ventilatory and cardiovascular limits were reached at a low level of approximately four METs, or four times the measured resting $\dot{V}O_2$. The measured resting $\dot{V}O_2$ in this patient probably was elevated by the testing situation, since the R was above one. The commonly used rule of thumb that 40 percent of the $\dot{V}O_2$ max or $MV\dot{V}$ can be sustained, suggests a steady state work tolerance for this patient lies near the 150 kpm/min work load, where the $\dot{V}O_2$ was 758 cc or 2 METs. This is consistent with only light work.

UNEXPLAINED DYSPNEA

Dyspnea is a subjective symptom that is difficult to measure and usually even harder to describe. The mechanisms of dyspnea are not well understood and appear to be different in various situations. For instance, dyspnea appears during exercise in patients when the work load of their respiratory muscles is increased, but also at rest when respiratory muscle work is normal as in pulmonary vascular obstruction. Patients with complete paralysis of respiratory muscles secondary to spinal cord injury experience dyspnea when there is no respiratory muscle work at all. No one theory to date seems to cover all situations in which dyspnea is a clinical problem.

The pattern of pulmonary and cardiac response to exercise can at least give strong clues that a recognizable pathological sequence is present to correlate with dyspnea.

Angina pectoris is a common cause of exertional dyspnea in a patient who seems perfectly normal when examined at rest. Unless heart failure is precipitated by exercise, the breathing pattern, minute ventilation, and gas exchange will be normal to the point of pain. Exercise may precipitate both the pain and diagnostic ECG changes discussed elsewhere in this volume. $\dot{V}O_2$ max may be reduced, but this varies with the physical condition of the patient.

EXERCISE-INDUCED BRONCHOSPASM (EIB)

EIB is another common cause of exertional dyspnea in a patient whose resting physical exam and lung function studies are normal or near normal. The history may be suggestive and the exercise test diagnostic. Exercise at 70 to 80 percent of the patient's $\dot{V}O_2$ max is reasonably likely to precipitate bronchospasm during or within 15 minutes after the test. Since therapy with beta-adrenergic aerosols or disodium chromoglycate are known to blunt or obliterate bronchospasm after exercise, these drugs must be withheld for 12 to 24 hours prior to a diagnostic exercise study. Spirometry is done before and at 5 minute intervals following exercise. Standardized exercise protocols for this purpose have been published, quantitating the exercise stimulus.[62] Strauss, McFadden, and Ingram have pointed out the importance of thermal heat loss in inducing EIB during exercise hyperpnea.[63] They suggest that eucapnic hyperventilation while the subject breathes subfreezing air works as well or better than exercise under usual laboratory conditions for precipitating EIB. Bronchoprovocation with cholinergic aerosols or histamine has also been used.

HYPERVENTILATION SYNDROME

In our experience, hyperventilation syndrome (HVS) is a common cause of dyspnea still unexplained after initial clinical evaluation. Dyspnea with various symptom combinations such as frequent sighing, air swallowing with eructations and flatulence, chronic fatigue, depression, anxiety, and inspiratory dyspnea at rest accentuated on exertion are suggestive of HVS. Lightheadedness, digital or perioral numbness and tingling and even syncope may be present, but are not often experienced by patients with the more chronic form of the syndrome. Sometimes simple voluntary hyperventilation at rest will reproduce the symptoms precisely, obviating the need for an exercise study. But often there are mild abnormalities such as minimal hypoxemia in an obese patient or minimal airflow obstruction, reduced vital capacity, or history of heart disease which complicate evaluation. Sometimes demonstrating adequate exercise tolerance to such a patient with HVS has a strongly reassuring value and helps to focus the patient's (and the referring physician's) attention on the underlying problem. Patients with HVS usually have a normal response to exercise with normal respiratory rates and blood gases, normal physiological dead space, and increase in diffusion capacity. Occasionally an early but transient excessive rise in blood pressure is noted. The maximal O_2 consumption may be lower than expected if the patient has become sedentary. Often such patients hyperventilate at the beginning of the test for the first few work loads, then gradually reduce ventilation to a level appropriate to O_2 consumption at the highest loads. Respiratory alkalosis is usually present at rest but resolves as work load increases. Gas exchange study reflects this by showing high $\dot{V}O_2/\dot{V}CO_2$ ratios (R > 1) early, then falling into the normal range and increasing again at anaerobic threshold. Oxygenation is normal or increased. The ECG may show nonspecific ST segment changes which also resolve. The "stopping symptom" in these patients is almost always leg pain rather than dyspnea, and the maximum ventilation achieved during exercise is well below 60 percent of the resting maximal voluntary ventilation (dyspnea index below 60 percent).

PULMONARY VASCULAR DISEASE

Rarely, pulmonary hypertension associated with collagen-vascular disease or idiopathic primary pulmonary hypertension may result in exertional dyspnea. Exercise in such patients results in increased pulmonary artery pressures, hypoxemia due to $\dot{V}/Q$ mismatch, rapid shallow breathing pattern, increased physiological dead space ($\dot{V}D/\dot{V}T$), and hyperventilation which persists through all work levels. During exercise, physical examination may elucidate accentuation of pulmonic valve closure reflecting increased pulmonary artery pressures. Tachycardia develops early and out of proportion to work load.

PULMONARY REHABILITATION

Comprehensive respiratory care for patients with pulmonary disease, particularly obstructive diseases, involves patient education, special bronchial hygiene techniques, bronchodilators and other medications, psychological support, physical reconditioning exercises and, when indicated, chronic home oxygen therapy. Chronic obstructive pulmonary disease is a heterogenous mixture of lung disease with varying severity, most commonly manifest in an older age group afflicted with other illness, i.e., vascular and heart disease, hypertension, diabetes, and orthopedic or other problems. Therefore, treatment must be tailored to individual patient needs. The equipment and details of home care therapy are complicated and cumbersome. Home care is often disruptive and, to many patients, embarrassing, particularly if oxygen is indicated. It is not surprising that a multidisciplinary approach to teaching and caring for these patients has developed. Physical therapists, respiratory therapists, cardiopulmonary technologists, respiratory care nurses, pharmacists, social workers, pastoral counselors, psychologists and psychiatrists, and pulmonary physicians and surgeons have formed "teams" in hospitals and clinics throughout the country to provide the needed services and continue clinical investigation. The American College of Chest Physicians Committee on Pulmonary Rehabilitation issued a lengthy definition of pulmonary rehabilitation in 1974, published in 1975[64] in *The Basics of Respiratory Disease* by the American Thoracic Society. The statement stressed as the paramount goal the attempt "to return the patient to the highest possible functional capacity allowed by his pulmonary handicap and overall life situation." Although therapy has not improved pulmonary function, all programs report significant subjective benefit to most patients, who experience an improved sense of well-being, measurably decreased anxiety, lessened dyspnea,[52] and increased activity and aerobic work capacity.

Controversy has arisen because some specific respiratory care techniques are lacking in clear efficacy such as inhalation of bland mists, intermittent positive pressure breathing (IPPB), certain breathing exercises, and postural drainage,[65] and there are no reports on control populations.

In 1964 Pierce reported improved work capacity following physical training in nine patients with severe chronic lung disease.[66] Subsequently, many rehabilitation programs have reported increased work tolerance in patients in physical training even without improvement in pulmonary function. Hale et al.[46] published a thoughtful critique of 12 such reports. Hale objected to the frequent use of symptom-limited $\dot{V}O_2$ max as an end point on which to analyze training, suggesting as did Nicholas[67] that improved motivation and willingness to tolerate dyspnea rather than true physiologic improvement could account for the changes. Patients can learn to perform better on the treadmill by lengthening their stride and improving their posture and economy of movement. Habituation may lead to reduced anxiety in the experimental situation,[68] resulting in lower heart and respiratory rates.[56,69,70] The benefits of physical training quickly fade if exercise is not continued, and most programs indicate the drop-out rate is high—approximately 50 percent or greater.[52,67] Oxygen therapy is indicated for hypoxic patients[71,72] and improves their ability to tolerate training.[53,55,73] The immediate psychological and physiological beneficial effects of oxygen therapy in severely hypoxic patients are difficult to separate from any additional training benefit the oxygen allows. Oxygen appears to improve endurance and duration of work tolerance at a given load,[55] but significant improvement in $\dot{V}O_2$ max has been unusual rather than common.[52]

If $\dot{V}O_2$ max in these patients is limited by low ventilatory capacity, perhaps the cardiovascular training effects can never be achieved. Normal subjects appear to require exercise at 50 percent of their $\dot{V}O_2$ max for 20 to 30 minutes three or four times weekly in order to develop recognizable conditioning[2] and similar work loads have been recommended for patients with coronary artery disease.[74] Some have suggested that the training effect may require exercise at 75 percent of $\dot{V}O_2$ max, measured in terms of anaerobic threshold.[75] For an average 50-year-old man, cardiovascular training might therefore require exercise at levels of 1.5 to 21 $\dot{V}O_2$. Patients with pulmonary disease could not be expected to train even close to such work levels. Belman[15] was unable to demonstrate increase in skeletal muscle enzymes in patients with chronic obstructive pulmonary disease trained for 6 weeks at a $\dot{V}O_2$ estimated to average about 0.75 l/min for the group. Training was done on a cycle ergometer and the load chosen for each patient was two-thirds to three-fourths the maximum load achieved in a preliminary incremental work test. The patients performed two 20-minute training periods four times each week. Of the 15 patients who exercised, nine improved their endurance and six did not. None of the patients decreased their ventilatory requirements or heart rates.

Pardy et al.[8] studied 12 patients with COPD who underwent respiratory muscle training by breathing 15 minutes twice daily through inspiratory resistances. The resistance chosen induced 40 percent of maximum inspiratory mouth pressure. Two months of such training improved treadmill exercise performance in seven of the 12 patients. Before training all but one of the seven had shown electromyographic evidence of diaphragm or scalene muscle fatigue during exercise, which was not found after inspiratory muscle training. This change suggested inspiratory muscle fatigue contributed to exercise limitation in these patients and that static inspiratory muscle training improved respiratory muscle endurance enough to permit greater exercise tolerance on the treadmill. Belman and Mittman[27] also found improved exercise performance in patients with COPD after inspiratory muscle endurance training. Further work and more patient studies are needed to determine the benefit of specific respiratory muscle training in COPD.

Pulmonary rehabilitation has to date not resulted in job returns for many patients despite psychological improvement and better exercise tolerance, maybe in part due to their age. Patients with the most severe dyspnea and airways obstruction get the least benefit[52] and most study groups are heavily weighted with such patients. COPD patients are known to have an annual decrement in FEV_1 two or three times greater than the normal 30 cc per year and no study has demonstrated a significant change in this.[76] Pulmonary rehabilitation does not seem to improve survival, except in the subgroup for whom oxygen therapy is indicated and used continuously at home. Earlier diagnosis by alert clinicians with office spirometers who are familiar with the long latency between onset of smoking and appearance of clinical symptoms may well be the key. Cigarette smoking is of course the most obvious preventable cause of respiratory disability. Even though it is currently not possible to predict which smokers will go on to respiratory disability and deaths, smoking should be discouraged vigorously. Meanwhile, comprehensive care of the disabled patient with obstructive lung disease should include all modalities that improve well-being. Exercise therapy is clearly beneficial, by whatever mechanism, in all but the most disabled.[52]

REFERENCES

1. Hermansen L: Lactate production during exercise. In *Muscle Metabolism During Exercise*. Pernow B, Saltin B (eds). New York, Plenum Press, 1971, 402.
2. Astrand PO, Rodahl K: *Textbook of Work Physiology*. 2nd ed. New York, McGraw-Hill, 1978.
3. Bennett FM, Reischl P, Grodins FS, Yamashiro SM, Fordyce WE: Dynamics of ventilatory response to exercise in humans. *J Appl Physiol* 1981; 51:194–203.
4. Wasserman K, Van Kessel AL, Burton GG: Interaction of physiological mechanisms during exercise. *J Appl Physiol* 1967; 22:71–75.
5. Asmussen E: Muscular exercise. In *Handbook of Physiology*. Fenn

WO, Rahn H (eds). Washington, DC, American Physiological Society, 1965.

6. Jones NL, McHardy GJ, Naimark A, Campbell EJ: Physiological dead space and alveolar-arterial gas pressure differences during exercise. *Clin Sci* 1966: 31:19–29.
7. Anderson P: Capillary density in skeletal muscle of man. *Acta Physiol Scand* 1975; 95:203.
8. Pardy RL, Rivington RN, Despas PJ, Macklem PT: The effects of inspiratory muscle training on exercise performance in chronic airflow limitation. *Am Rev Resp Dis* 1981; 123:426–433.
9. Cotes JE: *Lung Function, Assessment and Application in Medicine.* 4th ed. Oxford, England, Blackwell Scientific Publications, 1979.
10. Astrand PO: Quantification of exercise capability and evaluation of physical capacity in man. *Prog Cardiovasc Dis* 1976; 19:51–67.
11. Pollock ML: The qualification of endurance training programs in exercise and sports science reviews. In Wilmore JH (ed). New York, Academic Press, 1973.
12. Shepard RJ: *Endurance Fitness.* Toronto, University of Toronto Press, 1969.
13. Astrand PO, Cuddy TE, Saltin B, Stenberg J: Cardiac output during submaximal and maximal work. *J Appl Physiol* 1964; 19:268–274.
14. Wasserman K, Whipp BJ: Exercise physiology in health and disease. *Am Rev Resp Dis* 1975; 112:219–249.
15. Belman MJ, Kendregan BA: Exercise training fails to increase skeletal muscle enzymes in patients with chronic obstructive pulmonary disease. *Am Rev Resp Dis* 1981; 123:256–261.
16. Astrand I, Astrand PO, Hallback I, Kilbom A: Reduction in maximal oxygen uptake with age. *J Appl Physiol* 1973; 35:649–654.
17. Wasserman K, Whipp BJ, Koval SN, Beaver WL: Anaerobic threshold and respiratory gas exchange during exercise. *J Appl Physiol* 1973; 35:236–243.
18. Karlson J, Diamant B, Saltin B: Muscle metabolites during submaximal and maximal exercise in man. *Scand J Clin Lab Invest* 1970; 26:385–394.
19. Wasserman K, McIlroy MD: Detecting the threshold of anaerobic metabolism in cardiac patients during exercise. *Am J Card* 1964; 14:844.
20. Levison H, Cherniack RM: Ventilatory cost of exercise in chronic obstructive pulmonary disease. *J Appl Physiol* 1968; 25:21.
21. Milic-Emili G, Petit JM, Deroanne R: The effects of respiratory rate on the mechanical work of breathing during muscular exercise. *Intern Z Angew Physiol* 1960; 18:330.
22. Roussos CS, Macklem PT: Diaphragmatic fatigue in man. *J Appl Physiol* 1977; 43:189–197.
23. Leith DE, Bradley M: Ventilatory muscle strength and endurance training. *J Appl Physiol* 1976; 41:508–516.
24. Bradley ME, Leith DE: Ventilatory muscle training and the oxygen cost of sustained hyperpnea. *J Appl Physiol* 1978; 45:885–892.
25. Derenne J, Macklem PT, Roussos C: The respiratory muscles: mechanics, control and pathophysiology. Part I, *Am Rev Resp Dis*

1978; 118:119–133. Part II, *Am Rev Resp Dis* 1978; 118:373–390. Part III, *Am Rev Resp Dis* 1978; 118:581–601.

26. Peress L, McLean P, Woolf CR, Zamel N: Ventilatory muscle training in obstructive lung disease. *Bull Europ Physiopath Resp* 1979; 15: 91–94.

27. Belman M, Mittman C: Ventilatory muscle training improves exercise capacity in chronic obstructive pulmonary disease patients. *Am Rev Resp Dis* 1980; 121:273–280.

28. Gross D, Ladd HW, Riley EJ, Macklem PT, Grassino A: The effect of training on strength and endurance of the diaphragm in quadriplegia. *Am J Med* 1980; 68:27–35.

29. Keens TG, Krastins IR, Wannamaker EM, Levison H, Crozier DN, Bryan AC: Ventilatory muscle endurance training in normal subjects and patients with cystic fibrosis. *Am Rev Resp Dis* 1977; 116: 853–860.

30. Stremel RW, Huntsman DJ, Casaburi R, Whipp BJ, Wasserman K: Control of ventilation during intravenous CO_2 loading in the awake dog. *J Appl Physiol* 1978; 44:311–316.

31. Jones NL, Campbell EM, Edwards RHT, Robertson DG: *Clinical Exercise Testing*. Philadelphia, W.B. Saunders, 1975.

32. Rebuck AS, Jones NL, Campbell EJ: Ventilatory response to exercise and CO_2 rebreathing in normal subjects. *Clin Sci* 1972; 43: 861–867.

33. Gandevia B, Hugh-Jones P: Terminology for measurements of ventilatory capacity: A report to the thoracic society. *Thorax* 1957; 12: 290–293.

34. Gaensler EA, Wright GW: Evaluation of respiratory impairment. *Arch Envirn Health* 1966; 12:146–189.

35. Hughson RL, Kowalchuk JM: Influence of diet on CO_2 production and ventilation in constant load exercise. *Resp Physiol* 1981; 46:149.

36. West JB: *Ventilation/Blood Flow and Gas Exchange*. London, Blackwell Scientific Publications, 1979.

37. Turino GM, Bergofsky EH, Goldring RM, Fishman AP: Effect of exercise on pulmonary diffusing capacity. *J Appl Physiol* 1963; 18: 447.

38. Dejours P: Control of respiration in muscular exercise. In *Handbook of Physiology*. Fenn WO, Rahn H (eds)., Washington, DC, American Physiological Society, 1965.

39. Oren A, Wasserman K, Davis J, Whipp BJ: Effect of CO_2 set point on ventilatory response to exercise. *J Appl Physiol* 1981; 51:185–189.

40. Hermansen L, Eckblom B, Saltin B: Cardiac output during submaximal and maximal treadmill and bicycle exercise. *J Appl Physiol* 1970; 29:82–86.

41. Jones NL: Exercise testing in pulmonary evaluation: Rational methods, and the normal respiratory response to exercise. *New Engl J Med* 1975; 293:541–544.

42. Mostyn EM, Helle S, Gee JB, Bentivoglio LG, Bates DV: Pulmonary diffusing capacity of athletes. *J Appl Physiol* 1963; 18:687–695.

43. Fishman AP, Ledlie JF: Dyspnea. *Bull Physiopathol Resp* 1979; 15: 789–804.

44. Spiro SG, Hahn HL, Edwards RH, Pride NB: An analysis of the physiological strain of submaximal exercise in patients with chronic obstructive bronchitis. *Thorax* 1975; 30:415–425.
45. Gilbert R, Keighley J, Auchincloss JH: Disability in patients with obstructive pulmonary disease. *Am Rev Resp Dis* 1964; 90:383–394.
46. Hale T, Cumming G, Spriggs J: The effects of physical training in chronic obstructive pulmonary disease. *Bull Eur Physiopath Resp* 1978; 14:593–608.
47. Freedman S: Sustained maximal voluntary ventilation. *Resp Physiol* 1970; 8:230–244.
48. Smidt U, Worth H, Petro W: Ventilatory limitation of exercise in patients with chronic bronchitis and/or emphysema. *Bull Eur Physiopath Resp* 1979; 15:95–104.
49. Potter WA, Olafsson S, Hyatt RE: Ventilatory mechanics and expiratory flow limitation during exercise in patients with obstructive lung disease. *J Clin Invest* 1971; 50:910–919.
50. Jones NL: Pulmonary gas exchange during exercise in patients with chronic airway obstruction. *Clin Sci* 1966; 31:39–50.
51. Marcus JH, McLean RL, Duffell GM, Ingram RH: Exercise performance in relation to pathophysiologic type of chronic obstructive pulmonary disease. *Am J Med* 1970; 49:14–22.
52. Moser KM, Bokinsky GE, Savage RT, Archibald CJ, Hansen PR: Results of a comprehensive rehabilitation program: Physiologic and functional effects on patients with chronic obstructive pulmonary disease. *Arch Intern Med* 1980; 140:1596–1601.
53. Flenley DC, Calverley PM, Leggett RJ, Leitch AG, Wraith PK, Brash HM: Ventilatory response to hypoxemia during exercise. *Bull Eur Physiopath Resp* 1979; 15:53–55.
54. Wasserman K, Whipp BJ, Casaburi R, Golden M, Beaver WL: Ventilatory control during exercise in man. *Bull Eur Physiopath Resp* 1979; 15:27–51.
55. Bradley BL, Garner AE, Billiu D, Mestas JM, Foreman J: Oxygen-assisted exercise in chronic obstructive lung disease. *Am Rev Resp Dis* 1978; 118:239–243.
56. Vu-Dinti M, Lee HM, Vasquez P, Shepard JW, Bell JW: Relation of VO$_2$ max to cardiopulmonary function in patients with chronic obstructive lung disease. *Bull Eur Physiopath Resp* 1975; 15:359.
57. Hannhart B, Peslin R, Bohadana A, Teculescu D: Limitations ventilatoires de l'exercise chez la malade obstuctif. *Bull Eur Physiopath Resp* 1979; 15:75–89.
58. Ingram RH Jr, Miller RB, Tate LA: Ventilatory response to carbon dioxide and to exercise in relation to the pathophysiologic type of chronic obstructive pulmonary disease. *Am Rev Resp Dis* 1972; 105:541.
59. Ingram RH Jr, McFadden ER Jr: Respiratory changes during exercise in patients with pulmonary venous hypertension. *Prog Cardiovasc Dis* 1976; 19:109–115.
60. Pepine CJ, Wiener L: Relationship of anginal symptoms to lung mechanics during myocardial ischemia. *Circulation* 1972; 46:863–869.

61. Wasserman K: Breathing during exercise. *N Engl J Med* 1978; 298: 780–785.
62. Cropp GJA: The exercise bronchoprovocation test: Standardization of procedures and evaluation of response. *J Allergy Clin Immunol* 1979; 64:627–633.
63. Strauss RH, McFadden ER Jr, Ingram RH, Deal EC Jr, Jaeger JJ: Influence of heat and humidity on the airway obstruction induced by exercise in asthma. *J Clin Invest* 1978; 61(2):433–440.
64. Petty TL: *Pulmonary Rehabilitation: Basics of RD*. American Thoracic Society, New York, 1975.
65. Proceedings of the conference scientific basis of in-hospital respiratory therapy. *Am Rev Resp Dis* (suppl) 1980; 122:1.
66. Pierce AK, Taylor HF, Archer RK, Miller WF: Response to exercise training in patients with emphysema. *Arch Intern Med* 1964; 113:28–36.
67. Nicholas JJ, Gilbert R, Grobe R, Auchincloss JH Jr: Evaluation of exercise therapy program for patients with chronic obstructive pulmonary disease. *Am Rev Resp Dis* 1970; 102:1–9.
68. Paez PN, Phillipson EA, Masangkay M, Sproule BJ: The physiologic basis of training patients with emphysema. *Am Rev Resp Dis* 1967; 95:944–953.
69. McGavin CR, Gupta SP, Lloyd EL, McHardy GJR: Physical rehabilitation for the chronic bronchitis, results of a controlled trial of exercises in the home. *Br Med J* 1976; 1:822–823.
70. Shepard RJ: Learning, habituation, and training. *Intern Z Angew Physiol* 1969; 28:38–48.
71. Block AJ, Castle JR, Keitt AS: Chronic oxygen therapy. *Chest* 1974; 65:279–288.
72. Stewart BN, Hood CI, Block AJ: Long-term results of continuous oxygen therapy at sea level. *Chest* 1975; 68:486–492.
73. Pierce AK, Paez PN, Miller WF: Exercise training with the aid of a portable oxygen supply in patients with emphysema. *Am Rev Resp Dis* 1965; 91:653–659.
74. Hellerstein HK: Principles of exercise prescription. In *Exercise Testing and Exercise Training in Coronary Heart Disease*. Naughton JP, Hellerstein HK (eds). New York, Academic Press, 1973:129.
75. Davis JA, Frank MH, Whipp BJ, Wasserman K: Anaerobic threshold alterations caused by endurance training in middle-aged men. *J Appl Physiol* 1979; 46:1039–1046.
76. Hodgkin JE: Pulmonary rehabilitation. In *Current Pulmonology*. Simmons DS (ed). New York, Wiley & Sons, 1981.

7

Exercise in the Management of High Blood Pressure

Gerald F. Fletcher, M.D.

Considerable data are available on the role of physical activity in the management of high blood pressure. Since patients with high blood pressure are often asymptomatic, they are likely physically active anyway. In addition, those who are diagnosed as hypertensive often improve their blood pressure control with physical activity over and above the effect of antihypertensive drug therapy. Indeed, many who exercise properly and regularly may decrease their need for drugs or control their blood pressure with exercise alone. Therefore the *proper* use of *exercise* is important and should be considered in all subjects with high blood pressure.

Exercise has been employed for many years in the evaluation of high blood pressure. Limited data are available on the effects of exercise and hypertension in animals. Schaible et al.[1] studied treadmill training relations to cardiac function in rats with renal hypertension compared to controls. Half of the animals from each group were admitted to chronic running for 10 weeks. Cardiac function was studied in an isolated heart apparatus at controlled levels of left atrial pressure and aortic pressure. Improved cardiac function in the running rats versus the controls was related to increased muscle shortening and increased compliance. Thus

From: Fletcher GF: *Exercise in the Practice of Medicine*, 2nd Revised Edition. Mount Kisco, NY, Futura Publishing Co., Inc., © 1988.

treadmill training in hypertensive rats does not worsen cardiac function and may modestly improve it. Another animal study was done by Schaible et al.[2] regarding the physical training, cardiac function, and biochemistry in established hypertension in animals. In this group of animals, with regard to cardiac function and Ca^{2+}-M (ATPase), both were depressed in established hypertension after 10 weeks. Training subsequently normalized cardiac function and Ca^{2+}-M, thus implying that physical training may reverse abnormal cardiac function as well as biochemistry in established hypertension. Though the animal studies are limited, available data supports the beneficial effects of exercise.

With regard to studies in *blood pressure in normals with relation to exercise*, Newburger et al.[3] studied blood pressure and vascular reactivity in highly trained young swimmers. Resting blood pressure and its change with cold pressor test were measured in 20 highly trained female swimmers and in 130 untrained girls. The data suggested that strenuous endurance training is associated with higher systolic blood pressure and vascular reactivity; increased salt ingestion in this situation may be a factor. A more complete study in normal subjects was performed by Jennings et al.[4] regarding the effects of changes in physical activity on major cardiovascular risk factors. In this study, the effects of four levels of activity on heart rate and blood pressure were studied in 12 normal subjects. The randomized periods were 4 weeks of below-sedentary activity, 4 weeks of sedentary activity, 4 weeks of 40 minutes of bicycling three times weekly, and 4 weeks of similar bicycling seven times weekly. Exercise three times per week reduced resting blood pressure by 10/7 mmHg (p<.01) and by 12/7 mmHg after exercise seven times per week (p<.01). It seems therefore that exercise performed three times per week does lower blood pressure, but the same exercise seven times per week enhances physical performance further, with even greater decrease in blood pressure. Therefore, there are limited studies to suggest that normal blood pressure and vascular reactivities are affected by exercise, and this certainly should be considered in populations of healthy exercising subjects with regard to the potential benefit on controlling the dormant or latent hypertensive.

With regard to *exercise and high blood pressure*, in the 1960s, Levy and co-workers[5] studied hemodynamic responses to graded treadmill exercise in young, untreated, labile hypertensive patients. They used two groups. Group 1 was composed of 20 untreated, young, labile hypertensive patients and those in Group 2 were age-matched controls. In Group 1, the mean resting blood pressure was 114 mmHg which peaked to a mean of 127 mmHg with exercise. In Group 2 (the controls), mean resting blood pressure was 89 mmHg, peaking to a mean of 107 mmHg with exercise. The significant difference in blood pressure as noted at rest remained constant throughout exercise. Heart rate, cardiac output, and stroke volume did not differ significantly in these two groups at rest or with exercise. In 30 percent of the patients with high blood pressure (Group 1), exercise provoked a diastolic increase in blood pressure. Thus, this study questions the classification of labile hypertension based on resting cardiac data or resting hemodynamic data. All 20 patients in Group 1 were previously diagnosed as having labile hypertension. Ten of the 20 had a resting recumbent diastolic blood pressure of greater than 90 mmHg. These 10 patients maintained their diastolic hypertension during exercise and in addition, six of the 10 exceeded 90 mmHg. The other 10 patients previously diagnosed as labile hypertensives were not considered normal because of their diastolic recording at the time of the study but were considered to be truly labile hypertensive patients. *This study reflects the efficacy and value of exercise testing for the proper diagnosis of labile hypertension.*

Amery and co-workers[6] reported on muscle blood flow in normal and hypertensive subjects specifically with regard to the influence of age, exercise, and body position. At rest, uncomplicated and established essential hypertension is hemodynamically characterized by a normal cardiac output and increases in total peripheral resistance. During exercise in hypertensive patients, the total peripheral resistance decreases, but at all levels of exercise it is found to be greater in hypertensives than in normal subjects. The data herein described more specifically determine local muscle blood flow in hypertensive patients and age-matched normals, and were collected in the resting state and after maximal ischemic exercises in different body positions. The three groups in this study were selected according to age and hypertension: Group 1, 17–34 years, Group 2, 35–49, Group 3, 50–75 years. The mean blood pressure of the hypertensive group was 139.1 mmHg while the mean blood pressure of normals was 89.2 mmHg. Results are noted in Tables 1 and 2. Table 1 shows that with increasing age and after exercise there is a decrease in maximum muscle blood flow and an increase in vascular resistance. The same trend is seen in hypertensive patients but at a higher level. Table 2 shows that muscle blood flow decreases both in normals and in hypertensives

Table 1
Muscle Blood Flow and Resistance (Mean Values) after Maximum Ischemic Exercise Recumbent in Normal and Hypertensive Subjects**

Age (years)	Blood Flow After Exercise (ml/min/100 gm tissue)		Resistance After Exercise (units)	
	Normal	Hypertensive	Normal	Hypertensive
17−34	64.1 ± 19.6	69.2* ± 26.6	1.49 ± 0.51	2.38# ± 0.92
35−49	57.2 ± 13.1	58.5* ± 13.6	1.67 ± 0.53	2.46# ± 0.7
50−75	49.3 ± 9.3	55.6* ± 20.8	1.88 ± 0.30	2.72# ± 0.7

*P value >0.01 when compared to the normal group of the same age.
#P value <0.001 when compared to the normal group of the same age.
**Modified from Amery et al.[6]

Table 2
Muscle Blood Flow (Mean Values) after Maximum Ischemic Exercise in Recumbent and Standing Positions in Normal and Hypertensive Patients**

Body Posture	Blood Flow After Exercise (ml/min/100 gm tissue)	
	Normal	Hypertensive
Recumbent	60.9 ± 18.0	65.4 ± 29.1
Standing	50.3* ± 18.1	43.7* ± 13.3

*P < 0.001 when compared to the recumbent position in the same population, using the method of paired comparison.
**Modified from Amery et al.[6]

after exercise, changing from recumbent to sitting and standing positions. It is felt that the slight decrease in muscle blood flow and a slight increase in resistance with aging is very significant in the population of patients dealt with in cardiac rehabilitation, again emphasizing that in this age group, one may achieve a more beneficial effect with exercise in the supine or recumbent position.

Khatri and Cohn[7] reported on the mechanism of exercise hypotension after sympathetic blockade. Blood pressure measured immediately after a brief period of upright leg exercise was considerably lower than the resting supine pressure in 38 hypertensive patients treated with guanethidine or debrisoquin. The hemodynamics of this hypotension after exercise was studied in six hypertensive patients given guanethidine intravenously and in 16 patients treated with effective oral doses of guanethidine or debrisoquin. Both treatments blocked the reflex forearm vasoconstriction that normally occurs during leg exercise. Blood pressure rose from normal to above-normal levels during exercise and fell promptly to low resting levels when leg movement stopped. Upright leg exercise in the treated patients was accompanied by a large increase in cardiac output and a sharp fall in leg volume. Immediately after exercise, cardiac output fell moderately and leg volume rapidly increased. These studies suggest that alterations in the hemodynamic response to exercise induced by sympathetic blocking agents are due both to the inhibition of reflex arterial constriction and to large passive shifts of blood volume that occur in the upright position as a result of a blockade of venous reflex adjustments.

Hypotensive symptoms related to exertion probably result from the combined effects of gravitational pooling after exercise and a persistently low peripheral vascular resistance. These symptoms can probably be alleviated by reinstitution of leg exercise. It is suggested that immediately after upright leg exercise the blood pressure is more sensitive to mild degrees of adrenergic blockade than when patients are in the resting standing position. It is felt that post-exercise blood pressure may serve as a more reliable guide to adjustment in the dose of the sympathetic blocking agents in patients with hypertension. Based on this study, one should advise patients after any physical activity to recover while in the sitting or recumbent position. However, these problems may be eliminated if blood pressures are evaluated immediately post-exercise and medication doses are adjusted at this level.

Wong and co-workers[8] studied impaired maximal exercise performance in patients with hypertensive cardiovascular disease. They studied maximal responses to multistaged treadmill testing in four groups of hypertensive subjects: Group 1 was composed of 13 patients considered uncomplicated; Group 2, 15 patients with associated retinopathy; Group 3, 22 patients with left ventricular hypertrophy (LVH); Group 4, 11 patients with coronary heart disease. Each group also had age-matched controls as seen below:

Group	Patients		Control	
	Rest	Exercise	Rest	Exercise
1	174/104	201/97 mmHg	130/81	186/70 mmHg
2	165/101	202/103 mmHg	128/83	166/77 mmHg
3	180/107	235/107 mmHg	125/83	174/78 mmHg
4	158/100	194/104 mmHg	131/80	187/74 mmHg

This evaluation revealed that elevated blood pressure alone imposed no impairment to exercise performance in any of the groups. It was concluded that the major factors of impaired exercise capacity and restricted circulatory transport of oxygen to skeletal muscles in these hypertensive patients were the clinical manifestations of their end-organ disease (i.e., coronary disease). Based on this data, one should caution patients regarding their hypertensive end points to various activities or exercise; however, they should be just as aware of other end points such as chest discomfort or dyspnea.

In 1969, Sannerstedt[9] studied hemodynamic findings at rest and with exercise in mild arterial hypertension. Three groups on no medication were evaluated. Group 1 consisted of 59 normotensive subjects, Group 2 had 17 hypertensives with normal fundi, and Group 3, 16 hyperactives with grade one retinopathy. The grading of fundi was done according to the Keith-Wagner scale. All hemodynamic data were recorded at rest and after exercise. Group 2 had significantly higher rest oxygen consumption than Group 1. Group 3 had a greater oxygen consumption than Group 1 but it was not significantly different. This pattern continued during the exercise. During exercise the mean arterial pressure rose in all the hypertensives with Group 2 averaging an increase equal to Group 1. Group 3 showed a greater rise in mean arterial pressure during exercise. As the oxygen consumption increased during exercise, the cardiac output of Groups 2 and 3 increased significantly less than the controls of Group 1. The important points of these data are:

1. Hypertensive patients have greater oxygen consumption and higher mean arterial blood pressures at rest than do normotensives.

2. The mean arterial pressure of mild hypertensives increases with exercise but little more than normotensives.

3. Normotensives have a larger stroke volume with exercise while hypertensives have a higher heart rate. Normotensives would therefore have an overall greater cardiac output than hypertensives with exercise.

Therefore, since patients with mild hypertension exhibit a somewhat higher heart rate to various activities, this should be taken into consideration when suggesting activities for these patients and when designating the target heart rate.

Sannerstedt and co-workers[10] also studied five men with borderline latent systemic hypertension of the "hyperkinetic" type. These subjects were studied hemodynamically at rest and during dynamic exercise before and after a 6-week period of physical training. Tendencies to lower heart rate, cardiac output, and blood pressure, both at rest and with exercise, were observed after training. Systemic vascular resistance was unchanged. A trend towards increased widening of the arteriovenous oxygen difference at rest and during exercise was also noted after training. These findings indicate that physical conditioning of patients with latent high blood pressure of the hyperkinetic type contributes to a normokinetic circulation. Blood pressure was also normalized, thus achieving a more "economic" energy expenditure of the cardiovascular system with physical training.

Bhasin et al.[11] reported on the value of the blood pressure response to exercise in the recognition of latent or early borderline hypertension. All patients were evaluated by graded treadmill exercise tests. All had resting pressure of less than 140/90 mmHg. Exercise pressures were designated as normal, abnormal, or borderline. A peak pressure of less than 180/100 mmHg was normal and there were 218 patients in this category. A pressure greater than 210/110 mmHg was considered abnormal and there were 46 patients in this category. During the subsequent follow-up period of 16 to 48 months, 39 patients developed sustained hypertension requiring antihypertensive therapy. Patients demonstrating a hypertensive response to exercise testing showed a significantly greater incidence of developing subsequent hypertension. *Graded treadmill exercise, therefore, appears to be a simple and useful technique in the recognition of latent or borderline hypertension.*

Shah and co-workers[12] reported on the importance of exercise testing in assuring adequate control in essential hypertension. During exercise, significant differences were found in the increase in both systolic and diastolic pressures at every workload in the hypertensive group when compared to the control group ($<.005$ level). Eleven of the patients were retreated and repeat exercise tests at the same workload showed no significant statistical difference in blood pressure response to groups at that time. In conclusion, the data reveal that resting blood pressure in hypertensives does not predict blood pressure during activity, and exercise testing may be an effective measure of assuring adequate control. This is just another example revealing that exercise testing is a more accurate way of assuring adequate treatment of hypertension.

Recent developments in exercise and blood pressure control have involved specifically nutritional considerations. Bier et al.[13] have proposed the possibility that exercise of high intensity and long duration may alter dietary amino acid needs to an extent not previously appreciated. This may coincide with the fact that modest exercise regimens have proved beneficial in the non-drug treatment of various chronic diseases, particularly hypertension. La-Forge et al.[14] studied the cardiorespiratory effects of a 3-month home diet and exercise program in 33 coronary-prone policemen. The exercise prescription involved 4−5 days a week of 50 minutes of either rapid-pace variable-terrain walking, jogging, or bicycle riding at a heart rate which corresponded to 75−80% of the individual's maximum. Resting blood pressure did not change significantly; however, hypertensive officers lowered their blood pressures from 155/98 to 134/88 (p<.01). It was concluded that a 3-month home diet and exercise program can alter risk factors, particularly blood pressure in specific individuals. Geer et al.[15] studied exercise-induced changes in diastolic blood pressure in hypertension. They examined 61 hypertensive patients all receiving antihypertensives at the time of the study. Twenty-four patients had a peak diastolic blood pressure ≥110 mmHg. They concluded that a significant percentage of hypertensive patients develop substantial elevation in diastolic blood pressure with mild to moderate exercise although resting diastolic pressure is in the normal range. Nicholson et al.[16] studied the use of 24-hour ambulatory blood pressure monitoring and exercise testing in predicting the effect of long-acting beta blockade (atenolol) in the treatment of hypertension. Twelve patients with essential hypertension were evaluated before and after one month of treatment with atenolol 100 mg taken once daily. While the results showed the uniform hypotensive effect of atenolol, the data further suggest that blood pressure measurement during exercise may be a more reliable method of assessing the antihypertensive effect of beta blockers than rest measurements. Pacheco et al.[17] studied abnormal hemodynamic response to upright exercise in hypertension. They evaluated 15 subjects with untreated mild hypertension (diastolic pressures 90−105) and 16 normal controls at 50 percent of maximal VO_2. During maximal exercise, mean arterial pressure was significantly higher and the VO_2 significantly lower in the hypertensive group compared with the controls. The total peripheral resistance was also elevated at rest in the hypertensives, but the percent fall during exercise was similar to the controls. Therefore, although the total peripheral resistance is substantially elevated both at rest and during exercise, patients with mild hypertension retain considerable ability to vasodilate during submaximal exercise. This latter finding may address the effect of certain antihypertensive drugs affecting patients during exercise and perhaps suggests that diastolic alterations in some patients may be more significantly changed with vasodilator drugs. Floras et al.[18] studied cardioselective and nonselective beta-adrenoceptor blocking drugs in hypertension and their effect on blood pressure during physical activity in 35 patients. The increase in systolic blood pressure during bicycling was attenuated significantly by the cardioselective drugs atenolol (by 23 mmHg, or 38%) and metoprolol (21 mmHg, or 41%), but not by the nonselective agents pindolol and propranolol. Only bicycle exercise induced norepinephrine concentrations by 80%. The results suggest that beta-adrenoceptor blocking drugs will not attenuate increases in blood pressure during physical activities unless intense sympathoadrenal activation also occurs, as was seen in this group of patients in the exercise (bicycle) induced plasma norepinephrine increase. More currently, Kaplan[19] has emphasized the non-drug treatment of hypertension. He feels that as more people with mild hypertension are treated, non-drug therapies should be used more frequently and effectively. These include weight reduction and exercise. Such therapies have been inadequately used in the past, because of a lack of confidence in effectiveness and overconfidence in the effectiveness and safety of drug therapy. Non-drug therapies may provide enough antihypertensive effect to lower blood pressure of many patients with mild hypertension to a safe level without the need for antihypertensive drugs. Therefore, there are a number of recent studies confirming the benefit of properly prescribed exercise in the management of hypertensive patients.

More current data support a positive effect in the management of high blood pressure. Hagberg et al.[20] confirmed this effect in hypertensive adolescents, particularly on certain hemodynamic features. Paffenbarger et al.[21] reported one of the largest epidemiology studies in their follow-up of 14,998 Harvard alumni. They found that alumni who did not engage in vigorous sports play (defined as 1−2 hours per week of running, swimming, hardball, tennis, or cross-country skiing) were at 35% greater risk of developing hypertension independent of other risk factors. Cade et al.[22] reported the effects of exercise in 105 hypertensive patients. The patients on no medication decreased their mean pressure by 15 mmHg. Patients with severe hypertension also benefitted from exercise and some patients were able to discontinue or decrease their medication. Nelson et al.[23] studied the effect of changing levels of physical activity on blood pressure and hemodynamics in 13 patients with essential hypertension. They found that exercise lowered blood pressure by 11/9 mmHg with three times weekly activity and by 16/11 mmHg with seven times weekly activity.

In local experiences, exercise therapy has been shown to moderately reduce increases in blood pressure. So not only is exercise testing beneficial in the follow-up and diagnosis of hypertension, but physical training is helpful in reducing blood pressure and may contribute to an increase in capacity for exertion in hypertensive patients. Patients with uncomplicated high blood pressure usually have a normal exercise tolerance. As their hypertension increases in severity, however, and especially when target organs are involved such as the heart, the brain, or the kidneys, exercise should be considered quite carefully.

In discussing exercise and high blood pressure, it is appropriate to mention isotonic and isometric exercises. *Isotonic* has to do with the length of the entire muscle changing. Thus the muscle may become shorter or longer causing movement in the parts of the body where it is attached. This is synonymous with a *dynamic* contraction. *Isometric* changes occur when the length of the total muscle does not change and there is no movement in that particular part of the body. This is synonymous with a *static* contraction. Contractions of muscle fibers occur in isometric exercises and are responsible for the increase in the tension of the muscle. Isometric exercises are useful when the extremities should not or cannot be used in a dynamic maneuver. Such occurs if an extremity is in a cast.

Isotonic exercise has several advantages over isometric exercise. It requires movement in joints and is used to develop coordination and to increase functional capacity of other organs. It has also been observed that isotonic training of a muscle in one limb increases the strength of the similar muscle in the other side of the body. This does not occur in isometric exercise. In accord with this, it is also known that isometric exercises elevate blood pressure more than heart rate whereas isotonic exercises have more effect on elevation of heart rate.

Ewing and co-workers[24] studied static exercises in untreated systemic hypertension. They observed circulatory responses to sustained hand grip exercises at 30 percent of maximum voluntary contraction of forearm muscles in patients with untreated high blood pressure. Arterial pressures increased in all patients and often at a very high level. Two patterns of circulatory response were observed: In Group 1 there was an increase in cardiac index and heart rate with little or no change in systemic vascular resistance. These patients conform to a pattern of response that has been previously observed in normal subjects. Group 2 responded by an increase in systemic vascular resistance with minimal increase in heart rate and little or no change in cardiac index. All of the patients in Group 2 had either electrocardiographic or radiographic evidence of left ventricular hypertrophy, thus suggesting that the difference in response was due to an impaired left ventricular function. In four of these patients further measurements were performed at increments of 10, 20, and 50 percent of the maximum voluntary forearm muscle contraction. With this they demonstrated incremental increases in blood pressures. One pressure was recorded as 348/182 mmHg. It was concluded that the very high pressures obtained during static or isometric exercise are potentially harmful to patients with known high blood pressures, as cardiac failure or cerebral hemorrhage may be provoked. In accord with this, it is felt that patients with evidence of left ventricular hypertrophy who are engaged in various daily activities, including specific isometric or static exercises, should be cautioned accordingly.

Thus there are considerable data to support the use of exercise testing and training in the management of subjects with high blood pressure. Care must be utilized as these subjects are usually asymptomatic. In addition, those with end-organ disease, such as left ventricular disease, should be managed with even more care and concern. Dynamic exercise at *low levels* (walking or bike ergometry) in these individuals is usually both acceptable and safe.

PERIPHERAL VASCULAR DISEASE

Peripheral vascular disease—particularly that of the femoral arterial system (and distally)—has taken on greater clinical importance in recent years with the surge of interest in exercise habits in our public. This is especially true in patients with coronary atherosclerosis who have experienced infarction or who have had coronary bypass surgery. These subjects are often in supervised exercise programs, and as their exercise capacity increases with their training effect, their end point becomes claudication of the lower extremities.

In the 1960s, Garrison et al.[25] reported on the role of exercise in the physical examination of peripheral arterial disease. They emphasized the importance of palpation and auscultation of arteries and observation of the skin over the distal part of extremities in the diagnosis of arterial stenosis. They related that significant arterial insufficiency is common and that observation of post-exercise changes is frequently necessary to establish the diagnosis. (Current studies reaffirm this use of exercise.[26])

In accord with this, Alpert and co-workers[27] reported on exercise and intermittent claudication regarding blood flow in the calf muscles during walking. With the Xenon 133 clearance method, they studied 19 patients with obliterative atherosclerotic disease of the legs. All were suffering from intermittent claudication and were studied before and during a 6-month training program. The maximal walking distance and the calf muscle blood flow during walking were recorded at monthly intervals. A significant correlation was established between improvement in maximal walking distance and a tendency to have a more normal blood flow in the calf muscles. It was also found that calf muscle blood flow when walking was increased by physical training. The data suggest that functional factors (for example, better coordination of working muscles) as well as anatomic factors of increase in number or diameter of collateral vessels are involved in increasing collateral efficiency.

Jonason et al.[28] studied the effects of physical training on different categories of patients with intermittent claudication. They evaluated 68 patients. Eight of the patients had resting pain when recumbent (Group 1), 25 had initial walking distances of less than 500 meters (Group 2), 11 had initial walking distances of 500 to 1000 meters (Group 3), and 24 had coronary insufficiency (Group 4). The study revealed that effective training should be undertaken for at least 3 months. In some patients with rest pain, training caused relief of pain and surgical treatment was not necessary. Almost all patients without signs of coronary insufficiency increased walking distances compared to only 14 of the 24 patients with coronary insufficiency. Walking distances increased significantly in Groups 2 and 3 and no significant difference was found between the patients with proximal or distal arterial disease.

From the study, it appears that patients with intermittent claudication, not presenting with rest pain, will benefit from a physical training program. Since 14 of the 24 patients with coronary insufficiency increased their walking distance with physical training, it seems reasonable to prescribe physical training for patients with claudication and coronary insufficiency and evaluate the effect of the training on both of these manifestations of atherosclerosis.

Therefore, as we evolve more exercise programs for subjects with generalized atherosclerosis, it seems quite feasible to incorporate those with claudication. In some instances exercise prescription may necessitate use of upper extremity exercise or carefully prescribed swimming activities to avoid the discomfort of claudication that occurs with walking and running. Certainly available data and current experiences suggest an exercise benefit in this field of peripheral vascular disease.

REFERENCES

1. Schaible TF, Ciambrone C, Scheuer J: Treadmill training improves cardiac function in hypertensive rats. *Circulation* 1985; 72:486 (Abstract).
2. Schaible TF, Malhotra A, Ciambrone G, Scheuer J: Physical training improves cardiac function and biochemistry in established hypertension. *Circulation* 1984; 70:11−77 (Abstract).
3. Newburger JW, Sosenko JM, Lerrer TJ, Miettinen OS, Ellison RC: Blood pressure and vascular reactivity in highly trained young swimmers. *Circulation* 1979; 60:11−207 (Abstract).
4. Jennings G, Nelson L, Nestel P, Esler M, Korner P, Burton D, Bazelmans J: The effects of changes in physical activity on major cardiovascular risk factors, hemodynamics, sympathetic function, and glucose utilization in man: a controlled study of four levels of activity. *Circulation* 1986; 73(1):30−40.
5. Levy AM, Tabakin BS, Hanson JS: Hemodynamic responses to graded treadmill exercise in young untreated labile hypertensive patients. *Circulation* 1967; 35:1063−1072.
6. Amery A, Bossaert H, Verstraete M: Muscle blood flow in normal and hypertensive subjects, influence of age, exercise and body position. *Am Heart J* 1969; 78:211−216.
7. Khatri IM, Cohn JN: Mechanism of exercise hypotension after sympathetic blockade. *Am J Cardiol* 1970; 25:329−338.
8. Wong HO, Kasser IS, Bruce RA: Impaired maximal exercise performance with hypertensive cardiovascular disease. *Circulation* 1969; 39:633−638.
9. Sannerstedt R: Hemodynamic findings at rest and during exercise in mild arterial hypertension. *Am J Med Sci* 1969; 258:70−79.
10. Sannerstedt R, Wasir H, Henning R, Werko L: Systemic haemodynamics in mild arterial hypertension before and after physical training. *Clin Sci* 1973; 45(Suppl.): 145−149.
11. Bhasin SS, Khullar SC, Weissler AM: Response to exercise and cardiac effects of therapy, value of blood pressure response to exercise in the recognition of latent or early borderline hypertension. *Am J Cardiol* 1980; 45:489 (Abstract).

12. Shah A, Barndt R, DeQuattro V, Milgrom M: The importance of exercise testing in essential hypertension: A new approach to assure adequate blood pressure control. *Circulation* 1980; 62:III–37 (Abstract).
13. Bier DM, Young VR: Exercise and blood pressure: nutritional considerations. *Ann Internal Med* 1983; 98(Part 2):864–869.
14. LaForge RL, Favrot L, Smith SC, Brown S: Cardiorespiratory effects of a 3-month home diet and exercise program in coronary-prone police officers. *Clin Res* 1981; 29(2):216A.
15. Geer M, Brown J: Exercise-induced changes in diastolic blood pressure in hypertension. *Clin Res* 1984; 32(2):331A.
16. Nicholson JP, Pickering TG, Harshfield GA, Resnick LM, Laragh JH: The use of 24-hour ambulatory blood pressure monitoring and exercise testing in predicting the effect of long-acting beta-blockade (atenolol) in the treatment of hypertension. *Clin Res* 1984; 32(2):336A.
17. Pacheco JP, Fan F, Wright R, Horowitz L: Abnormal hemodynamic response to upright exercise in hypertension. *Circulation* 1985; 72: 111–465 (Abstract).
18. Floras JS, Hassan MO, Jones JV, Sleight P: Cardioselective and nonselective beta-adrenoceptor blocking drugs in hypertension: A comparison of their effect on blood pressure during mental and physical activity. *JACC* 1985; 6(1):186–195.
19. Kaplan NM: Non-drug treatment of hypertension. *Ann Intern Med* 1985; 102:359–373.
20. Hagberg JM, Goldring D, Ehsani AA, et al: Effect of exercise training on the blood pressure and hemodynamic features of hypertensive adolescents. *Am J Cardiol* 1983; 52:763–768.
21. Paffenbarger RS Jr, Wing AL, Hyde RT, et al: Physical activity and incidence of hypertension in college alumni. *Am J Epidemiol* 1983; 117:245–257.
22. Cade R, Mars D, Wagemaker H, Zauner C, Packer D, Privette M, Cade M, Peterson J, Hood-Lewis D: Effect of aerobic exercise training on patients with systemic arterial hypertension. *AJM* 1984; 77(5): 785–790.
23. Nelson L, Esler MD, Jennings GL, Korner PI: Effect of changing levels of physical activity on blood-pressure and haemodynamics in essential hypertension. *The Lancet* 1986; 473–479.
24. Ewing DI, Irving JB, Kerr F, Kirby BJ: Static exercise in untreated systemic hypertension. *Br Heart J* 1973; 35:413–421.
25. Garrison GE, Floyd WL, Orgain FS: Exercise in the physical examination of peripheral arterial disease. *Ann Intern Med* 1967; 66:587–593.
26. Carter SA: Arterial auscultation in peripheral vascular disease. *JAMA* 1981; 246:1682–1686.
27. Alpert JS, Larsen OA, Lassen NA: Exercise and intermittent claudication. Blood flow in the calf muscle during walking studied by the xenon-133 clearance method. *Circulation* 1969; 39:353–359.
28. Jonason T, Jonzon B, Ringquist I, Oman-Rydberg A: Effect of physical training on different categories of patients with intermittent claudication. *Acta Med Scand* 1979; 206:253–258.

8

Exercise and Hematology

Gerald F. Fletcher, M.D.

INTRODUCTION

Exercise has long been known to affect certain elements of circulating blood. The more traditional observations have been confined to circulating blood cells and leukocytes. Several studies have suggested that athletes tend to have an increase in blood volume.[1-5] In addition, slightly lower hemoglobin concentrations have been noted at rest in well-trained persons although these findings have not been uniformly confirmed.[1,6-10] A study by Ross and Atwood[11] revealed decreases in hematocrit and hemagloblin (13% in one group) during the first 2 weeks but not the third week of increasingly severe exertion. It was felt that plasma expansion was likely the chief cause of this phenomenon. In a note by Ernst,[12] the role of enhanced blood fluidity is proposed as a cause for the decrease in hematocrit in athletes. In addition, training has been shown to increase red cell 2,3-diphosphoglycerate.[13,14] The latter may well have a very significant effect on delivery of oxygen to both skeletal muscle and cardiac muscle.

Runners' anemia has been a well-known entity for some time and there have been several other proposed mechanisms. Inhibition of erythropoiesis has been considered by Dressendorfer et al.,[15] as has decreased iron absorption by Ehn et al.[16] At this

From: Fletcher GF: *Exercise in the Practice of Medicine*, 2nd Revised Edition. Mount Kisco, NY, Futura Publishing Co., Inc., © 1988.

point, however, there is no clear, single explanation for the exercise decrease in hematocrit, and all considerations must be included.

Marked leukocytosis occurs with strenuous exercise. White blood cell counts as high as $22.0 \times 10^9/l$ have been found in a runner after doing a 100 yard dash in 11 seconds, and $35.0 \times 10^9/l$ on completing a quarter-mile run in less than a minute.[17] The increment of cells is usually made up of segmented neutrophils but lymphocytosis may be prominent as well. Such leukocytosis decreases to normal in less than an hour and, in the case of the neutrophils, is due to a shift of cells from marginal sites to the circulation.[18,19]

This leukocytosis is thought to occur in the absence of the spleen, and therefore the spleen is not likely a major site of cell margination. Leukocyte counts above $20.0 \times 10^9/l$ (mainly neutrophils) are often seen in runners completing a marathon of 26 miles in 2 1/2 to 3 hours; however, there is disagreement as to whether or not a shift to the left, suggesting mobilization of marrow neutrophils, occurs in this circumstance.[17] Post-marathon leukocytosis subsides slowly over a number of hours and probably reflects a redistribution of granulocytes in the blood combined with mobilization of cells. The magnitude of the leukocytosis associated with exercise appears to depend primarily on the intensity of the activity rather than upon its duration.[20]

Of recent interest has been the mechanism of exercise-enhanced lymphocyte cytotoxicity. Hirsen et al.[21] studied peripheral mononuclear cells in normal subjects before and after treadmill exercise and found that exercise increased lymphocyte natural killing and antibody-dependent cell-mediated cytotoxicity. The data suggest that this change is due at least in part to mobilization of effector cells in peripheral blood and may have implications concerning specific lymphocyte traffic and conditions under which human peripheral lymphocytes are obtained for study.

PLATELET ACTIVITY

More interestingly of late, especially with the current data on platelet activity and coronay artery disease, is the presence of thrombocytosis following exercise.[22,23] This thrombocytosis is unaffected by splenectomy[24] and may be the result of the release of platelets from the lung.[25] Following either epinephrine administration or exercise, the platelet count usually returns to normal within 30 minutes. Exercise increases ADP-induced platelet aggregation and platelet adhesion to glass beads.[26]

There is currently a great deal of research activity and interest in the role of blood platelets in promoting intravascular thrombosis. Clinically, the utility of this information lies in the prevention or retardation of thrombosis by altering platelet activity through several mechanisms, including exercise. The final result and recommendations are still pending, but nationwide multicenter trials have suggested a beneficial effect of antiplatelet drug therapy in presenting recurrent myocardial infarction (Paris study)[27] as well as transient ischemic attacks.[28] Although the pathogenesis of these effects is not clearly established, data are being collected and scientifically applied in an attempt to understand the clinical phenomena.

With specific reference to coronary artery disease, Steele et al.[29] and Doyle et al.[30] demonstrated shortened platelet survival in patients with angiographically documented coronary artery disease. Steele et al.[29] reported shortened platelet survival by the standard chromium 51 labeling technique in 68 percent of 104 men with coronary disease prior to therapeutic interventions (medical or surgical), including nitroglycerin. They also demonstrated a correlation between aortocoronary graft occlusion and platelet survival time. Thirty-six of 55 men examined after coronary bypass procedures had one or more grafts occluded, and 35 of the 36 demonstrated shortened platelet survival. In addition, the average platelet survival for the 35 was significantly shorter than that for the 19 patients whose grafts had remained patent.

Doyle et al.[30] also noted shortened platelet survival in coronary disease patients and correlated the chromium 51 labeling technique with assays of platelet-specific proteins, namely platelet factor 4 and beta-thromboglobulin, as indicators of intravascular platelet activity. These proteins, along with others, are released from the platelet alpha granule following platelet adherence and comprise part of the "release" reaction. Increased levels of these platelet proteins are postulated to indicate stimulated platelet activity. Others are currently attempting to refine these assays in an effort to provide more sensitivity and specificity in the determination of platelet activity.

Realizing the role of the platelet in thrombosis and the importance of being able to accurately quantitate its activity in the setting of atherosclerotic vascular disease, Mehta et al.[31] have

shown an aortic-to-coronary sinus concentration gradient of platelets and decreased aggregation activity in platelets from coronary
sinus blood in patients with coronary atherosclerosis. Similarly,
Rubenstein et al.[32] reported significantly elevated transmyocar-
dial aortic-to-coronary sinus measurements of beta-thromboglobulin levels in patients with documented coronary artery spasm by
cardiac catheterization versus patients with normal coronary arteries. This information strongly suggests blood platelet consumption or activation in atherosclerotic plaques and implies again that
antiplatelet therapy may be beneficial, at least in secondary
prevention.

The alpha granule of the platelet is also known to
Platelet activity in promoting intravascular thrombosis may
also have important applications in the primary prevention of
atherosclerosis. The alpha granule of the platelet is also known to
contain a protein termed platelet-derived growth factor or mitogenic factor. Ross et al.[33] have demonstrated that with stress of
endothelial injury this substance stimulated the migration of
smooth muscle cells from the media to the intima and is also
mitogenic for smooth muscle cells and fibroblasts. This action
results in formation of new connective tissue at the site of vessel
injury. At the site of injury created by chronic hyperlipidemia
(presumably the "fatty streak"), platelet-derived growth factor is
also felt to stimulate the deposition of lipid within these recently
accumulated connective tissue elements, both intracellularly and
extracellularly. As pointed out by Harker and Ritchie,[34] the process can obviously be progressive and additive to result in the
propagation of atherosclerotic plaques. Likewise, regulation of
hyperlipidemia in control of platelet activity could provide a deter-
rent to atherogenesis via the mechanisms postulated in these
preliminary studies.

The relationship of *exercise* to platelet activity has been defined, at least in patients with coronary artery disease. Green et
al.[35] demonstrated increases in platelet factor 4 following exercise
in 11 of 20 patients with positive exercise tolerance tests. Eighteen
of 20 patients with negative exercise tests had no post-exercise
increase in platelet factor 4 level over the resting levels.

Platelet release during exercise and coronary disease has been
further studied by Steele et al.[36] These investigators found that
with maximum exercise testing in 22 men with coronary artery
disease (at the point of angina), there was an increased release of
beta-thromboglobulin and platelet factor 4 but no definite increase
in thromboxane. These patients were compared to 16 normal con-

trols who, with exercise, did not have an increase in these platelet factors. In addition, the patient population was restudied after sulfinpyrazone administration and data suggested that this medication decreased the release of platelet factors. The results suggest that increased platelet release occurs during exercise in patients with coronary artery disease, but sulfinpyrazone decreases this release and that the release correlates with the intensity of exercise.

Another study was done by Steele et al.[37] on the release of beta-thromboglobulin during isometric exercise and coronary disease and the relationship of platelet-suppressing agents. Results suggested that there was an exaggerated phase of beta-thromboglobulin release by platelets during isometric exercise in patients with coronary artery disease and that beta-thromboglobulin release is inhibited both at rest and during exercise by aspirin, sulfinpyrazone, and phenoxybenzamine.

Williams et al.[38] studied platelet aggregation following cardiac rehabilitation in a small group of seven men who were post-infarction and who had completed a 6-month cardiac rehabilitation program of exercise training. In samples of platelets drawn at rest, aggregation induced with levoepinephrine was strikingly reduced following the conditioning program in all subjects. Total aggregation fell from 50 ± 26 percent to 11 ± 5 percent after training. They felt that possible mechanisms for reduced aggregation by levoepinephrine after exercise training might include platelet alpha-receptor desensitization, reduced cholesterol content of platelet membranes, or altered platelet kinetics. The latter study is limited in value because of small numbers but does stimulate thought regarding alterations of platelet activity with exercise conditioning.

More current studies have been done in platelet factor 4 activity before and after exercise testing in trained coronary heart disease patients.[39] Platelet factor 4 (PF-4) activity was investigated in 50 trained (≥6 months of medically supervised exercise) patients with identified coronary heart disease. Thirty-five patients were classified as post-myocardial infarction and 17 were post-aortocoronary bypass graft. Blood samples were collected immediately before and immediately following treadmill exercise testing using careful venipuncture technique. Assay was done by the radioimmunoassay procedure of Abbott Laboratories (commercial kit preparations).

There were no significant differences in platelet factor 4 activity before and after exercise testing either within or between groups (myocardial infarction vs. post-aortocoronary bypass graft) in the absence of clinical myocardial ischemia. It was concluded that lack of platelet factor 4 activity increases during exercise testing in this group of trained coronary heart disease patients may reflect stabilization of platelet activity through the training process. More studies are being done to further clarify the role of exercise training in altering platelet activity.

FIBRINOLYSIS

Just as platelet activity is stimulated during exercise, the fibrinolytic system is also activated. With regard to fibrinolysis, Menon et al.[40] reported as early as 1967 on the effect of strenuous, graded exercise and fibrinolytic activity. They noticed an increased fibrinolytic activity after strenuous exercise in 58 trained athletes but a lesser degree with moderate exercise in ten volunteers. The increase in activity was found to persist for at least one hour after exercise. They concluded, in addition, that to obtain the beneficial effects of exercise and prevent thromboembolism, it is not necessary to involve the endangered part of the body. Exercise of the arms, for instance, may benefit a leg encased in plaster.

In 1968, Cohen et al[41] studied alterations of fibrinolysis and blood coagulation induced by exercise and the role of beta-adrenergic receptor stimulation in five healthy volunteers. On one day placebo and on another day propranolol was administered before exercise. Exercise significantly enhanced fibrinolysis and also caused factor 8 increases from two to four times resting values. No significant change was noted in other coagulation factors. The administration of propranolol did not affect the enhanced fibrinolysis but did prevent the increase of platelet factor 8. Thus, while exercise seems to increase platelet factor 8 activity by beta-receptor stimulation, this mechanism is not responsible for the associated increase in fibrinolysis.

Epstein et al.[42] reported an impaired fibrinolytic response to exercise in patients with type 4 hyperlipoproteinemia. Seven normal subjects and eight patients with type 4 hyperlipoproteinemia were studied. Exercise greatly increased the fibrinolytic activity in six of the seven normals. A similar increase took place in only one of the eight patients. These data may indicate that normal fibrinolytic activity is impaired in patients with type 4 lipid abnormalities.

Korsan-Bengtsen and Wilhelmsen[43] reported blood coagulation and fibrinolysis in relation to the degree of physical activity during work and leisure time. They studied a sample of 722 men and concluded that there is a diurnal rhythm of fibrinolysis which is not linked to physical activity and that physically active men have shorter clotting times of plasma than less active men. They reported no differences in other variables of blood clotting and fibrinolysis between morning and afternoon samples or between groups with different activity.

Rosing et al.[44] reported the impairment of the diurnal fibrinolytic response in man with reference to the effects of aging, type 4 hyperlipoproteinemia, and coronary artery disease. They found that the marked diurnal increases in fibrinolysis observed in young normal subjects were significantly reduced in a large percent of older normal subjects and in most of these with coronary artery disease or type 4 lipid abnormalities. Although not conclusive, their findings were compatible with the hypothesis that an impairment in the responsiveness of the fibrinolytic system may be related to the development of coronary artery disease.

Khanna et al.[45] reported from India studies of the effect of submaximal exercise on fibrinolytic activity in ischemic heart disease. These authors studied 20 patients with ischemic heart disease and eight healthy controls. There was a significant increase in the fibrinolytic response in both groups, but it was significantly less in the ischemic groups (36.2 percent compared to 55.9 percent in the control group). The diminished response in this ischemic disease may favor predisposition to thrombotic episodes.

Davis et al.[46] reported the fibrinolytic and hemostatic changes during and after maximal exercise in males. They found that in maximal exercise fibrinolytic activity increased as well as white blood cell count and platelet count. Collen et al.[47] reported from Belgium on the turnover of fibrinogen, plasminogen, and prothrombin during exercise in man. The data supported the concept that plasminogen activation and plasmin-induced fibrinogen degradation occur to some extreme in man following strenuous exercise.

More recently Williams et al.[48] demonstrated augmentation of stimulated fibrinolytic response to venous occlusion in patients following physical conditioning. They felt that one of the beneficial effects of habitual exercise may be stimulation of the fibrinolytic system. This would certainly seem potentially beneficial in the setting of occlusive vascular disease.

SUMMARY

In the field of hematology, therefore, the role of exercise seems to be most involved with the fibrin-fibrinolysis system and platelet activity. This relates to and may be quite instrumental in delaying or affecting the process of atherogenesis. The effectiveness of current management of atherosclerosis lies predominantly in primary prevention with alteration of certain risk factors—namely high blood pressure, smoking, and abnormal blood lipids and sedentary life-style. The role of blood coagulation is of constantly increasing importance in this area, especially as new drugs are available and utilized to alter platelet activity.

REFERENCES

1. Oscai LB, Williams BT, Hertig BA: Effect of exercise on blood volume. *J Appl Physiol* 1968; 24:622−624.
2. Saltin B, Grimby G: Physiological analysis of middle-aged and old former athletes: Comparison with still active athletes of the same ages. *Circulation* 1968; 38:1104−1115.
3. Saltin B, Hartley LH, Kilbom A, Astrand I: Physical training in sedentary middle-aged and older men. II. Oxygen uptake, heart rate, and blood lactate concentration at submaximal and maximal exercise. *Scand J Clin Lab Invest* 1969; 24:323−334.
4. Cook DR, Gualtier WS, Galla SJ: Body fluid volumes of college athletes and non-athletes. *Med Sci Sports* 1970; 1:217−220.
5. Montage JH, Metzner HL, Keller JB, Johnson BC, Epstein FH: Habitual physical activity and blood pressure. *Med Sci Sports* 1972; 4: 175−181.
6. Clausen JP: Circulatory adjustments to dynamic exercise and effect of physical training in normal subjects and in patients with coronary artery disease. *Prog Cardiovasc Dis* 1976; 18:459−495.
7. Astrand PO, Rodahl K: *Textbook of Work Physiology.* New York, McGraw-Hill, 1970.
8. Bass DE, Buskirk ER, Iampietro PF, Mager M: Comparison of blood volume during physical conditioning heat acclimatization and sedentary living. *J Appl Physiol* 1958; 12:186−188.
9. Herrlich HC, Raab W, Gigee W: Influence of muscular training and of catecholamines on cardiac acetylcholine and cholinesterase. *Arch Int Pharmacodyn Ther* 1960; 129:201−215.
10. Reuschlein PS, Reddan WG, Burpee J, Gee JBL, Rankin J: Effect of physical training on the pulmonary diffusing capacity during submaximal work. *J Appl Physiol* 1968; 24:152−158.
11. Ross JH, Atwood EC: Severe repetitive exercise and haematological status. *Postgrad Med J* 1984; 60:454−457.
12. Ernst E: Changes in blood rheology produced by exercise. *JAMA* 1985; 253:2962−2963.
13. Shappell SD, Murray JA, Bellingham AJ, Woodson RD, Deter JC,

Lenfant C: Adaptation to exercise: role of hemoglobin affinity for oxygen and 2, 3-diphosphoglycerate. *J Appl Physiol* 1971; 30: 827–832.

14. Klausen K, Rasmussen B, Clausen JP, Trap-Jensen J: Blood lactate from exercise extremities before and after arm or leg training. *Am J Physiol* 1974; 227:67–72.

15. Dressendorfer RH, Wade CE, Amsterdam EA: Development of pseudoanemia in marathon runners during a 20-day road race. *JAMA* 1981; 246:1215–1218.

16. Ehn L, Carlmark B, Hoglund S: Iron status in athletes involved in intense physical activity. *Med Sci Sports Exercise* 1980; 12:61–64.

17. Garrey WE, Bryan WR: Variations in white blood cell counts. *Physiol Rev* 1935; 15:597–638.

18. Athens JW, et al: Leukokinetic studies. III. The distribution of granulocytes in the blood of normal subjects. *J Clin Invest* 1961; 40:159–164.

19. Athens JW, et al: Leukokinetic studies. IV. The total blood, circulating and marginal granulocyte pools and the granulocyte turnover rate in normal subjects. *J Clin Invest* 1961; 40:989–995.

20. Farris EJ: Blood picture of athletes as affected by intercollegiate type sports. *Am J Anal* 1943; 72:223.

21. Hirsen DJ, Hsu CCS, Malham LM, Su SJ-Y: Mechanism of exercise enhanced lymphocyte cytotoxicity. *Clin Res* 1983; 31:732A (Abstract).

22. Sarajas HSS, et al: Thrombocytosis evoked by exercise. *Nature* 1961; 192:721–722.

23. Wachholder K, et al: Der Einfluss Korperlicher Arbeid auf die Zahl der Thrombocyten und auf deren Haftneigung. *Acta Haematol* 1957; 18:59–79.

24. Dawson AA, Ogston D: Exercise-induced thrombocytosis. *Acta Haematol* 1969; 42:241–246.

25. Bierman HR, et al: The release of leukocytes and platelets from the pulmonary circulation by epinephrine. *Blood* 1952; 7:683–692.

26. Prentice CRM, et al: Studies on blood coagulation, fibrinolysis and platelet function following exercise in normal and splenectomized people. *Br J Haematol* 1972; 23:541–552.

27. Persantine and aspirin in coronary heart disease. The persatine-aspirin reinfarction study Research Group. *Circulation* 1980; 62:449–461.

28. Canadian Cooperative Study Group: A randomized trial of aspirin and sulfinpyrazone in threatened stroke. *NEJM* 1978; 299:53–59.

29. Steele P, Rainwater J, Vogel R, Genton E: Platelet-suppressant therapy in patients with coronary artery disease. *JAMA* 1978; 240: 228–231.

30. Doyle DJ, Chesterman CN, Cade JF, et al: Plasma concentration of platelet-specific proteins correlated with platelet survival. *Blood* 1980; 55:82–84.

31. Mehta J, Mehta P, Pepine CJ: Platelet aggregation in aortic and coronary venous blood in patients with and without coronary disease. 3. Role of tachycardia stress and propranolol. *Circulation* 1978; 58: 881–886.

32. Rubinstein MD, et al: Increased platelet activity in the human coronary circulation in coronary atherosclerosis and spasm. *Circulation* 1980; 62:III-276 (Abstract).
33. Ross R, et al: A platelet-dependent serum factor that stimulates the proliferation of arterial smooth muscle cells in vitro. *Proc Natl Acad Sci* 1974; 71:1207−1210.
34. Harker LA, Ritchie JL: The role of platelets in acute vascular events. *Circulation* 1980; 62:13.
35. Green LH, Seroppian E, Handin RI: Platelet activation during exercise-induced myocardial ischemia. *NEJM* 1980; 302:193−197.
36. Steele PP: Platelet release during exercise in coronary disease. *Clin Res* 1981; 29:80A (Abstract).
37. Steele PP: Platelet suppressants inhibit release of beta-thromboglobulin during isometric exercise in coronary disease. *Clin Res* 1981; 29:214A (Abstract).
38. Williams RS, Eden S, Andersen J: Reduced epinephrine-induced platelet aggregation following cardiac rehabilitation. *J Cardiac Rehab* 1981; 1:127.
39. Bullock G, Watt EW: Platelet factor-4 activity before and after exercise testing in trained coronary heart disease patients. Abstract, Presented at 1981 Scientific Session of American Heart Association, Georgia Affiliate.
40. Menon IS, Burke F, Dewar HA: Effect of strenuous and graded exercise on fibrinolytic activity. *Lancet* 1967; 1:700−703.
41. Cohen RJ, Cohen LS, Epstein SE, Dennis LH: Alterations of fibrinolysis and blood coagulation induced by exercise and the role of beta-adrenergic-receptor stimulation. *Lancet* 1968; 2:1264−1266.
42. Epstein SE, Brakman P, Rosing DR, Redwood DR: Impaired fibrinolytic response to exercise in patients with type-IV hyperlipoproteinemia. *Lancet* 1970; 2:631−634.
43. Korsan-Bengtsen K, Wilhelmsen L, Tibblin G: Blood coagulation and fibrinolysis in relation to degree of physical activity during work and leisure time: A study based on a random sample of 54-year-old men. *Acta Med Scand* 1973; 193:73.
44. Rosing DR, Redwood DR, Brakman P, Astrup T, Epstein SE: Impairment of the diurnal fibrinolytic response in man: Effects of aging, type IV hyperlipoproteinemia and coronary artery disease. *Circ Res* 1973; 32:752−758.
45. Khanna PK, Seth HN, Balasubramanian V, Hoon RS: Effect of submaximal exercise on fibrinolytic activity in ischemic heart disease. *Br Heart J* 1975; 37:1273−1276.
46. Davis GL, Abildgaard CF, Bernauer EM, Britton M: Fibrinolytic and hemostatic changes during and after maximal exercise in males. *J Appl Physiol* 1976; 40:287−292.
47. Collen D, Semeraro N, Tricot JP, Vermylen J: Turnover of fibrinogen, plasminogen and prothrombin during exercise in man. *J Appl Physiol* 1977; 42:865−873.
48. Williams RS, Logue EE, Lewis JG, et al: Physical conditioning augments the fibrinolytic response to venous occlusion in healthy adults. *N Engl J Med* 1980; 302:987.

9

Exercise, Infection, and Immunity

Harvey B. Simon, M.D.

EXERCISE, INFECTION, AND IMMUNITY

Many athletes believe that exercise can enhance their "resistance" to infection; indeed, popular lore holds that good physical conditioning will help prevent the infectious process, but that being "run-down" or "out of shape" increases vulnerability to these common problems. Whereas exercise does have many important cardiovascular, metabolic, and musculoskeletal health benefits which have been scientifically validated, the effects of exercise on infection and immunity have been studied in much less detail.

HOST-DEFENSE MECHANISMS: A BRIEF OVERVIEW

Man lives in a sea of microbes; an intricate and elegant series of host-defense mechanisms is remarkably effective in protecting healthy individuals from infection with these organisms. To understand how exercise may affect immunity, it is important to understand the components of the immune system.

From: Fletcher GF: *Exercise in the Practice of Medicine*, 2nd Revised Edition. Mount Kisco, NY, Futura Publishing Co., Inc., © 1988.

Nonspecific Mechanisms and Anatomic Barriers

The first line of defense against infection is a series of anatomical and physiological barriers which prevent penetration of microorganisms from the outside world into vulnerable body tissues. These are nonimmunologic defense mechanisms; they do not depend on prior exposure to specific organisms, and they are designed to provide nonselective protection against a broad range of microbes rather than defending against a specific pathogen. Despite their simplicity, however, these mechanical barriers play an extremely important role in preventing infection.

The skin and mucous membranes are the most important anatomic barriers to infection. An intact epidermis provides a tough mechanical barrier to bacterial penetration; in addition, the low moisture content of the stratum corneum is inhospitable to most bacteria, and various fats and acids secreted by sebaceous and sweat glands possess antibacterial activity. Whereas the mucous membranes are less intrinsically tough than skin, they do provide some protection against the numerous bacteria that normally reside in the upper respiratory tract, gastrointestinal tract, and genitourinary tract. More importantly, the mucus itself can entrap bacteria. In the respiratory tract, entrapped organisms can be expelled by ciliary movement which continually moves the carpet of mucus toward the oropharynx. The squeeze, cough, gag, and bronchoconstrictor reflexes provide additional protection to the respiratory tract. The respiratory tract is also protected by antibacterial substances present in its secretions. These include both nonspecific factors such as lysozyme, alpha-antitrypsin, and lactoferrin and a specific immunoglobulin, secretory IgA.

In the gastrointestinal tract, gastric acidity is an important barrier to exogenous bacteria, and normal peristalsis helps expel organisms, preventing bacterial overgrowth. Other nonspecific factors that may help prevent infection include free drainage of body cavities (sinus, gallbladder, urinary tract), an intact lymphatic network, and normal arterial and venous circulatory systems.

Lymphocytes

Lymphocytes are the primary cells in the immune response. All lymphocytes derive from pluripotential stem cell in the bone marrow. During embryogenesis, lymphocytes differentiate into two major types, B-lymphocytes and T-lymphocytes; subtypes are present within each group, and a third population of lymphocytes ("null" cells) do not belong to either group.

B-lymphocytes differentiate in the bone marrow. They can be recognized by the presence of immunoglobulins on their cell surfaces, and they comprise 5 to 15 percent of the circulating blood lymphocytes. When stimulated by specific antigens, B-cells proliferate and differentiate into nondividing plasma cells, which in turn secrete immunoglobulins. Other B-cells serve as memory cells, retaining the capacity to recognize foreign antigens for indefinite periods after the primary immune response.

T-lymphocytes differentiate in the thymus, and can be recognized by surface receptors which allow them to form rosettes with sheep red blood cells. About 80 percent of circulating lymphocytes are T-cells, but within the T-cell population there are several important subgroups. Fifteen to 60 percent of T-lymphocytes contain the surface protein T4. These T4 cells have several important functions in promoting the immune response: they stimulate the production of antibody by B-lymphocytes, they induce cytotoxic T-cells, and they release mediators called lymphokines which stimulate macrophages and enhance delayed hypersensitivity or cell-mediated immunity. Hence, these T4 lymphocytes are also called helper or inducer T-cells. In contrast, 25 to 35 percent of circulating T-lymphocytes contain the surface protein T8. These T8 cells help regulate the immune response by providing negative feedback: they supress various functions of B- and T-lymphocytes. Cytotoxic T-cells, which kill virus-infected or tumor cells, also belong to the T8 subset. Hence these T8 lymphycytes are also called suppressor or cytotoxic T-cells.

Antibodies

B-lymphocytes and plasma cells secrete five classes of immunoglobulins. IgG is the immunoglobulin present in the serum in the highest concentration, and is the major antibody produced following antigenic challenge. IgG is very important in host-defense against infection: IgG can opsonize or coat microorganisms so that they can be efficiently phagocytized and killed, it can neutralize viruses, and it can neutralize bacterial toxins. IgM is the largest immunoglobulin, and is produced earliest in the immune response. IgM is much shorter-lived than IgG and is produced only during the primary response following initial exposure to the antigen. Even so, IgM can help fight infection: it can agglutinate and lyse bacteria. IgA is the predominant immunoglobulin in the body's external secretions, including tears, saliva, and secretions of the respiratory and GI tracts. Also present in blood, IgA helps defend against infection by interfering with the adherence of organisms to mucosal surfaces, by neutralizing viruses, and by opsonizing organisms (through the so-called alternate complement pathway). IgE is normally present in serum in trace amounts, but is increased in patients with allergies and parasitic infections. IgD is also present in tiny quantities; its function remains unknown.

Complement

At least 20 proteins in the blood interact together in the complement system. Produced by the liver and by macrophages, these proteins circulate as inactive precursor molecules. Complement activation can be initiated by various stimuli including antigen-antibody complexes and by bacterial cell wall polysaccharides. Once activated complement proteins interact with each other in a cascading fashion to activate the entire system by either of two pathways (the "classical" and "alternate" pathways). Activated complement proteins play many roles in the host response to infection, including opsonizing micro-organisms to enhance phagocytosis, producing direct membrane damage to bacteria and fungi, stimulating chemotaxis of polymorphonuclear and mononuclear phagocytes, and mediating acute inflammation at the tissue level.

Polymorphonuclear Leukocytes

Originally derived from a pleuripotential stem cell, polymorphonuclear leukocytes (PMNL) differentiate subsequently from myeloid stem cells in the bone marrow. They are the most important phagocytic cells in the defense against bacterial infection. PMNLs are short-lived cells, but are present in huge numbers in the bone marrow, peripheral blood, and in the "marginal pool" (a reserve of PMNLs adherent to walls of post-capillary venules). Within minutes of bacterial invasion, they are mobilized from the circulation to the inflammatory site in a process called chemotaxis. The major function of polymorphonuclear lymphocytes is to phagocytize or ingest micro-organisms, which are then killed and digested. PMNLs are not immunologically specific or selective, but phagocytosis is greatly enhanced if the organisms are opsonized or coated by a specific antibody and by various serum proteins belonging to the complement sequence (see above). Acting with antibody and complement, polymorphonuclear lymphocytes are crucial to host defense against acute pyogenic pathogens, including most bacteria.

Monuclear Phagocytes

Mononuclear phagocytes include both blood monocytes and tissue macrophages of the reticuloendothelial system; marrow myeloid stem cells differentiate into blood monocytes which appear to travel through the circulation to the tissues where they mature into macrophages. Once dismissed as mere scavenger cells, it is now clear that the body's 200 billion mononuclear phagoctyes are a complex and essential component of the immune response.

Mononuclear phagoctyes have three important roles: (1) they process antigens and present them to lymphocytes to faciliatate induction of the immune response; (2) they produce and secrete biologically important materials, including enzymes complement proteins, prostaglandins, and other mediators, and interleukin-1 which can further stimulate the immune responses (discussed later); and (3) they are phagocytic cells which migrate to sites of inflammation and infection more slowly than polymorphonuclear lymphocytes, but still ingest and kill micro-organisms. The phagocytic capacity of macrophages can be greatly enhanced if these cells are activated by helper T-lymphocytes which have been stimulated by antigens. Activated macrophages may aggregate to form granulomas, and are crucial to host defenses against intracellular parasites including viruses, mycobacteria and fungi, and certain bacteria and parasites.

Interferons

The interferons are a group of naturally occurring proteins produced by host cells in response to viral infections and other stimuli. Interferons exert antiviral effects against a wide spectrum of viruses; the antiviral action of interferons occurs within hours and can persist for days. A variety of effects on tumor cells and on immunologic functions are also mediated by interferons. Three distinct interferon proteins are produced by human cells. Peripheral blood leucocytes and other lymphoid cells produce interferon-α, which has been used to treat viral infections and neoplasia. Interferon-β is derived from fibroblasts, and interferon-γ is produced by immunologically stimulated helper T-lymphocytes.

Interleukin-1

Interleukin-1 (IL-1) is a protein produced by mononuclear phagocytes in response to endotoxin, immune complexes, phagocytosis, and other stimuli (including exercise; see below) IL-1 has three major actions: (1) IL-1 is an immunostimulator, increasing both T-lymphocyte activity and the production of antibody by B-lymphocytes; (2) IL-1 mediates the acute phase response which characterizes so many infections and inflammatory states, including leukocytosis, hepatic synthesis of fibrinogen, and other acute phase proteins, fibroblast proliferation and collagen production, and muscle catabolism; and (3) IL-1 produces fever by traveling in the circulation to the thermal control center in the anterior hypothalmus, where it increases prostaglandin levels, thereby resetting the "thermostat" upwards.

Fever

IL-1 produces immunostimulation and inflammation as well as fever; the immunostimulatory activity of IL-1 is in fact increased at elevated temperatures. Although it is tempting to speculate that these events help fight infection, there is still no direct proof that fever is beneficial in fighting infection in man. Quite apart from the immunostimulatory activity of IL-1, fever *per se* may also be beneficial by directly injuring thermolabile microorganisms and by lowering serum iron levels. Whereas fever can enhance recovery from infection in certain experimental animals, the importance of fever in clinical infection in man is uncertain.

THE EFFECTS OF EXERCISE ON
IMMUNE PARAMETERS

I have previously reviewed the immunology of exercise,[1] citing studies performed through 1983. Table 1 extends these observations for studies published through 1986. In all 14 studies,

Table 1
Effects of Exercise on Various Host-Defense Parameters

Study	Ahlborg & Ahlborg[2] (1970)	Hedfors et al.[3] (1976)	Yu et al.[4] (1977)	Eskola et al.[5] (1978)	Busse et al.[6] (1980)
Number of subjects	8	15	8	16	13
Exercise	Bike, maximal	Bike—15 minutes	Treadmill 10 minutes	Run 7 km 42 km	13 km (trained subjects) maximal treadmill (untrained)
Granulocytes Total Count	I	I	—	I	Trained,6 NC Untrained 7 See Below
Function	—	—	—	—	—
Immunoglobulins	—	—	—	—	—
Complement	—	—	—	—	—
Lymphocytes Total Count	I	I	I	NC	—
B-Cells	—	I	I	—	—
T-Cells	—	I	I	—	—
Function	—	Transformation D Cytotoxicity I	—	Transformation D Antibody Production NC	—
Other	Leukocytosis blunted by propanolol	—	Lymphocytosis blocked by prednisone	Serum cortisol I	Granulocyte response to isoproterenol and plasma catecholamine I in untrained subjects

Continued

Study	Green et al.[7] (1981)	Hanson & Flaherty[8] (1981)	Robertson et al.[9] (1981)	Soppi et al.[10] (1981)	Tomasi et al.[11] (1982)
Number of Subjects	20	6	9	29	8
Exercise	None Marathoners tested at rest	13 km run	Bike, maximal	Bike, maximal	Cross-country ski racing
Granulocytes					
Total Count	NC	NC	I	I	—
Function	Phagocytosis NC Killing NC	—	—	—	—
Immunoglobulins	NC	NC	—	—	—
Complement	NC	NC	—	—	—
Lymphocytes					
Total Count	NC	NC	I	I	—
B-Cells	NC	NC	—	NC	I
T-Cells	NC	NC	I	NC	NC
Function	Transformation NC	Increased antibody dependent cytotoxic effector cells (K lymphocytes)	Transformation I	Transformation I	—
Other			Changes transient-leukocytes back to baseline in 15 mins. Serum cortisol I		

Study	Cannon & Klugel[12] (1983)	Cannon & Dinarello[13] (1984)	Viti et al.[14] (1985)	Watson et al.[15] (1986)
Number of Subjects	14	3	8	46
Exercise	Bike, submaximal 1 hour	Unspecified	Bike, submaximal 1 hour	Walk-jog (15 week training)
Granulocytes				
Total Count	—	—	—	—
Function				
Immunoglobulin	—	—	—	—
Complement	—	—	—	—
Lymphocytes				
Total Count	—	—	—	
B-Cells				
T-Cells				NC
Function				I
Other	Increased Interleukin-1	Increased Interleukin-1	Increased plasma-interferon	T Cell Mitogenesis I Cytotoxicity D No change in number of monocytes No differences in subjects studied on β-blockers

I = incrased; D = decreased; NC = no change.
Modified from reference 1.

healthy adult volunteers served as subjects; only seven of the 203 subjects were women.

The fitness level of the study subjects varied widely. In many investigations,[2-4,9,15] unconditioned individuals were utilized, and in some studies[12,13] the fitness level of the subjects was not specified. In contrast, several studies[6,10,15] put their subjects through a supervised training program using aerobic exercise (biking or running) for 6 to 15 weeks measuring VO_2 max to document the training effect. Finally, in four of the studies, highly trained marathon runners[5-7] or cross-country ski racers[11] were studied.

The exercise protocols also varied greatly in these studies, ranging from a modest work load of 15 minutes of submaximal exertion on a bike ergometer[3] to marathon running[5] and cross-country skiing.[11] In general, the subjects in these investigations served as their own controls, as various immunologic parameters were measured before and after exercise to determine the effects of acute exercise. In one study,[15] immunological parameters were measured in the resting state before and after a 15 week training program, and in one investigation[7] marathon runners were studied at rest and were compared with untrained control subjects.

The host-defense parameters that were measured in these studies also varied greatly, ranging from simple determinations of leukocyte counts to sophisticated measurements of lymphocyte subsets and function. Because these studies were performed over a 16-year period, the laboratory techniques that were utilized also vary greatly. In two studies, the effects of β-blockade were investigated, and the effects of isoproterenol and prednisone were measured in one study each. Finally, most of the studies were quite small, with three to 46 subjects (mean 14.5) in each study group.

In view of the many disparities, it is not surprising that the results of these investigations also display considerable variability, and in some cases are contradictory. Nevertheless, a review of these studies can begin to paint a picture of the effects of exercise on host-defense mechanisms. In addition, because the immunological response to exercise has been studied much less carefully than other areas of exercise physiology, important questions for future study can be delineated.

Nonspecific Mechanisms and Anatomical Barriers

Little attention has been paid to the effects of exercise on nonimmunological host-defense mechanisms, and indeed these effects are probably minimal. Even noncontact sports can result in trauma which can disrupt the integrity of the cutaneous barrier to infection. In some cases, exposure (ranging from sunburn to frostbite) can lead to a serious breach of this barrier. Much more often, perspiration can damage the skin by producing maceration; superficial fungal infections (see later in chapter) may result from these problems, but cellulitis and other bacterial infections are much less frequent.

Many athletes observe increased rates of respiratory mucous production during exercise, especially in cold weather. Actual mucociliary clearance has not been measured, but it is possible that increased clearance could help fight respiratory infections by removing micro-organisms. On the other hand, Tomasi and co-workers[11] reported a decrease in salivary IgA levels following cross-country ski races of 20 to 50 km; the magnitude of this decrease was substantial, with post-race values less than 25 percent of normal. The duration of the decline was not studied, but since pre-race levels in these highly trained skiers were also significantly low, repeated endurance exercise in cold temperatures may well result in persistently low secretory IgA levels. While the mechanism of this decline is unknown, depletion of nasal fluid or impaired function of mucosal plasma cells due to decreased temperatures could be responsible. Whereas depletion of secretory IgA could predispose athletes to respiratory infections, the clinical significance of these findings has not been investigated.

Some athletes report increased gastric acidity or increased intestinal motility (the "runner's trots") during or after exercise. Theoretically, both phenomena could help combat intestinal infections, but studies have not been performed, and it seems unlikely that these factors are clinically important.

Lymphocytes

Lymphocytes are the primary cells in the immune response; not surprisingly, they are also the most important link in the relationship between exercise and immune function. Of the seven studies that measured the acute effects of exercise on the total lymphocyte count, five reported an increase (see Table 1). Although both T- and B-cells increase after exercise, T-lymphocyte counts seem to be elevated more significantly. Many other immunological studies, unrelated to exercise, have shown that T-cells are the most readily mobilized class of hyman lymphocytes, and in this respect, the effects of exercise seem similar to those of very different immunological stimuli. It is not known if exercise affects T4 (helper) and T8 (suppressor) cells differently. An additional investigation[15] measured the effects of long-term conditioning on lymphocyte counts at rest and found that the number of mature T-lymphocytes was significantly increased. Whereas these results imply that conditioning produces a long-term increase in T-cells, Robertson and co-workers[9] found that exercise-induced T-cell lymphocytosis persisted for less than 15 minutes. Because their study measured only the acute effects of exercise in unconditioned subjects, however, these studies are not actually contradictory; both observations could fit the hypothesis that conditioning increases base-line T-cell counts, and that acute exercise produces a further increase which is transitory. Clearly, additional studies will be needed to elucidate this possibility.

The mechanism of exercise-induced lymphocytes is unknown. β-blocking agents do not prevent the effect,[15] suggesting that it is largely independent of adrenergic mechanisms. In contrast, corticosteroids do prevent the exercise-induced lymphocytosis.[3] Perhaps the lymphocytosis produced acutely by strenuous exertion is transient because plasma cortisol levels rise with exercise.[5,9]

If the effects of exercise on lymphocyte counts are complex, its effects on lymphocyte function are even less clear-cut. Five studies investigated the influence of exercise on lymphocyte transformation, or mitogenesis, *in vitro*; three report an increase after acute exercise or long-term conditioning,[15] whereas two report a decrease[3,5] after acute exercise, with recovery to normal within 24 hours.[5] Green and co-workers[7] found normal lymphocyte transformation in marathon runners studied at rest. The results of cytotoxicity testing are also divided, with two studies showing an increase[3,8] and one a decrease.[15]

Because of the central role of the lymphocyte in the immune response, further studies of lymphocyte function in athletes are warranted. In particular, T-cell subsets and function should be investigated. Until such studies are available, it is impossible to know if exercise produces clinically relevant changes in lymphocytes. Based on the present, incomplete data, I doubt that exercise-induced changes in lymphocytes alter host-defense mechanisms to a clinically important extent.

Antibodies

Very few studies have examined the effects of exercise on serum immunoglobulin levels. Two studies of runners[7,8] report normal serum immunoglobulin levels. As discussed earlier, Tomasi and co-workers[11] measured secretory IgA levels in eight highly trained Nordic ski racers; salivary IgA levels were significantly depressed, and fell further after a strenuous race. It is not known if these changes result from exposure to cold ambient temperatures, strenuous exertion, or both. Serum immunoglobulin levels were measured in the skiers but are not reported in the study.

Although data on immunoglobulins and exercise are extremely limited, it seems unlikely that serum immunoglobulin levels are altered by exercise. Studies of specific antibody titers, however, would be of interest to confirm this belief. Lower secretory IgA levels could predispose to respiratory tract infections; clearly, further studies of cold- and warm-weather athletes are needed to resolve this question.

Complement Levels

Two studies have reported serum complement levels in endurance athletes, both before[7] and after[8] exercise. In both, the results were normal. Although conclusions based on studies of only 26 subjects must be somewhat tentative, it seems unlikely that the serum complement system is responsible for any alterations in the host-defense mechanisms of athletes.

Polymorphonuclear Leukocytes

For at least 30 years, it has been known that exercise produces a rise in serum leukocyte counts. Seven of the more recent studies summarized in Table 1 measured white blood cell counts before and after exercise; five of these investigations document a significant exercise-induced granulocytosis. In the negative studies, Hansen and Flaherty[8] failed to demonstrate granulocytes in six well-conditioned men who ran 8 miles at a brisk pace; Busse et al.[6] also found normal post-exertion leukocyte counts in six trained athletes who ran 13 km, but they found that treadmill running did produce significant granulocytosis in seven unconditioned subjects. These findings might suggest that training blunts the leukocytosis of exercise, which could be explained by lower post-exercise catecholamine levels in trained athletes. However, Eskola et al.[5] found that exercise did produce a significant leukocytosis in highly trained marathon runners, and Soppi et al.[10] found that exercise produced a leukocytosis both before and after 6 weeks of physical conditioning.

Only one study[7] investigated granulocyte function in athletes; both phagocytosis and killing were normal in 20 marathon runners. These athletes were studied only at rest, at which time their total leukocyte counts were within the normal range.

The mechanisms of exercise-induced leukocytosis have not been studied in detail, but four factors probably contribute to this effect. Strenuous exercise rapidly causes significant shifts in extracellular fluids, producing hemoconcentration which can elevate the concentrations of formed elements in the blood. Exercise elevates catecholamine levels, and epinephrine in turn mobilizes granulocytes from the marginal pool. Indeed, Ahlborg and Ahlborg[2] found that propranolol blunts the leukocytosis of exercise, suggesting that adrenergic mechanisms do play an important role. Cortisol mobilizes granulocytes from the marrow pool and also slows their egress from the circulation; cortisol levels are also increased by exercise. Finally, exercise increases interleukin-1 levels (see later), and IL-1 can stimulate granulocytosis.

Whereas exercise produces a leukocytosis, it is unlikely that these elevated granulocyte counts play a significant role in enhancing host-defense against infection. Robertson and co-workers,[9] have demonstrated that the leukocytosis of exercise is transient, with granulocyte counts returning to normal within 45 minutes before rising again at 2 hours. Moreover, the granulocytes of highly trained athletes appear to be functionally identical to the white blood cells of sedentary individuals.[7]

Mononuclear Phagocytes

Neither blood monocyte counts nor mononuclear cell function in exercise have been studied in detail. However, the fact that interleukin-1 levels rise with exercise (see later) implies that mononuclear phagocytes are indeed activated by physical exertion. Further studies in this area would be of interest.

Interferons

In a study of eight untrained men, Viti and colleagues[14] found that 1 hour of submaximal exercise on a bicycle ergometer elevated plasma interferon-α levels from 3 to 7 IU. Peripheral blood leukocytes are a source of interferon-α, and these observations may reflect the leukocytosis of exercise; unfortunately, white blood cell counts were not reported in this study. Although those exercise-induced changes in interferon levels were statistically significant, I doubt that they are biologically significant to host-defense mechanisms: these elevations are brief, lasting less than 2 hours, and of minimal magnitude, since viral infections produce interferon levels which may be 10- to 20-fold higher.

Interleukin-1 and Fever

Cannon and Kluger[12] have studied the effects of exercise on the production of "endogenous pyrogen" in man. Fourteen subjects exercised on bike ergometers for 1 hour at 60 percent of their maximal aerobic capacity. Both immediately after exercise and 3 hours later, elevated circulating levels of endogenous pyrogen could be demonstrated in several bioassays. In addition, blood mononuclear phagocytes collected from five of the subjects after exercise also released endogenous pyrogen after incubation *in vitro*, whereas monocytes harvested from these subjects prior to exercise did not.

It is now clear that endogenous pyrogen is identical to interleukin-1. Indeed, in a smaller study using an immunological assay (the mitogenic response of mouse thymocytes) Cannon and Dinarello[13] have shown that exercise elevates circulating IL-1 levels.

Although these observations are based on very small studies, they are the most provocative and potentially important link between exercise and host-defense mechanisms. First, IL-1 is an immunostimulator, increasing the activity of both T- and B-lymphocytes; hence exercise-induced production of IL-1 might account for the lymphocyte activation reported in other exercise studies, and could potentially enhance host-defense mechanisms in athletes. Second, IL-1 mediates the acute phase reponse to infection and inflammation; in this capacity, it produces leukocytosis and could therefore be a contributing factor in the leukocytosis of exercise. Finally, IL-1 produces fever; fever can enhance recovery from infection in some experimental animals, but the effects of fever *per se* on clinical host-defense in man remains uncertain.

The observations of Cannon, Kluger, and Dinarello also have interesting implications for work physiology. Body temperatures are regularly elevated as a result of intense exercise and sports.[16] However, the hyperthermia of exercise has been regarded as entirely different from the fever of infection in terms of its pathogenesis.[17,18] In infection and other inflammatory states, IL-1 acts on the anterior hypothalmus to elevate the set-point of the body's "thermostat." Neural control mechanisms then produce vasoconstriction, cessation of sweating, and increased heat production by skeletal muscle until body temperature rises to the new set-point. In contrast, the hypothalmic set-point is unchanged in exercise hyperthermia; body temperature is elevated simply because intense exercise generates heat faster than it can be dissipated by thermal control mechanisms. The extreme pyrexia that accompanies heart stroke, thyroid storm, and certain other disease states is also thought to result from excessive heat production, impaired heat dissipation, or both.[19]

Clearly the studies of Cannon, Kluger, and Dinarello should lead to re-examination of this hypothesis. It should be noted that they studied only a modest number of individuals, and that they did not measure the body temperature of their subjects. In addition, the demonstration of IL-1 in the circulation of febrile humans has been quite difficult.[17] Hence, I believe that these fascinating observations should be confirmed before we conclude that exercise hyperthermia involves the production of IL-1, much less immunologic enhancement. Indeed, it seems likely that exercise hyperthermia may depend on both excessive heat production by metabolically active skeletal muscle and on IL-1 production; the relative importance of these two mechanisms, as well as the possible contribution of each to host-defense mechanisms, will require further study.

Endorphins and Neuroendocrine Mechanisms

In the past few years, an increasing body of evidence has suggested that there are complex interactions between the central nervous system and the immune system. The influence of psychosocial stress on the immune system and on susceptibility to infections, neoplasia, and autoimmune disorders is the subject of ongoing experimental and clinical study. Although much remains to be learned, it appears that a variety of neuroendocrine hormones including corticosteroids, endorphins, interferon, interleukin-1 and catecholamines may mediate bidirectional interactions between the central nervous system and the immune system.[20]

Most studies have focused on psychosocial stress or adversive physiologic stimuli (such as electric shocks) in studying neuro-immunologic interactions. Although exercise is a very different form of stress, many of these same neuroendocrine transmitters are stimulated by exercise. Studies of exercise, neuroendocrine mechanisms, and immunity would be of interest.

EXERCISE, SPORTS, AND INFECTIOUS DISEASES

Whereas the studies of exercise and host-defense mechanisms demonstrate that strenuous exertion can produce potentially important alterations in a number of these mechanisms, they do not answer the fundamental question of whether or not habitual exercise alters host resistance to infection. To answer this all-important question, clinical studies would be needed. Popular lore is full of anecdotal reports of people who claim improved "resistance" to infection when they exercise for fitness. Some athletes, however, also report increased vulnerability to infection when they overtrain or "get run down." Clearly, these anecdotes are of little scientific merit. Unfortunately, to my knowledge no clinical studies of exercise and infection have been reported. Indeed, controlled trials of exercise in independently living populations are exceedingly difficult. Many large studies of exercise and coronary artery disease have been performed and others are in progress; it would be interesting to include questions about exercise and infection in such surveys in the future. Objective measurements would be necessary; perhaps employee absenteeism due to febrile and respiratory infections could serve as a reasonably objective endpoint. Closer prospective observations of smaller population groups might also be used to study the relationship of exercise and infection. A possible approach would be to observe the rate and severity of common respiratory infections in matched pairs of individuals who have similar epidemiologic exposures, such as college athletes and their sedentary roommates.

Can exercise adversly affect infection in man? Again, although direct clinical observations are lacking, the popular lore holds that exposure to cold decreases "resistance" to infection. If this were true, winter sports might predispose to respiratory infection. However, careful study of cold exposure on rhinovirus infection in man failed to demonstrate any such effect.[21] In a very different animal study, forced swimming did increase the severity of myocarditis in mice with experimental coxsackie virus B-3 infections.[22] These studies were performed with young, vulnerable animals experimentally inoculated with a cardiotropic virus and then forced to swim in heated water. Clearly, this model is very unlike human exercise, and indeed myocarditis is an uncommon mechanism of sudden death in athletes;[23] nevertheless, these observations should have a sobering effect on athletes who have systemic viral illnesses.

Clinical Infections

Skin infections are relatively common in people who exercise regularly. Trauma is the major predisposing factor and can sometimes lead to serious bacterial infections in which microorganisms are directly inoculated into traumatized skin. Cellulitis and lymphangitis can result, but fortunately these are not common in athletes. When these processes do occur, they require therapy with parenteral antibiotics and usual ancillary measures including rest and elevation of an affected limb. Clearly, continued exercise is not possible until healing occurs.

Much more common but much less serious skin infections in athletes are caused by fungi. Here, moisture and maceration allow infection by superficial dermatophytes to occur. Since these molds do not live free in nature but are spread from person-to-person, shared locker-room facilities play an epidemiological role in the spread of these infections. Although these processes can be unsightly and uncomfortable, they are confined to the superficial layers of the epidermis and are rarely serious. However, they can be a focus for secondary bacterial infection and should therefore be treated promptly.

Because infection with superficial dermatophytes is so common in athletes, several varieties pay tribute to the athlete in their common names. Tinea cruris is an infection of the inguinal region which is known also as "jock itch." Tinea pedis involves the interdigital areas of the foot and is called "athlete's foot." Both of these processes respond promptly to topical antimycotic agents such as tolfinate, miconazole, or clotrimazole. Rarely, refractory cases may require oral therapy with ketoconozole. Meticulous drying is very important in preventing and treating these processes as well.

A less-common viral infection of skin which is reported in athletes is herpes gladiatorum, which occurs when herpes virus type I is inoculated directly into the skin in a nonimmune individual. Contact sports such as wrestling have been implicated. Typical herpetic vesicles are the key to diagnosis. Although the therapy of herpes gladiatorum has not been studied specifically, it seems likely that orally administered acyclovir would be symptomatically helpful without affecting viral latency.

Respiratory infections are no different in people who exercise regularly than in sedentary individuals. Upper respiratory infections due to viruses generally do not require interruption of exercise schedules. In fact, some individuals report symptomatic relief probably due to the increased mucus flow associated with exercise. A word of caution may be in order, however, about the use of typical cold remedies since many of these contain sympathomimetic agents which could theoretically cause tachycardia, which might be undesirable during exercise. Lower respiratory tract infections may predispose to bronchospasm which can further be exaggerated by exercise, particularly in cold weather. It would seem prudent for people with lower respiratory tract infections to avoid strenuous exertion until recovery has occurred. If fever is present, the same guidelines for a systemic infection should be followed.

Systemic infections should also be managed in the athlete as they would be in sedentary individuals. Because of the potential concern of myocarditis, it would seem prudent to advise against strenuous exertion if fever and myalgias are present, particularly with viral processes. Physicians practicing sports medicine are well aware, however, of the difficulties in stopping a committed athlete from working out. Because of this, I generally link advice against strenuous exertion with suggestions for alternate, more gentle activities such as stretching exercises until recovery has occurred.

Infectious mononucleosis is a systemic viral infection that is relatively common in high school and college-age athletes. When fever, lymphadenopathy, pharyngitis, and fatigue are present, even the committed athlete will not be inclined to exercise strenuously and the physician should certainly caution against strenuous exertion. However, I am not aware of scientific data supporting the value of the traditional recommendation for bed rest, even during the acute phases of mononucleosis, and I generally allow ordinary daily activities to the limits of tolerance. In fact, I believe that prescriptions for prolonged bed rest are responsible for deconditioning, which can give rise to protracted fatigue even after active viral infection has subsided. This syndrome of "post-infectious asthenia" has, in my experience, responded to a program of graded aerobic exercise and reassurance. I suspect that at least some cases of "chronic" mononucleosis may in fact be little more than deconditioning caused by protracted rest.

Many patients with mononucleosis develop splenomegaly; because of the risk of splenic rupture, contact sports should be avoided until splenomegaly resolves.

Immunization for Athletes

In general, immunization requirements of people who exercise regularly are no different from those of sedentary individuals.[24] Tetanus immunization should be kept up in all adults with boosters every 10 years, but this is often neglected by internists. Because of the risk of trauma, it is particularly important to maintain tetanus immunizations in athletes. If trauma does occur and immunization has not been maintained, tetanus immune globulin may be advisable; Table 2 outlines the recommended management of wounds.

Another immunization which may be helpful in college-age athletes is measles vaccine. Individuals born after 1957 may not have contracted natural measles and may therefore lack immunity. Since the effective live vaccine was not produced until 1967, people born between 1957 and 1967, people who received the earlier inactivated vaccine, or those who received live vaccine before their first birthday may not be protected. Measles outbreaks have occurred in college students and can be prevented by immunizing vulnerable individuals. Unless natural infection or immunity can be documented, measles vaccine should be given, since it produces no ill effects in previously immune individuals.

Although active young athletes are hardly in the population group who are usually targeted for influenza vaccination, it is reasonable to consider influenza vaccine for such individuals providing that the supply of vaccine is sufficient to first meet the needs of elderly and chronically ill patients. Influenza vaccine may be particularly helpful for athletes playing fall or winter team sports, since close contact among these people can result in rapid spread of influenza and impact adversely on the entire season. For this reason I have recommended influenza vaccination for the New

Table 2
Summary Guide to Tetanus Prophylaxis in Routine Wound
Management—United States, 1985[a]

History of Adsorbed Tetanus Toxoid (Doses)	Clean, minor Wounds		All other Wounds[b]	
	Td[c]	TIG	Td[c]	TIG
Unknown or < three	Yes	No	Yes	Yes
≥ three[d]	No[e]	No	No[f]	No

[a]For details, consult the original text.
[b]Such as, but not limited to, wounds contaminated with dirt, feces, soil, saliva, etc.; puncture wounds; avulsions; and wounds resulting from missiles, crushing, burns and frostbite.
[c]For children under 7 years old; DTP (DT, if pertussis vaccine is contraindicated) is preferred to tetanus toxoid alone. For persons 7 years old and older, Td is preferred to tetanus toxoid alone.
[d]If only three doses of *fluid* toxoid have been received, a fourth dose of toxoid, preferably an adsorbed toxoid, should be given.
[e]Yes, if more than 10 years since the last dose.
[f]Yes, if more than 5 years since last dose. (More frequent boosters are not needed and can accentuate side effects.)
Source: *Morbidity and Mortality Weekly Reports* 34:422, 1985.

England Patriots, and I believe that many other teams follow similar practices. The close contact among teammates may require special isolation precautions if one member of a team develops a communicable disease.

CONCLUSION

Exercise produces a variety of changes in host-defense mechanisms. Because of the complexity of these host-defense mechanisms and of exercise physiology, these effects have not been fully elucidated, and further studies in this area are needed. Of particular interest are the effects of exercise on the production of interleukin-1 and the augmentation of immune mechanisms that may result.

Because clinical studies in exercise and infectious illnesses are not available, we do not know if the immunological changes that have been documented are of clinical significance. My own speculation is that some of these changes may cancel each other out, and that the overall effect may prove to be slight. Clearly, further studies are necessary, but these may prove difficult.

Clinical infections in people who exercise regularly can in general be managed as they would be in sedentary people. It seems prudent to advise against strenuous exertion when fever, myalgias, and systemic symptoms are present; very gentle exercises such as stretching can be substituted in the committed athlete until recovery has occurred.

Guidelines for immunization in athletes are the same as those for sedentary people. Particular attention should be paid to tetanus immunization, and measles and influenza vaccinations should be considered in appropriate circumstances.

Professor J.N. Morris, a pioneer in the study of exercise and health, has concluded that "vigorous exercise is a natural defense of the body, with a protective effect on the aging heart against ischemia and its consequences."[25] Until further studies become available, we are unable to conclude that exercise has a similar protective effect on the body's natural defense against infection.

REFERENCES

1. Simon HB: The immunology of exercise: A brief review. *JAMA* 1984; 252(19):2735–2738.
2. Ahlborg B, Ahlborg G: Exercise leukocytosis with and without beta-adrenergic blockade. *Acta Med Scand* 1970; 187:241–246.
3. Hedfors E, Holm G, Ohnell B: Variations of blood lymphocytes during work studied by cell surface markers, DNA syntheseis and cytotoxicity. *Clin Exp Immunol* 1976; 24:328–335.
4. Yu DTY, Clements PJ, Pearson CM: Effect of corticosteroids on exercise-induced lymphocytosis. *Clin Exp Immunol* 1977; 28:326–331.
5. Eskola J, Ruuskanen O, Soppi E, et al: Effect of sport stress on lymphocyte transformation and antibody formation. *Clin Exp Immunol* 1978; 32:339–345.
6. Busse WW, Anderson CL, Hanson PG, et al: The effect of exercise on the granulocyte response to isoproterenol in the trained athlete and unconditioned individual. *J Allergy Clin Immunol* 1980; 65(5):358–364.
7. Green RL, Kaplan SS, Rabin BS, et al: Immune function in marathon runners. *Ann Allergy* 1981; 47(2):73–75.
8. Hanson PG, Flaherty DK: Immunological responses to training in conditioned runners. *Clin Sci* 1981; 60:225–228.
9. Robertson AJ, Ramesar KCRB, Potts RC, et al: The effect of strenuous physical exercise on circulating blood lymphocytes and serum cortisol levels. *J Clin Lab Immunol* 1981; 5:53–57.

10. Soppi E, Varjo P, Eskola J, Laitinen LA: Effect of strenuous physical stress on circulating lymphocyte number and function before and after training. *J Clin Lab Immunol* 1982; 8:43–46.
11. Tomasi TB, Trudeau FB, Czerwinski D, Erredge S: Immune parameters in athletes before and after strenuous exercise. *J Clin Immunol* 1982; 2(3):173–178.
12. Kluger MJ: Endogenous pyrogen activity in human plasma after exercise. *Science* 1983; 220:617–619.
13. Cannon J, Dinarello C: Interleukin-1 activity in human plasma. *Fed Proc* 1984; 43:462.
14. Viti A, Muscettola M, Paulesu L, et al: Effect of exercise on plasma interferon levels. *J Appl Physiol* 1985; 59(2):426–428.
15. Watson RR, Moriguchi S, Jackson JC, et al: Modification of cellular immune functions in humans by endurance exercise training during β-adrenergic blockade with atenolol or propranolol. *Med Sci Sports and Exercise* 1985; 18(1):95–100.
16. Simon HB: Sports medicine. In *Scientific American Medicine*. Rubenstein E, Federman D (eds). New York, Scientific American, 1986, pp 1–26.
17. Dinarello C, Wolff SM: Molecular basis of fever in humans. *Am J Med* 1982; 72:799–819.
18. Stitt JT: Fever versus hyperthermia. *Fed Proc* 1979; 38(1):39–42.
19. Simon HB: Extreme pyrexia in man. In *Fever*. Lipton JM (ed). New York, Raven Press, 1980, pp 213–224.
20. Hall NR, McGillis JP, Spangelo BL, Goldstein AL: Evidence that thymosins and other biologic response modifiers can function as neuroactive immunotransmitters. *J Immunol* 1985; 135(2):806s.
21. Douglas GR, Lindgren KM, Couch RB: Exposure to cold environment and rhinovirus common cold. *NEJM* 1968; 279(14):742–747.
22. Gatmaitan BG, Chason JL, Lerner AM: Augmentation of the virulence of murine Coxsackie virus B-3 myocardopathy by exercise. *J Exp Med* 1970; 131:1121–1136.
23. Simon HB: Immunizations and chemotherapy for viral infections. In *Scientific American Medicine*, Rubenstein E, Federman D (eds). New York, Scientific American, 1986.
24. Simon HB: Sports medicine. In *Scientific American Medicine*. Rubenstein E, Federman D (eds). New York, Scientific American, 1986.
25. Morris JN, Pollard R, Everitt MG, Chave SPW: Vigorous exercise in leisure-time: Protection against coronary heart disease. *Lancet* 1980; 2:1207–1210.

10

Exercise in Endocrinology

Gerald F. Fletcher, M.D.

INTRODUCTION

There is continued emphasis on the intrinsic endocrine response to exercise. This involves several subsets of endocrine anatomic physiology, namely the adrenal, pancreatic, and central nervous systems. The brain has historically been a focus of discussion with regard to pituitary axial neuroendocrine relationships and the role of the hypothalamus has been explored. Of great interest, however, with regard to exercise has been the endorphin system (intrinsic intracerebral opiates) and the role of these substances in high intensity, high frequency exercise. The so-called "runner's high" has often been attributed to elaboration of the endorphins and some investigators have addressed the problem quite specifically.

Of all endocrine disorders, however, diabetes mellitus is probably the most common and the management of this disease requires specific knowledge and control of the patient's physical activity. This is not to say that diabetics should not exercise, but rather that diet and insulin dosage need careful regulation and "tailoring" for the patient with regard to their level of physical activity. Data continue to evolve on glucose metabolism and in diabetic endocrinology and will likely serve to stimulate more investigation in this very important field of medical practice.

From: Fletcher GF: *Exercise in the Practice of Medicine,* 2nd Revised Edition. Mount Kisco, NY, Futura Publishing Co., Inc., © 1988.

ANIMAL RESEARCH

Data have recently been published in preliminary form regarding glucose metabolism in relation to physical exercise in animals. Zawalich and associates[1] reported on a physical training effect in decreasing beta cell sensitivity to glucose and decreasing liver glucokinase in the rat. Sprague Dawley rats (N-8) were placed in wheel cages in which they ran 4−6 miles per day for 3−6 weeks. Intravenous glucose tolerance tests were done and insulin secretion from perifused islets and glucokinase activity in liver were compared with a sedentary control group. They found that in the trained group, blood glucose levels during glucose tolerance tests were comparable to controls; however, in the trained, both basal and stimulated plasma insulin levels were reduced by 28 percent and 39 percent, respectively ($p < 0.05$). Their conclusions were that physical training in rats leads to decreased beta cell sensitivity to the stimulatory effects of glucose and that training also results in a reduction in liver glucokinase comparable to other insulin-deficient states such as starvation and diabetes. These changes in insulin secretion and in the rate limiting enzyme for glucose uptake in liver provide an explanation for the failure of physical training to improve glucose tolerance despite augmented muscle sensitivity to insulin.

Reaven et al.[2] have studied how long insulin sensitivity is enhanced with exercise training. In order to determine how long this effect of exercise training persists after cessation of exercise, rats exercise trained for 2−3 months were removed from their exercise cages for 0, 1, 3, and 7 days and insulin action was assessed with an indirect and a direct method. An insulin resistance index was significantly lower ($p < 0.001$) in rats immediately off exercise (5 hours), although insulin resistance values had increased in rats off exercise 1 and 3 days. The overall results showed that mean steady state plasma glucose levels (mg/dl) were significantly lower in rats off exercise for 0, 1, and 3 days. In contrast, steady state levels in rats off exercise for 7 days had increased to control values. These findings indicate that the enhanced insulin sensitivity due to exercise training disappeared rather quickly, when rats cease to run.

Davis and associates[3] studied the differential effects of acute exercise training on glucose metabolism by muscle. To determine whether exercise training modifies the effect of an acute bout of exercise on the glucose metabolism in muscle, rats were exercise trained for 4 weeks by swimming or they remained sedentary. Epitrochlearis muscles were studied and it was found that, although muscle glycogen was increased by exercise training, the amount of glycogen utilized during acute exercise was similar in trained and in sedentary rats. Basal glucose uptake and glucose utilization were unaffected by acute exercise or exercise training. Basal rate and insulin sensitivity of glycogen synthesis were unaffected by training alone but acute exercise increased the basal rate and the insulin sensitivity of glycogen synthesis more in sedentary than in trained rats. It was concluded that the effects of acute exercise and exercise training on glucose uptake and glucose utilization by muscle are additive and the increase in muscle glycogen with training reduces the stimulation in glycogen synthesis after acute exercise. Therefore, a number of basic studies are now available regarding glucose metabolism and insulin activity in animals relative to exercise activity. Such investigations to date further substantiate the state of increased sensitivity to insulin in the trained state but are inconclusive with regard to the metabolism and uptake/utilization of glucose with regard to exercise.

HUMAN RESEARCH

In humans, a number of studies have evolved with regard to exercise and various aspects of endocrinology. These have been in the subsets of *pancreatic (glucose)*, *pituitary*, and *testicular* function.

Glucose Metabolism

Soman et al.[4] reported on increased insulin sensitivity and insulin binding to monocytes after physical training. Their data revealed that increases in insulin sensitivity correlated directly with increases in oxygen consumption. This was statistically significant at the $p < 0.05$ level. Binding of insulin to monocytes increased by 35 percent after physical training primarily because of the increase in concentration of insulin receptors. The data indicate that physical training increases tissue sensitivity to insulin in proportion to the improvement in "physical fitness." Physical training may therefore have a role that is independent of effects on body weight in the management of insulin-resistant states such as obesity and maturity-onset diabetes. Nadeau et al.[5] reported on the long-term effects of physical training on glucose metabolism and showed a significant correlation between an estimate of insulin receptors and percentage of body fat. These studies suggest that insulin needs are diminished after intensive physical training which may be accounted for by reduced body fats and increased insulin receptors. Therefore, one must take into consideration patients who are diabetic requiring insulin when they begin an exercise program. Perhaps they will need less exogenous insulin in their follow-up management.

Passa et al.[6] studied influences of muscular exercise on plasma levels of growth hormone in diabetics both with and without retinopathy in two groups of 10 male, non-obese, insulin-dependent subjects. Group 1 had severe retinopathy and Group 2 had no retinopathy. Plasma growth hormone level was determined during moderate, controlled muscular exercise. Growth hormone levels in Group 1 (the severe retinopathy group) were increased but not in Group 2 (the diabetics without retinopathy). This study suggests that in muscular exercise there is an abnormal growth hormone secretion in insulin-dependent diabetics with microangiopathy. (Growth hormone is known to have a diabetogenic action.) The authors found increases in growth hormone in diabetics with retinopathy while they are exercising but not so in diabetics without retinopathy.

In 1979 Saltin et al.[7] reported on physical training and glucose tolerance in middle-aged men with chemical diabetes. In this survey, the men who were normoglycemic but had a pathological oral glucose tolerance test had an increased risk for developing diabetes. In the obese men, insulin levels during the oral glucose tolerance test were reduced by physical training. This study demonstrated that middle-aged men with a pathological oral glucose tolerance test are likely physically unfit and have a decreased oxygen consumption level when compared to age-matched normals. Whether or not weight was decreased with training, the improvement in oral glucose tolerance testing was significant after the training. Improvement in oral glucose tolerance test occurred in the group not having dietary changes but in those who had physical training.

Brief reports are available regarding exercise, diabetes, and glucose metabolism. Felig et al.[8] studied hypoglycemia in endurance exercise and found that increased motivation delays exhaustion in presence of frank hypoglycemia. Wallberg et al.[9] found, in a small group of insulin-dependent diabetics, that physical exercise enhances insulin sensitivity but in itself did not improve blood glucose regulation. From the cardiac standpoint, Bakth et al.[10] studied the effects of exercise training on electrical vulnerability in the diabetic heart. They postulated that during an arrhythmogenic stimulus, an increased availability of glucose may reduce the tendency to arrhythmia in the trained state, probably through alterations in ion transport. Schneider et al.[11] reported an abnormal cardiorespiratory response to exercise in noninsulin-dependent diabetics which is felt to represent a clinically silent diabetic neuropathy not previously appreciated.

In humans, considerable data have been reported in the last several years on glucose metabolism and insulin reactivity. Gavin et al.[12] examined the effects of endurance training on insulin receptor binding glucose disappearance rates, fasting plasma sugar, and peripheral immunoreactive insulin in uremic patients. The patients studied either jogged or cycled three times weekly with controls with no exercise and both were evaluated initially and at 6 months. There was an increase of VO_2 max by 39 percent in the exercisers compared to 6.5 percent in the controls. Total insulin receptor binding was 30–42 percent higher in the exercisers and the difference was due to a 3- to 10-fold increase in apparent receptor affinity with no change in receptor number. Thus, endurance training resulted in decreased serum peripheral immunoreactive insulin and an increase in glucose disappearance rates. The authors felt that the mechanism for this improvement in insulin sensitivity may in part be mediated by increased insulin receptor affinity.

Ahlborg et al.[13] in 1983 studied glucose utilization in healthy subjects; six were exercised on an arm ergometer and six on a leg ergometer. Arterial blood glucose fell significantly by 0.46 mm in 17 during leg exercise but remained unchanged with arm exercise. Total splanchnic glucose output was 77 percent greater with arm than with leg exercise. They concluded that, as compared to leg exercise, *arm exercise* resulted in (1) greater utilization of blood glucose as oxidative fuel, (2) greater splanchnic production of glucose, and (3) a very stable arterial blood glucose concentration.

In a 1984 review, Koivisto and Felig[14] discussed the clinical implications of exercise in diabetics. They concluded that in normal human subjects, exercise training results in increased insulin sensitivity and binding to receptors and may improve glucose tolerance in adult-onset diabetes. They felt also that, in juvenile-onset diabetes, exercise may reduce insulin needs. However, whether or not augmented insulin sensitivity in exercise-trained diabetics is mediated as increased insulin binding is unclear.

Yale et al.[15] questioned whether or not the recovery period after strenuous exercise is a physiological response. To determine the possible mechanism for the sustained elevation of glucose and insulin after strenuous exercise in the post-absorptive state, eight lean and 12 obese untrained subjects were exercised to exhaustion at 80 percent VO_2 max on an isocaloric diet. The results suggested that post-exercise hepatic insulin resistance continues longer in the obese than in the lean subjects and that these responses are well preserved during hypocaloric diets. Osei[16] studied *blood pressure responses* in Type 1 diabetes. Portable blood pressure monitoring was done in 12 Type 1 diabetics and in 12 age-matched nondiabetic controls. Mean ambulatory pressures and heart rates were significantly higher in diabetics than in controls. In addition, there was a positive relationship between ambulatory and peak exercise mean arterial pressure in the diabetics but not in the controls. Mean peak exercise blood pressures were significantly higher in the diabetics with proliferative retinopathy versus those without. These findings suggest defects in the autonomic and autoregulatory mechanisms that maintain normal blood response in diabetic patients. Rodnick et al.[17] studied the effects of exercise training on *in vivo* and *in vitro* glucose uptake in humans. Mean percent body fat was lower and maximal aerobic capacity higher in trained subjects. *In vivo* glucose uptake at basal insulin was similar in the two groups, but the incremental response to hyperinsulinemia was increased in the trained group. Basal glucose uptake by isolated adipocytes was similar in the two groups, but both the incremental and maximal increases in glucose uptake in response to insulin were higher in the exercise trained group. They concluded that the ability of insulin to stimulate glucose uptake both *in vivo* and *in vitro* is increased in the exercise-trained state and this is associated with the degree of conditioning as estimated by VO_2 max. The fact that maximal insulin-stimulated glucose uptake by isolated adipocytes from trained subjects was also increased suggests that exercise training leads to a post-binding change in the glucose transport system which could be responsible for the increased insulin sensitivity of these individuals.

Therefore, considerable recent data (largely in abstract form) are available with regard to the effects of exercise training on glucose metabolism particularly with reference to the diabetic state. The data suggest that exercise training increases insulin sensitivity and insulin receptor binding and may improve glucose tolerance and reduce insulin requirements. These changes can be influenced by muscle groups involved, i.e., arm versus leg activity.

With the current interest in physical activity and the diabetic state, Flood[18] has outlined 10 steps to assure success with minimal hazard in such patients:

1. *Evaluate the patient's overall status.*
   This is particularly true for cardiovascular reasons and is most pertinent for older individuals and for those whose diabetes is of long duration. Such an examination should elucidate any conditions that might preclude exercise or necessitate modification in the guidelines.
2. *Encourage proper training and conditioning.*
   Torn muscles, strained ligaments, blisters, and other annoying problems can bring to a halt an evolving exercise program. In this regard, the diabetic beginning physical activity is really no different that his/her nondiabetic counterpart. The one exception is *care of the feet*, which does assume a greater magnitude of importance since certain individuals will have either neuropathy or peripheral vascular disease, and foot trauma in this setting can lead to more serious complications.
3. *Consider the type of diabetes.*
   As a generalization, individuals with insulin-dependent diabetes tend to be younger, have fewer general health problems, and tend to have more "mechanical" problems associated with the management of their diabetes on a day-to-day basis. Conversely, the noninsulin-dependent diabetic tends to be in an older group that may have more health problems but have a type of diabetes that is basically simpler to manage and requires fewer adjustments on a day-to-day basis.
4. *Be sure the current level of diabetic management is adequate.*
   It is a common misconception that exercise can be used as a crutch to simply "burn up sugar" and that the diabetic patient can use bursts of exercise to compensate for lack of dietary discretion. In fact, the physiologic response to exercise in-

cludes the mobilization of hepatic glucose; subsequently, ketone bodies will accumulate, causing an apparent paradoxical deterioration in the diabetic state.

5. *Work with the patient to establish a sound basic program.*
This step is simply a logical follow-up on the potential problem listed previously. Certain elementary questions must be answered in the affirmative or action must be taken to initiate fundamental aspects of diabetic management if an exercise plan is to be employed successfully. The simple addition of exercise without proper attention to other variables may lead to episodes of hypoglycemia or frank deterioration in control.

6. *Encourage detailed record keeping.*
Questions pertinent to specific dietary changes or insulin adjustments necessary to maintain balance as an exercise program advances are subject to extreme individual variation and become a matter of total guesswork unless there are records documenting changes in glycemia as the adjustments are made. If a variety of manipulations to the diabetic regimen are contemplated, the answer to the question "which works best?" can only be arrived at if the records are detailed and sophisticated enough to make comparisons.

7. *Be prepared to revise the diet.*
As a generalization, brief episodes of vigorous exercise are best handled by dietary manipulation, whereas exercise of prolonged duration is better compensated by adjustment of the insulin dosage. Exercise that is both vigorous and of long duration (marathoning, backpacking, etc.) frequently requires supplementary caloric intake as well as a decrease in the dose of insulin.

8. *Be prepared to revise the insulin dosage.*
With regard to day-to-day changes in insulin dose, only about one-third of runners find it necessary to make daily changes in their insulin dosage.

9. *Guard against hypoglycemia.*
The vast majority of patients who are willing to observe urine or blood tests and be alert for early signs of hypoglycemia are able to successfully participate in an exercise program with minimal risk. Patients should be encouraged to have access to rapidly absorbed oral carbohydrate and should also have some form of visible identification so that they might be assisted should they experience an insulin reaction severe enough to require the assistance of others. It must be stressed, however,

that reactions of this severity are distinctly unusual in those patients who have observed the proper precautions. Insulin injected into a depot above an actively exercising group of muscles may be more rapidly absorbed and it may be prudent to avoid injecting into these areas on days of exercise.

10. *Encourage regularity.*

Most studies of diabetic athletes have shown that changes in their diet and insulin regimen necessary to maintain the proper balance generally occur early in their exercise program. Those individuals who can incorporate a given amount of exercise into their daily routine usually achieve a new steady state and report only minimal variations once their regimen has been established.

Considerable benefits are apparent in exercising diabetics. This is seen both in increased insulin sensitivity and often in control of the clinical state without use of insulin. Care must be taken in insulin-dependent diabetics as less exogenous insulin is needed in the exercising state. If such care is not taken, hypoglycemic reactions may ensue and the exercise safety of the diabetic may be impaired.

Pituitary and Testicular Function

Limited studies are available regarding exercise and effects on the pituitary-testicular axis. Vigersky et al.[19] investigated pituitary-testicular axis function in 10 marathon runners who ran more than 50 miles per week and compared them to nine sedentary, age-matched nonobese, nonsmoking controls. The basal, peak and integrated gonadotropin responses were:

	LH (mIU/ml or mIU/ml/min)			FSH (mIU/ml or mIU/ml/min)		
	basal	peak	area ($\times 10^{-3}$)	basal	peak	area ($\times 10^{-2}$)
Marathoner	8.6	41.6	2.7	15.1	23.6	5.6
Control	6.8	51.5	3.4	10.4	19.2	6.1

Semen parameters (two analyses on each individual) with regard to density, total count, motility, and normal forms were no different in marathoners and sedentary controls. Therefore, these data suggest no significant abnormalities are present in the pituitary or testicular axis of men who engage in vigorous exercise programs.

Murray et al.[20] studied the effect of prolonged submaximal exercise on testosterone levels in untrained insulin-dependent diabetic males. They utilized nine diabetic subjects and 10 healthy male controls during 45 minutes of bike ergometry exercise at 50 percent VO_2 max. Mean testosterone and free testosterone levels were higher in the diabetics than in the controls. Testosterone and free testosterone increased during exercise in both groups but were higher in the diabetics. There was no significant relation between the testosterone levels and VO_2 max in either group. The authors concluded that both serum and free testosterone increase during moderate exercise in diabetics independent of change in leuteinizing hormone and that androgen levels during exercise do not correlate with conditioning states as indicated by VO_2 max. MacConnie et al.[21] studied the effects of strenuous exercise on the reproductive organs of five male marathon runners. They found no changes in leuteinizing hormones but found that plasma testosterone concentration increased significantly at 40 minutes of exercise and remained elevated for 2 hours. They concluded that plasma elevation of testosterone with exercise probably represents changes in clearance rather than increased secretion.

CONCLUSION

Therefore, the role of exercise remains important in the subspecialty of endocrinology. The practical application seems to be primarily in the management of diabetes mellitus. In this role, proper exercise may, with diet and weight loss, eventually eliminate the need for exogenous insulin in many patients. The future role of exercise and endocrinology will likely involve specific neurohumeral responses, prostaglandin pathophysiology, and more elucidation of endorphin metabolism and physiology. Specific correlations of adrenal catecholamine responses with exercise will likely be clarified and protocols through which exercise may moderate this response will be employed in exercise programs.

REFERENCES

1. Zawalich W, Maturo S, Felig P: Physical training: Decreased beta cell sensitivity to glucose and decreased liver glucokinase in the rat. *Clin Res* 1982; 30:407A.

2. Reaven GM, Dolkas CB, Mondon CE: Enhanced insulin sensitivity with exercise training: How long does it last? *Clin Res* 1983; 31:395A.
3. Davis TH, Harter HR: Fetal differential effects of acute exercise and exercise training on glucose metabolism by muscle. *Clin Res* 1985; 33:427A.
4. Soman VR, Koivisto VA, Diebert O, Felig P, DeFronzo RA: Increased insulin sensitivity and insulin binding to monocytes after physical training. *N Engl J Med* 1979; 301:1200–1204.
5. Nadeau A, Rosseau-Migneron S, Boulay M, LeBlanc J: Long-term effects of physical training on glucose metabolism. *Clin Res* 1977; 25:702A (Abstract).
6. Passa P, Gauville C, Canivet J: Influence of muscular exercise on plasma levels of growth hormone in diabetics with and without retinopathy. *Lancet* 1974; 2:72–74.
7. Saltin B, Lingared F, Houston M, Horlin P, Nygaard E, Gad P: Physical training and glucose tolerance in middle-aged men and chemical diabetes. *Diabetes* 1979; 28(Suppl. 1):30–32.
8. Felig P, Cherif MSA, Minagawa A, Wahren J: Hypoglycemia in endurance exercise: Primacy of motivation rather than blood glucose in determining exercise performance. *Clin Res* 1981; 29:577A (Abstract).
9. Wallberg H, Gunnrasson R, Henrikkson J, DeFronzo R, Ostman J, Felig P, Wahren J: Physical training in diabetes; Dissociation between changes in insulin sensitivity and blood glucose regulation. *Clin Res* 1981; 29:577A (Abstract).
10. Bakth S, Moore R, Lee WK, Oldewurtel HA, Regan TJ: Electrical vulnerability in the diabetic heart: Effects of exercise training. *Clin Res* 1981; 29:439A (Abstract).
11. Schneider SH, Ruderman N, Khachadurian A, Amorosa L: Abnormal cardiorespiratory response to exercise and physical training in noninsulin-dependent diabetes mellitus. *Clin Res* 1981; 29:682A (Abstract).
12. Gavin JR, Goldbert AP, Hagberg J, Delmez JA, Geltman E, Harter HR: Endurance exercise training improves insulin sensitivity in uremia. *Clin Res* 1982; 30:393A.
13. Ahlborg A, Wahren J, Felig P: Role of specific muscle groups in determining the metabolic response to exercise: Enhanced glucose turnover in arm as compared to leg exercise. *Clin Res* 1983; 31:543A.
14. Koivisto VA, Felig P: Exercise in diabetes: Clinical implications. *Cardiovas Rev Rep* 1984; 5:399–404.
15. Yale JF, Leiter LA, Marliss EB: Recovery from strenuous exercise: A period of physiological insulin resistance? *Clin Res* 1984; 32:524A.
16. Osei K: Exaggerated ambulatory and exercise-induced blood pressure response in Type 1 diabetic patients. *Clin Res* 1985; 33:833A.
17. Rodnick K, Swislocki A, Foley J, Reaven GM: Effect of exercise training on in vivo and in vitro glucose uptake in humans. *Clin Res* 1986; 34:105A.
18. Flood TM: Ten steps to a successful exercise program. *Resident and Staff Physician* (August) 1981; 31s–38s.
19. Vigersky RA, Smallridge R, Wigutoff S, Ferguson EW: Effect of

physical conditioning on the pituitary-testicular axis. *Clin Res* 1983; 31:275A.
20. Murray FT, Vogel RB, Zauner CW, Thomas R: The effects of prolonged submaximal exercise on testosterone levels in untrained insulin-dependent diabetic males. *Clin Res* 1984; 32:404A.
21. MacConnie S, Backan A, Broderick W, Lang L, Magal E, Beitins I: The effects of strenuous exercise on the reproductive hormones in male marathon runners. *Clin Res* 1985; 33:311A.

11

Exercise in Obstetrics and Gynecology

Edwin Dale, Ph.D.

INTRODUCTION

Since the previous edition of this book there has probably been no other area in which the impact of exercise on the practice of medicine has been greater than that which concerns those entities specific to the female, i.e., pregnancy and menstruation. Long considered as contraindications to the performance of strenuous physical exercise by women, these two uniquely female physiological events and the relationship of exercise to them has been the subject of many clinical and scientific investigations during the past decade. As the results of these studies became available, hypotheses, theories, thoughts, and ideas were presented and examined. Some were rejected, others were accepted as part of contemporary medical management, and still others are now awaiting confirmation or are being studied further. In this chapter, a review of literature from the mid-1970s through the current year is given and guidelines are presented for the physician in dealing with the contemporary medical/scientific phenomenon of exercise in obstetrics and gynecology.

From: Fletcher GF: *Exercise in the Practice of Medicine*, 2nd Revised Edition. Mount Kisco, NY, Futura Publishing Co., Inc., © 1988.

OBSTETRICS

Pregnancy, in the past, has been considered by many physicians (and their patients) as a time of "pampering" and "confinement" of the mother and her fetus. In fact, obstetricians during the first half of the 20th Century calculated an estimated date of confinement (EDC) as the date for predicting delivery of the child. However, with the increased awareness of and participation in various types of physical fitness and exercise, especially jogging, many women during the past 10 years expressed dissatisfaction with "confinement" and essentially stated they wished to continue, or even begin, exercise programs during their pregnancies. Confronted with this revolution, obstetrical health care providers were faced with many questions, for example: What are the effects of exercise on the mother? The fetus? What type of exercises can be carried out? How much? What are the legal and ethical issues of exercise prescription? Is exercise during pregnancy safe, necessary, or desirable in improving the quality of labor and delivery or the outcome of pregnancy?

Interestingly, the historical perspective provides some basis and many thoughts relating maternal fitness and pregnancy outcome. The following examples illustrate this point. In biblical times, Hebrew working slave women had easier (more rapid) labor than their less physically active Egyptian mistresses: "they are lively, and are delivered ere the midwife came to them" (*Exodus* 1:19). Aristotle, in the Third Century B.C., attributed difficult childbirth to a sedentary life-style. In more modern times the pendulum has swung in both directions with the philosophy of the 18th Century to encourage exercise, albeit with strong limitations. In 1892, Stacpoole wrote "when you neglect, risk, or injure your own health during pregnancy, you do a direct injustice to and commit a real crime against your baby." This statement obviously suggested a more moderate approach to work and exercise during pregnancy. The 19th Century also brought forth the first scientific attempts at examining the relationship of maternal activity and pregnancy outcome. These studies continue into the present time.

Entering the 20th Century, the themes of moderation in exercise and the need for fresh clean air were the dominant recommendations, despite the absence of any scientific proof for either. The amount of exercise that the prospective mother should take could not be stated precisely, but what was definitely said was that she should stop the moment she began to feel bad. Further, "walking is the best kind of exercise . . . most women who are pregnant find that a 2 to 3 mile walk daily is all they enjoy and few are inclined to indulge in 6 miles, which is generally considered the upper limit." Additional restrictions included prohibitions against horseback riding, tennis and, interestingly, excessive walking. Throughout the 1930's, there were attempts to permit increased physical activity of pregnant women. The major contributions of this period were Vaughn's prenatal exercises emphasizing squats as a method of strengthening the perineal musculature, Read's progressive specific breathing patterns, and the psychoprophylactic method of childbirth being proclaimed by Lamaze, which also appeared during this decade. A more complete account of the historical perspective is found in a recent book.[1] Exercise advice for 1940–1960 differed little from the conservative 1920's with all the previous admonitions and emphasis on moderation and regular walking in the open air.

Within the past two decades, however, more and more women began participating in many different sports activities and physical fitness programs, at all levels of fitness and competition. The views of earlier years were considered old-fashioned and outmoded and were rejected by many. Today many women want to know if they can continue their sports activity during pregnancy and others ask if an exercise program will enhance their pregnancy outcome or shorten labor and delivery. Much of today's exercise emphasis is on aerobic dancing, cycling, and running as part of essential health maintenance.[2,3] It is difficult to determine what proportion of American women exercise during their pregnancies. In a recent publication, it was estimated that some 85 million people are involved in fitness programs and 25 million jog regularly.[4] Women of reproductive age constitute a significant portion of the active American public. In 1982, the *Mortality-Morbidity Weekly Report* (MMWR) reported that a survey of California women aged 18–34 showed only 10.8 percent admitted to a sedentary life-style.[5] Also, many women work outside the home during their pregnancies. In the period 1970–73, 42 percent of all pregnant women were reported to be in the work force. In view of the current trend toward increased physical fitness, we must be aware of where our patients are "coming from" and where they want to go in terms of expediting their pregnancies, labors, and deliveries.

Maternity care providers are often confronted with issues of safety and maternal/fetal effects of exercise during pregnancy as they attempt to counsel their pregnant patients on the advisability of exercise. The literature available on exercise during pregnancy is varied. Much is anecdotal and appears in popular magazines.[6-8] Women read about Olympic gold medalists competing in the first trimester of their pregnancy or of women competing in 10K's or half-marathons in the latter half of pregnancy. Health care providers also read these success stories of exceptional athletes in their own professional journals.[9] Much of the early research on exercise during pregnancy was done on the exceptional athlete.[10-13] The question is, What about the "everyday" athlete who is pregnant? What specific information does one give her concerning the advisability of beginning or continuing her exercise program during pregnancy? The available literature consists mainly of animal studies and research concerning the physiological responses to exercise in human subjects, and will be discussed in the following sections.

Before describing the physiological changes that occur during pregnancy and the impact of exercise upon these adaptations and some of the animal model experiments that have provided basic physiological information, it is important to state the concerns of the obstetrical health care provider and to present certain absolute and relative contraindications to exercise during pregnancy.

Concerns of the Effects of Exercise in Pregnancy

The volume of research concerning exercise during pregnancy has grown in the past few years. Many questions remain because the studies have been performed on small numbers of subjects or have had technical or ethical problems associated with the research process. Furthermore, there are questions about the application of results of animal studies to humans with regard to fetal effects.[14]

A summary of concerns about the effects of exercise during pregnancy include the following:

1. Fetal hypoxia is a major concern. Specifically, maternal hyperventilation reflects increased maternal oxygen demand during exercise, and the possibility that blood flow would be shunted from the uterus in favor of actively exercising skeletal muscle must be considered.

2. Generation of metabolic acids and alterations in energy and fat metabolism may also affect the fetus.

3. During exercise, a pregnant woman may experience hyperthermia which increases oxygen requirements and in early pregnancy is associated with neural tube defects, mental retardation, and seizures.

4. Fetal well-being and obstetric outcome may be influenced by repetitive mechanical stress of the gravid uterus on maternal skeletal and soft tissues.

5. As pregnancy progresses, orthopedic injuries may increase due to changes in maternal balance and softening of ligaments and joints.

More research concerning fitness of the pregnant female concurrent with fetal heart rate testing is needed to satisfy these concerns. Longitudinal studies of infant growth and development would also be informative.

Many of the concerns stated above have been shown by the recent studies to have little foundation, e.g., exercise-induced hyperthermia. Others will require additional study and some remain controversial, such as alteration in fetal heart rate in response to exercise.

Additionally, it is important to keep in mind that the human studies and their results have been conducted in generally healthy patients without underlying disease complications such as diabetes or hypertension. The impact of exercise on pregnancies with metabolic complications has not been reported. Bearing in mind that, in addition to cardiopulmonary and musculoskeletal changes during pregnancy, there are also profound carbohydrate and endocrine changes which occur as well. How a pregnancy compromised by pathology in one or both of these systems would respond to increased exercise has not been addressed in the current literature.

Finally, there are certain absolute and relative contraindications to exercise during pregnancy. These are presented below. Others may be individualized by the obstetrical health care provider.[1]

Absolute Contraindications
- Suspected fetal distress
- Risk of premature labor
- Incompetent cervix
- Intrauterine growth retardation
- Heart disease
- Infection

Relative Contraindications
- Diabetes mellitus
- Obesity, inactivity
- Hypertension
- Anemia
- Malpresentation of fetus

Severe hypertension
No prenatal care
Thrombophlebitis
Rh disease

With these concerns as background, let us now examine the physiological changes occurring during pregnancy and show how these normal adaptations are impacted by additional responses to exercise occurring simultaneously.

Physiological Response to Exercise During Pregnancy

Exercise imposes additional requirements on the respiratory, cardiovascular, musculoskeletal, and metabolic systems beyond those changes already established because of pregnancy. As pregnancy is a state of intimate interaction between mother and fetus, and which may be disturbed by physiological stresses which would be inconsequential to a nongravid woman, several aspects of exercise cause concern for possible effects on the fetus.

Cardiopulmonary

The circulation of a pregnant woman may be characterized as hyperdynamic. The heart rate is increased, the pulse is rapid and bounding, and there is increased blood flow to several organ systems and to the rapidly enlarging uterus. Total blood volume increases by 35 percent or more during pregnancy, and cardiac stroke volume increases to accommodate this increase in circulating blood. Since both heart rate and stroke volume are increased, it follows that cardiac output is elevated in pregnant women. Cardiac output increases approximately one-third above resting nonpregnant levels. The major portion of the increase has occurred by 8 to 10 weeks after the last menstrual period.[15]

Exercise elicits a greater increase in cardiac output in the pregnant woman. This occurs not only because she is moving a greater body weight; the cardiac output increase for a standard amount of exercise is greater during pregnancy than in the nonpregnant state. In response to moderate exercise, the corresponding increase in cardiac output is progressively smaller as pregnancy nears term. This progressive decline in cardiac reserve may be attributed to obstruction of the vena cava secondary to the enlarging uterus which contributes to peripheral pooling of blood.[16]

During pregnancy, the respiratory center in the medulla becomes further sensitized to carbon dioxide. The change is effected by increased circulation of progesterone during pregnancy. The result is a lowering of carbon dioxide tension in maternal blood by approximately 25 percent. The sensation of breathlessness with mild exercise which is frequently reported by pregnant women is probably a manifestation of increased sensitivity to carbon dioxide. Other respiratory changes that impact upon pregnancy include a rise in minute volume which at term is about 40 percent above nonpregnant levels. The increase in minute volume is brought about by an increase in tidal volume and not by increase in respiratory rate. Minute ventilation during exercise also increases during the latter months of pregnancy. The rate of increase remains proportional to the work load on a bicycle ergometer. These alterations indicate that during pregnancy, metabolic efficiency of the body remains the same, but energy cost of a given work load is increased. As a result of increase in body weight during pregnancy, more oxygen is required to exercise during pregnancy. Therefore, a pregnant woman reaches maximal exercise capacity at a lower level of work than in the nonpregnant state.[15]

The alterations in cardiopulmonary functioning produced by pregnancy have been studied in relation to exercise. Guzman and Caplan[17] found no difference in the physiological response to exercise in pregnancy. However, they found that the pregnant woman reached her maximum work capacity at a lower level of work than in the nonpregnant state.

Knuttgen and Emerson[18] also studied 13 pregnant women and found that exercise did not constitute a severe physiological stress during pregnancy when weight-bearing, lifting, or walking was not involved. Where body weight impacts on the cost of exercise, as in treadmill walking, the increased cost during pregnancy is proportional to the increase in body weight. Similar cardiorespiratory responses were also noted in a study by Artal et al.[19]

Musculoskeletal

Alterations in the musculoskeletal system may also affect a pregnant athlete's performance. Estrogen and the ovarian hormone, relaxin, induce softening of connective tissue ligaments and joints predisposing them to stress and strain. The resulting relaxation of the fibrous ligaments and cartilage is particularly apparent in increased mobility of the pelvic joints which can be painful and impact on the ability to perform exercise.

The enlarging uterus also accentuates lumbar lordosis which affects balance and center of gravity. Exercises that require rapid movement and coordination may predispose the pregnant woman to a fall.

Approximately 30 percent of all pregnant women experience weakening of the central fibrous tissue seam between the rectus abdominus muscles of the abdomen. This can result in a separation called the diastasis recti. Abdominal strengthening exercises need to be modified to prevent further separation if the diastasis is larger (greater than three fingerbreaths). Until the diastasis lessens during the postpartum period, exercise such as full bent-leg sit ups or leg lifts would be detrimental.

In general, exercise brings about similar physiological alterations. Changes are most pronounced for the cardiovascular and respiratory systems and less marked for the musculoskeletal and endocrine systems. If pregnancy and exercise are combined, there is a doubled physiological impact. This fact suggests that if a prospective mother has not been involved in an exercise program prior to pregnancy, she should not be encouraged to begin one during her pregnancy, except for walking.

Animal Studies

Understandably, animal experiments have provided the most precise information available regarding fetal effects from maternal exercise. Several studies using pregnant ewes with both fetal and maternal catheters inserted have produced similar results. Orr et al.[20] found that treadmill exercise in pregnant ewes did not change maternal mean arterial pressure while cardiac output and iliac blood flow increased. Emmanouilides et al.[21] found that fetal responses generally followed the maternal cardiovascular and pulmonary changes including steady arterial pressure and increasing heart rate. The female ewes hyperventilated, producing a respiratory alkalosis with increased pH and decreased CO_2. These same biochemical findings were present in the fetus along with a reduction in PO_2. The authors suggest this hypoxemia was due to a reduction in the uterine blood flow during maternal exercise.

In another study utilizing pregnant ewes, Clapp[22] found significant detrimental changes in maternal and fetal parameters as maternal exhaustion approached. As maternal exhaustion was reached, the fetal PO_2 decreased significantly, maternal rectal temperature rose 1.4°C, uterine blood flow decreased 28 percent, umbilical flow fell 10 percent, and maternal systemic lactic acid developed. Clapp speculated that fetal hypoxia was a result of exercise redistribution of cardiac output away from the splanchnic bed, systemic catecholamine release, respiratory alkalosis, and hyperthermia. These are factors which have been documented to reduce uterine blood flow by 25 percent.

Hyperthermia is another area of consideration of maternal exercise effects on the fetus. Edwards[23] conducted research concerning the effects of hyperthermia in animals. Induction of hyperthermia (body temperature of 40–41°C) in mice resulted in maternal mortality, resorbed or aborted fetuses in 50 percent of the cases, and vertebral anomalies in over 30 percent of the surviving offspring. In human studies, Parker[24] found a trend towards increased meningomyelocele in newborn deliveries of women who exercised vigorously during the first trimester of pregnancy and who suffered heat stress.

Studies utilizing the pregnant ewe model have provided some of the best information concerning physiological response to exercise. Lotgering et al.[25,26] have published data on oxygen consumption, uterine blood flow, and blood volume as well as information about blood gases, temperatures, and the fetal cardiovascular system in these animals. A clinical extension of these and other data appears in a recent review by Longo and Hardesty.[27] Emphasis here is on the maternal blood volume, hypothesis of control, and clinical considerations. Again, the recent publication by Artal and Wiswell[1] provides over 180 references as well as a section describing experimental methodology that may be of interest both to the reader and to the laboratory researcher.

Human Studies

The effects of exercise on the human fetus are not as easy to evaluate as in the animal studies. The assumption is made that the condition of the mother is not complicated by hypertension, diabetes mellitus, anemia, or other metabolic diseases, which in themselves affect management of the pregnancy. The few reported studies of exercise during pregnancy are limited to small numbers of subjects and all deal with healthy volunteers. In an early study, Hon and Wohlegemuth,[28] using a five-step climbing program, monitored fetal heart rates before and after exercising in 10 normal and 16 high-risk pregnancies. After exercising, 20 to 26 subjects had no remarkable changes in their monitor patterns. Three of the remaining had minor changes and three fell into bradycardia, tachycardia, or an irregular pattern.

Using the bicycle ergometer, Pomerance, Gluck, and Lynch[29] monitored fetal heart rates before and after exercising in 54 normal pregnancies. A post-exercise change in fetal heart rate of more than 16 beats per minute defined a suspicious test. Four of five subjects with suspicious tests had signs of distress during labor after normal exercise testing.

Hauth et al.[30] evaluated moderate exercise in seven pregnant women who routinely ran 4.5 miles per week prior to and during their pregnancies. In the third trimester, nonstress tests were performed immediately after a 1.5 mile run. All nonstress tests remained reactive although fetal tachycardia was present. All women delivered healthy infants at term.

Dressendorfer[31] studied the acute responses of the fetal heart rate using five trained swimmers who performed graded cycling exercise in a semi-Fowler's position at 32–39 weeks' gestation. The fetal heart rate averaged 142 beats per minute before exercise and gradually increased during exercise to a peak of 149 beats per minute. Maternal heart rate reached 146 beats per minute during the same time period. Dressendorfer suggested their findings portrayed a normal fetal heart response to dynamic work of submaximal effort. The aerobic exercise that raised maternal heart rate was approximately 80 percent of the maximum and did not produce fetal bradycardia or tachycardia.

Sibley et al.[32] studied the influence of aerobic swimming on levels of maternal physical fitness and the influence of each swimming period on maternal and fetal circulatory parameters. Thirteen low-risk pregnant women were divided randomly between experimental and control groups. Experimental subjects participated in a 10-week swim conditioning program while controls did not participate in any form of aerobic conditioning. Fitness levels for both groups were measured via respiratory gas analysis during graded exercise testing on a treadmill prior to and following the swimming program. Experimental subjects were able to maintain their initial fitness levels while the control group could not. Additionally, maternal blood pressure, pulse, and fetal heart tones remained, for all subjects, within clinically acceptable limits during the swim conditioning program and treadmill testing.

In a retrospective questionnaire study involving 67 healthy, experienced runners who continued jogging during pregnancy, Jarrett and Spellacy collected data on pre-pregnancy health status, pregnancy and delivery information, and running experience during pregnancy. No correlation was found between running mileage and infant weight or gestational age. The incidence of fetal and maternal complications was low. There was a prematurity rate of 4.4 percent and one reported spontaneous abortion (1.5 percent). The information gathered suggested that jogging during pregnancy by conditioned runners is not harmful to the infant.[33]

Research conducted at Emory University has examined the clinical course of pregnancy and fetal and neonatal outcome in young women who continued to run or jog during their pregnancy. The majority of runners decreased their mileage as their pregnancy progressed. Acute illnesses such as nausea, vomiting, fatigue, joint pain, ligament pain, uterine contractions, fear of harm to the fetus, and awkwardness were listed as reasons for a decrease of running distance. Also, training speeds decreased from 10.7 km/hr (5.6 min/km) to 8.0 km/hr (7.5 min/km). The mean increase of maternal body mass was 11.2 kg for runners and 12.9 kg for nonrunner controls. Length of labor in the runners ranged from 8 hours 20 minutes to greater than 20 hours, as contrasted to controls whose labor ranged from 4 hours to 27 hours. Use of analgesics and anesthesia during labor and delivery was similar in both groups. All runners had episiotomies, except for those who had cesarean sections. Similar information was recorded for the controls. Infant birth "weights" averaged 3.39 kg for runners and 3.45 kg for controls.

Studies of simultaneous maternal and fetal heart rates during treadmill exercise demonstrated a transient fetal bradycardia in three technically acceptable tracings. This decline continued for 2 to 3 minutes, at an intensity of effort likely in submaximal training. Recovery of the fetal heart rate to a normal range of 120 to 160 beats/minute occurred after the 3 or 3½ minute mark of exercise, before attainment of the target heart rate for the mother. These results suggest that moderate maternal exercise has no harmful effects on fetal heart activity.[34]

Other recent studies include those of Clapp and Dickstein,[35] whose data showed that women who continued to exercise at or near preconception levels during pregnancy gained less weight

(4.6 kg), delivered earlier (8 days), and had lighter-weight off-spring (500 g) than those who stopped exercising prior to 28 weeks' gestation. This latter group gained more weight (2.2 kg) but also delivered smaller birth-weight infants at the same gestational age than did the sedentary controls.

Investigation of thermoregulation during aerobic exercise in pregnancy by Jones et al.[36] demonstrated that mean resting skin temperatures increased whereas mean resting core and vaginal temperatures did not change. Core temperatures did not exceed 39°C during weight-bearing exercise stress in four aerobically conditioned pregnant women studied in a climate controlled environment during each trimester and post partum. Heat storage (heat content/kg) was not increased as a result of exercise with advancing gestational age. The authors interpret their findings as being consistent with the hypothesis that thermal balance is maintained with advancing gestation when exercise prescriptions are appropriately modified for conditioned women.

The question of effect of exercise on uterine activity during the last 8 weeks of pregnancy was addressed by Veille et al.[37] Two exercise forms, weight-bearing (running) and nonweight-bearing (stationary bicycle) were utilized. Results of a study of 17 women show no increase in uterine activity as measured before and after exercise. Additionally, both maternal and fetal heart rates increased during exercise with the fetal heart rate significantly increased during the first 15 minutes post-exercise but returning to baseline with the next 15 minute recovery period. No change in maternal blood pressure was recorded.

In a larger study by Collings and Curet,[38] 25 pregnant women without recognizable complications underwent fetal heart rate evaluations during an exercise program targeted between 61 and 73 percent maximal capacity. The results confirmed previous findings by these authors of an acceleration of fetal heart rate in response to exercise. The exercise sessions consisted of 10 minutes of warm-up flexibility followed by 30 minutes of continuous aerobic activity. Walking, jogging, and stationary cycling were the chosen modes of activity. The exercise form was directed by acceptable prescriptions for the appropriate state of conditioning.

A summary of the results of several investigations is shown in Table 1. It is apparent from the data that the question of alteration of fetal heart rate pattern in women with healthy uncomplicated pregnancies employing different exercise forms is unresolved at this time.[39]

Table 1
Fetal Heart Rate: Summary of Data

Author	Date	Pre-Exercise	During	Post-Exercise	Change
Dressendorfer[31]	1980	135–152	149 ± 5	NR	Increased
Hauth[30]	1982	140–155	NR	155–204	Increased
Dale[34]	1982	133	108	131	Decreased-Normal
Collings[38]	1983	144	147	147	Unchanged
Artal[19]	1984	140	90	140–190	Decreased-Increased
Collings[38]	1985	140	NR	149	Increased

NR = Not Recorded

A final consideration should be given to the work status of a pregnant woman. In a recent editorial, Chamberlain addresses this question and raises several meaningful points. His general conclusions are that health care personnel pay much attention to diet and prenatal (home) environment but do not regard work outside the home. In the workplace, hazards of transportation, radiation, chemicals, boredom, fatigue, etc. also require evaluation and assessment of their role in the pregnancy outcome. Currently, advice by the practicing physician is overly cautious as physicians are uncertain of the basic and clinical data standards available to them.[40]

A review of the literature described above suggests certain recommendations which may be presented both to physicians and to their patients. Before giving these recommendations, it is important to note that agreement is not necessarily unanimous and that recommendations therefore carry no guarantee of favorable outcome or maintenance of fitness during the pregnancy. Legal discussions are beyond the realm of this chapter but should be kept in mind when describing exercise prescriptions.

Practical Recommendations and Guidelines

The three trimesters of pregnancy carry specific recommendations. For the first trimester, hot baths, whirlpools, and saunas are to be avoided. The mother should not begin a strenuous exercise program after she is knowingly pregnant. It is not necessary for her to make any radical changes in her ongoing exercise program, but rather she should continue them. Finally, she should not take any medications during pregnancy unless necessary for treatment of medical illness and prescribed by a physician.

In the second trimester, unless directed by a physican, she should not resort to any type of special diets; exceptions are made in the cases of maternal hypertension and/or diabetes mellitus. She should avoid foods high in calories and low in nutritive value. A well-balanced diet is usually prescribed and when followed will be of advantage for both mother and developing fetus. A mother-to-be should also remember that exercise in pregnancy is not done for weight control, but rather is done in order to preserve muscle tone, hopefully to make the period of labor and delivery easier on both mother and baby and hasten return to desired or optimal physical fitness following delivery.

In the third trimester, she should avoid exercises that may compromise blood flow, particularly to the venous return. She should avoid long periods of standing and/or lifting heavy objects. It is desirable to avoid activities that might initiate uterine contractions and to avoid any activities that may lead to a potential imbalance by the mother which may cause a fall. Activities that require a rapid change of direction such as tennis or soccer, or activities that may result in a fall such as horseback and/or motorcycle riding, are to be avoided. Ideal exercises that may be conducted throughout pregnancy include certain yoga exercises, swimming, at least until near-term, but certainly not after rupture of the membranes, and, most ideally, walking with good posture.

Post-Partum Exercises

Depending on the type of delivery and normalcy of delivery events, an exercise program may be, and in fact should be, resumed as soon after delivery as is felt comfortable by both mother and attending physician or nurse-midwife. Even before she leaves the hospital the mother can begin to restore muscular tone to abdomen and pelvis. Restoration of muscle tone will prevent the possibility of urinary incontinence and prolapse of the uterus, and may possibly enhance the return to satisfactory sexual activity. Exercise will also promote blood flow and prevent stasis causing varicose veins, leg cramps, edema, and thrombus formation. The improved circulation will promote healing of traumatized pelvic tissues and strengthening of uterine and pelvic ligaments and tendons. An added factor, while not scientifically documented, may be that exercise could be useful in reducing or diminishing the post-partum depression that accompanies some pregnancies. The benefits of exercise have always been known to improve self-image and this would be very useful for the mother during the post-partum period. During this period, the Kegel exercises are certainly recommended as they were before delivery. Exercises that strengthen the pelvic floor, particularly the pubococcygeal muscles, will be of greatest benefit. The major exercises to be avoided in the post-partum period are those which employ a knee-chest position. This position has been implicated in several maternal deaths and may be associated with air embolism or neurologic changes.

In May 1985, the American College of Obstetricians and Gynecologists (ACOG), in response to a number of requests from physicians and patients, presented guidelines for exercise during pregnancy.[41] At the same time, AGOC published two video tapes entitled *Pregnancy Exercise Program* and *Post-natal Exercise Program*. While there has been great demand for these tapes, there has not been complete agreement on whether the guidelines or the video tapes for the patients meet the needs of pregnant women. A discussion of the opposing views appears in a recent publication.[42]

Guidelines and recommendations based on studies and reviews by Mullinax and Dale are given below.[43] Again, it must be emphasized that these are theoretical guidelines which must be individualized for the pregnancy under consideration. Like the ACOG guidelines, these recommendations are not intended to be applicable to all normal pregnancies, complicated pregnancies, women who are well trained or those who are poorly trained. They aim merely to guide and should not be construed as basis for litigation in cases of poor outcome.

The following are general guidelines for counseling pregnant women who wish to maintain or develop physical fitness:

1. Contraindications to exercise during pregnancy are those conditions that increase the risk for disrupting the pregnancy or decreasing utero-placental reserve. Those conditions include: pregnancy-induced hypertension, diabetes, history of premature labor/delivery, placenta previa, threatened abortion, postdatism, multiple gestation, and smoking during pregnancy.

2. Exercise in the heat should be avoided throughout pregnancy. Hot tub and sauna bathing should be limited to 5–15 minutes.[39]

3. Any activity that utilizes large muscle groups (running, cycling, aerobic dancing, tennis) should be decreased in intensity, speed, and frequency as pregnancy advances. Advising the pregnant woman to switch from running to walking or from aerobic dancing to swimming (weight-bearing to nonweight-bearing activity) would be an example.

4. Water skiing is to be avoided throughout pregnancy. Forceful entry of water into the uterus has been reported to cause miscarriage.[44]

5. It is recommended that women stop scuba diving as soon as they realize they are pregnant.[45] Many factors related to this activity pose potential hazards for the pregnant woman and her fetus. These include: increased risk of decompression sickness during pregnancy, teratogenic effects of hypercapnea and hyperoxia, and exposure to marine animal venoms that may produce adverse effects in the fetus.

6. Competition at an anaerobic pace is to be avoided throughout pregnancy.

7. Participation in contact sports is not advisable throughout pregnancy because of the danger of falls and blows to the abdomen. This includes snow skiing (downhill).

8. Racquet sports and those sports that require good balance and coordination (mountain climbing, gymnastics) must be avoided or modified during pregnancy. As weight increases during pregnancy, the center of gravity changes. The resulting lordosis of the spinal column as well as softening of ligaments and joints in response to progesterone may alter coordination and predispose one to a fall.

9. Brisk walking affords the same cardiovascular benefits as running and is less stressful to the joints. Aerobic capacity can be improved safely during pregnancy by a regular program of physical exercise performed at least 30 minutes three times per week or more.

10. For the nonathlete who wishes to begin exercise during pregnancy, prenatal exercise programs designed for low intensity of effort with a warm-up and cool-down period are recommended. These programs should be taught by qualified personnel with backgrounds in physical fitness and training. The activity should be done gently over time with endurance and strength built slowly. The American College of Obstetricians and Gynecologists have developed a Pregnancy Exercise Program (available in videotape and audiovisual) that is available for the public use.

11. Exercising to the point of exhaustion or chronic fatigue is detrimental to both the woman and the fetus. Pregnancy is not the time to work on a personal record in a 10K or to begin training for a marathon.

12. Pregnant women who wish to continue their weight-lifting routines need to be advised to alter those exercises that may strain the lower back (i.e., dead lifts, bent rows, squats). Straining and using the Valsalva maneuver to push heavy weight is not advisable. Many exercises using certain equipment for upper body and leg strength building can probably be continued with modification (i.e., lighter weight, fewer repetitions with no straining).

13. Postpartum fitness is improved when pregnant women enter their labor and delivery experience in good physical condition. Following an uncomplicated labor and delivery, many women can begin exercising again prior to the 6 weeks check-up. Gradual return to exercise should be emphasized with special attention given to fatigue levels, pain, and bleeding patterns. For example, if a woman resumes attending an aerobic dance class, and the lochia returns again as bright red, the period of involution has not ended, and physical activity should be curtailed until the lochia disappears.

The final, but perhaps also the first recommendation is that *the decision to exercise during the course of pregnancy is one that must be made by consultation between parent(s) and obstetric health team* and should be based on considerations of maternal health, exercise form, duration, and intensity and how each of these factors may relate to fetal outcome. A major concern voiced throughout the years is the effect of maternal exercise upon fetal well-being. To date, there is no evidence to prove that a healthy mother guarantees a healthy fetus. Nevertheless, a mother who has a strong health orientation in terms of exercise and diet, is a nonsmoker, and does not consume large quantities of alcohol will certainly deliver a baby that is healthier than a baby born of a mother who continues to smoke cigarettes and consumes large amounts of alcohol and/or other drugs and medications during her pregnancy. There is no suggestion that exercise during pregnancy is detrimental to fetal growth and development, nor is there evidence of reduced fetal mass, increased perinatal or neonatal mortality, or physical or mental retardation as sequelae to strenuous exercise performed during pregnancy. Because of the newness of this field, we must await future studies to determine the impact upon childhood development, although it appears safe to speculate that the parents' health orientation will most likely carry over to their children.

A number of popular books emphasize Kegel-type exercises and yoga as being helpful to the mother. It is important that the attending physician and/or nurse-midwife be familiar with these exercises so that he/she can discuss them with the patient, stressing why certain exercises will be helpful and why others should not be done. Whether the mother exercises strenuously or merely engages in daily recreational activity, the program does not have to be altered drastically during pregnancy. The pregnancy itself often serves to make the necessary adjustments in the exercise program. Exercise can be carried out alone, in a group, or with friends. It can be undertaken with the confidence that a healthy mother is the woman most likely to deliver and nurture a healthy baby.

GYNECOLOGY

Even more dramatic than the research endeavors attempting to answer the questions concerning exercise during pregnancy have been those efforts directed toward understanding the impact of exercise on the menstrual cycle of women who exercise. Within the past decade, the observation of altered menstrual cycle patterns has evolved from the realm of anecdotal reports to become the subject of a large number of investigations involving hundreds of subjects. These will be reviewed subsequently. More challenging than documentation of alteration of menstrual cyclicity have been the research efforts directed toward determining the causal mechanism(s) of menstrual dysfunction. The postulated mechanisms and their evidence will be considered in the sections that follow. Finally, what are the physiologic effects of menstrual disruption and the accompanying hormonal changes? Are injuries, infertility, and osteoporosis the legacy of exercise? These and other issues from the current literature will be presented for consideration by the practicing physician.

While the historical record is vague regarding the effects of strenuous labor in the homes and fields on the menstrual flow of our female ancestors, it should be noted that alteration of menses (including prolonged absence) has been associated with pregnancy, starvation, incarceration, and other stress-related aspects of life for many years.[46] It was not however, until the 1960's and 1970's that a relationship between menstruation and athletic performance was suggested. The early studies of Erdelyi[10] and Zaharieva[13] at the Olympic Games in 1960 and 1972 provided the first demonstration of what is presently termed "athletic amennorhea." The terms "athletic-associated" and "athletic-induced amennorhea" have also been employed as well as similar terminology using the word *exercise* in place of the word *athletic* in order to describe menstrual cycle changes in these women.

Before proceeding to a review of the literature dealing with the incidence and the presumed mechanisms of the etiology of menstrual dysfunction, it is important to provide some clinical and endocrinologic background for this phenomenon. Whereas the chapter on exercise in obstetrics and gynecology in the previous edition of this book dealt primarily with documentation of the extent of menstrual dysfunction associated with exercise, this chapter will be more concerned with studies of endocrine mechanisms operative in the etiology of this clinical entity. By way of background, certain information needs to be presented concerning clinical manifestations. Initially, the very existence of menstrual dysfunction associated with or induced by athletic (fitness) training is a subject of controversy and dispute. The available data suggest a range from no higher incidence among athletes[47] than in the sedentary population up to 50 percent[48] for women participating in fitness programs who exhibit some form of menstrual alteration. Although several endocrine and other physiological mechanisms have been postulated as causative in this amennorhea, none have been proven. It may be that a single etiologic factor which is the result of several different mechanisms is operating synergistically in response to the life-style, training, and nutritional background of the patient herself. Much of the reason for lack of precise information concerning this entity comes from the fact that many different specialists have contributed to the background studies from which the data base has been obtained. For example, among others, coaches,[49] physicians,[47] exercise physiologists,[48] and nurses[50] all have made original contributions to the literature. Definitions and terminology applicable to descriptive studies have themselves not been uniform and in agreement; for example, amenorrhea and "acyclic," oligomenorrhea and "irregular" ("very irregular") and eumenorrhea which may be "regular" or "cyclic" have all appeared in various publications and have often been used interchangeably. The definitions have also been complicated by equating menstruation with an antecedent ovulaton or assuming that a "normal" menstrual interval, 21–37 days, is synonymous with normal endocrine function. To set the stage for understanding the incidence data, postulated endocrine and nonendocrine mechanisms, and management outline presented below, a discussion of amenorrhea is now presented.

Endocrine Background and Review of Literature

Amenorrhea, absence of menstruation, is a clinical term indicating a sequence of events leading to disruption of reproductive function probably associated with anovulation. The etiology(ies) of amenorrhea may be multiple and variable and provide a challenge to the practitioner of medicine. Primary amenorrhea is the delay of menarche beyond age 16. Secondary amenorrhea is absence of menses in women who had previously menstruated. The information provided here is concerned exclusively with the latter. The former is not the usual experience seen in practice and is managed by an additional set of protocols not necessary in general evaluation of exercise-associated amenorrhea.

For purposes of the discussion below, the following terms and definitions will be employed.

Secondary amenorrhea (acyclic): menstrual cycles with an interval of greater than 90 days in women who had previously exhibited normal or eumenorrheic cycles.

Eumenorrhea (regular, normal or cyclic): menstrual cycles that occur at intervals of 21–37 days usually accompanied by pain or cramping near or at the onset of next menses. Menstrual flow is described as moderate for 3–5 days duration.

Oligomenorrhea (irregular): menstrual cycles are described with 38–89 day intervals without regard to flow characteristics or duration.

Secondary amenorrhea is generally classified into three major categories: anatomical, ovarian, and chronic anovulation syndrome. The anatomic pattern etiologic to secondary amenorrhea is usually related to a specific defect such as Ashermann's syndrome and, as such, is not related to exercise. The ovarian type may include premature failure or resistant ovary syndrome. Other genetic defects associated with ovarian development, such as

Turner's syndrome, often result in primary amenorrhea and are beyond the scope of this review. Premature menopause is, however, a diagnostic possibility which needs to be kept in mind along with pregnancy and post-pill amenorrhea as differentials in the diagnosis of secondary amenorrhea in women who exercise.

The most common presentation of secondary amenorrhea is that described as chronic ovulation syndrome. This diagnosis is generally made in women who present with disruption of cyclic menses and in which the reproductive system is considered to be nonfunctional. This pattern is probably induced through a defect operative in the central nervous system (CNS)-hypothalamic-pituitary neuroendocrine control system or a defect in the ovarian follicle leading to either inappropriate metabolism of steriod hormones or luteal dysfunction if ovulation does occur. Chronic anovulatory amenorrhea is generally subdivided into the following site-specific defects: (1) hypothalamic, (2) pituitary, (3) inappropriate feedback, and (4) other endocrine or metabolic alterations.[51] Each of these is briefly described below. Amenorrhea associated with or induced by exercise in women of reproductive age may have its etiology in any or several of these sites.

1. Hypothalamic anovulatory patterns result from disruption of the CNS-hypothalamic nucleus leading to abnormal gonadotropin-releasing hormone (GnRH) production and/or secretion. This disturbance results most commonly from malnutrition, anorexia nervosa, or interference by neurotransmitters, e.g., dopamine.

2. Anterior pituitary dysfunction is essentially hyper- or hypogonadotropinism secondary to biochemical defects in follicle stimulating (FSH) or luteinizing (LH) hormone production or secretion. These defects may be secondary to lesions in the higher centers or local phenomena, e.g., pituitary tumor. The patterns of pituitary gonadotropin production and secretion generally fall into one of three classes:

a. *Hypogonadotropic.* FSH and LH both less than 10 mIU. (milli-international units of the 2nd International Reference Preparation, World Health Organization). This is seen in patients with anorexia nervosa, amenorrhea coupled with galactorrhea, severe gonadotropin deficiency leading to hypogonadism, and CNS-hypothalamic disorders.

b. *Eugonadotropic.* FSH and LH both above 7 mIU to as high as 20 mIU and in which one of these is equal to or greater than 10 mIU. Women exhibiting these values and amenorrhea usually have an associated hypothalamic defect.

    c. Elevated LH patterns. LH is usually greater than 25 mIU. Generally includes women with inappropriate steroid hormone feedback, e.g., polycystic ovarian syndrome.

    3. Steroid hormone feedback-associated amenorrhea could stem from failure at the gonadal level (inappropriate synthesis), e.g., corpus luteum defect or perhaps failure of synthesis in an extra gonadal site, e.g., peripheal fat. The defect may be enzyme-specific, such as failure of conversion of androstenedione to estrone or estrone to estradiol-17B.

    Anovulatory patterns caused by other endocrine or metabolic disease states are generally more evident to the practitioner and include malnutrition, adrenal hyperfunction or Cushing's disease, thyroid dysfunction, and disorders of prolactin production and secretion. All of these entities contribute to an anovulatory pattern and disruption of reproductive function. Because some of these may be life-threatening, they cannot be dismissed from the diagnostic work-up by attributing the amenorrhea to a simplistic etiology of running or other fitness endeavor.

    With this endocrine background, we can now proceed to consideration of the proposed mechanism for "athletic amenorrhea." Before proceeding to the currently postulated mechanisms, it is prudent to review the incidence of the phenomenon under discussion. Following the discussion of etiologies, we shall return to the presentation of a management plan.

Incidence and Review of Literature

    Until 1978 most of the reports of alteration of menstrual cyclicity were based on anecdotal reports or from information gathered by survey from variously selected groups of athletes. These included the Erdelyi,[47] Zaharieva,[13] and Foreman[49] reports cited in the earlier edition. From that time to the present, a number of studies based on questionnaire-type surveys given to obliging "athletes" from a variety of different levels of training and competition and covering an even wider age span and range of menstrual patterns have been administered, responded to, and analyzed with the results published in a variety of professional and lay journals. As one might imagine, the results have reflected the great variety of investigators and their interests and knowledge as well as that of the physiological divergences among the respondents.

Feicht et al.,[48] in their survey of women on collegiate track and field and cross-country teams, reported the frequency of amenorrhea to be positively correlated with the number of miles run per week. They also observed that amenorrheic athletes were significantly better in performance time for middle distance events than their eumenorrheic counterparts. Finally, these authors could show no body-weight difference between the two groups of runners as being significant and suggested that stress might be a contributing factor. A 1979 two-part survey and laboratory evaluation by Dale, Gerlach, and Wilhite[52] was the first large study attempting to relate or define a number of causal variables in a group of women who were involved in strenuous exercise programs. As shown in Table 2, there were significant differences in the menstrual data between women who ran greater than 30 miles per week and those who did not exercise regularly. In their attempt to

Table 2
Correlation of Menstrual Pattern and Parity
with Intensity of Distance Running*

	Controls (N = 54)	Runners (N = 90)
Age at menarche	12.22	12.88
Menstrual data	N = 54	N = 90
10–13 menses/year	52 (96%)	59 (66%)
6–9 menses/year	2 (4%)	9 (10%)
0–5 menses/year	0 (0%)	21 (24%)
Average no. of menses/year	11.85 ± 0.92	9.16 ± 4.04
History of previous pregnancy	23/54 (43%)	52/90 (58%)
Current oligo/amenorrhea	2/54 (4%)	30/89 (34%)
Parous, oligo/amenorrhea	0/23 (0%)	11/52 (21%)
Parous, average no. menses/year	11.97 ± 1.05	10.07 ± 3.38
Nulliparous, oligo/amenorrhea	2/31 (6%)	19/37 (51%)
Nulliparous, average no. menses/year	11.69 ± 0.70	8.27 ± 4.46

*Reprinted with permission from The American College of Obstetricians and Gynecologists. *Obstetrics and Gynecology,* 1979; 54(1):49.[52]

explain the possible etiology of exercise-associated amenorrhea, Dale et al.[53] offered total (low) body weight, percent body fat, and intensity of exercise as antecedent to gonadotropic and steroid hormone changes leading to the reported oligo/amenorrheic pattern in their subjects. It was considered that "there is probably no single amount of training, weight loss, or percentage of adipose tissue that will induce amenorrhea in every woman. Instead, every woman probably has a different oligo/amenorrheic threshold which may be correlated to these and other currently unknown factors."

From the results of a questionnaire survey of 885 women, Speroff and Redwine[54] stated that the predominant factors in developing menstrual irregularity and amenorrhea were total body weight and weight loss. Young women who weigh less than 115 pounds and who lost more than 10 pounds after they started running were the most likely to present with exercise-associated amenorrhea. The suggestion was made that amenorrhea associated with simple weight loss is due to a hypothalamic dysfunction, and since the hypothalamus regulates appetite, thirst, and water conservation, temperature, sleep, autonomic balance, and endocrine function, it is not surprising to see abnormal change in these areas. These particular areas must also be evaluated in women runners with amenorrhea as it (amenorrhea) may not necessarily have been induced by strenuous exercise.

In order to ascertain appropriately if exercise-associated amenorrhea is a distinct entity, Schwartz[55] and co-workers conducted a descriptive study in which amenorrheic runners were compared to regularly menstruating runners and nonrunning control subjects. Body composition, psychological profiles, dietary habits, and peptide and steroid hormone levels were examined. Their data indicate there were no differences in age at study or age of menarche between the various groups. The amenorrheic runners did have a higher incidence ($p < 0.01$) of menstrual irregularity prior to running, they weighed less ($p < 0.01$) than other runners and controls, had a lower percentage of body fat ($p < 0.005$), and also were the fastest of the runner groups ($p < 0.05$). These amenorrheic runners also claimed a greater weight loss ($p < 0.001$) subsequent to running than did regularly cycling individuals. In the psychological profiles, there were no differences with regard to depression, anxiety, or obsessive/compulsive tendencies. The amenorrheic runners did associate more stress ($p < 0.001$) with their running endeavors than did the eumenorrheic ones. Runners had a higher caloric intake than nonrunners and the amenorrheic runners derived less of their calories from protein than did regularly cycling runners or controls. Luteinizing hormone levels were higher (p<0.05) for amenorrheic than for cycling runners in follicular phase, and thyroid-stimulating hormone levels were lower (p<0.05). For the estrogens, estrone/estradiol ratios were higher (p<0.01) in runners and runners with amenorrhea showed increased levels of dehydroepiandrosterone sulfate. All of these data demonstrate that "some of the same factors known to exist in amenorrheic nonrunners, namely, altered diet, weight loss, and stress, are also present in amenorrheic runners. However, these findings suggest that exercise-associated amenorrhea is an entity distinct from hypothalamic amenorrhea."

From another survey, evaluation of a large number (n=353) of women who competed in either the 1980 Boston Marathon or a Bonnie Bell 10 km race, Lutter and Cushman[56] found that 69.4 percent menstruated regularly, 19.3 percent menstruated at irregular intervals, and 3.4 percent had been amenorrheic during the previous year. Although there was a statistically significant trend toward fewer menstrual periods in runners with low body weight and high training mileage, less than 25 percent of subjects with amenorrhea had both low body weight and high training mileage. Thus, it is suggested that other factors must be sought to explain the alteration of menstrual function which occurs in these subjects. In addition, 14 women had both low body weight and high mileage and yet seven of these individuals continued to menstruate regularly. The authors suggest that physicians seek explanations other than running when evaluating female runners with menstrual dysfunction.

In order to have a better understanding of the association of exercise and secondary amenorrhea, Baker et al.[57] undertook a study to (1) correlate the incidence of this dysfunction with menstrual age, age at study, mileage and parity, and (2) to correlate these factors further with plasma measurements of androgens, estrogens, gonadotropins, prolactin and sex-hormone binding globulin (SHBG). The results of this study are summarized briefly here and discussed in detail in relation to exercise and endocrine changes in the previous chapter. Twenty-three subjects, 18–42 years of age, with normal menses prior to running were studied. Six became amenorrheic (AM) before the study began, three during the course of study, and 14 remained regular (REG). Amenorrhea was greater in those women less than 30 years of age, in the nulliparous, and interestingly, in those who ran 40 miles/week or less. Menarchal age was higher in the AM group (13.8 vs. 12.2 years). Plasma estradiol, SHBG, and LH were lower in AM than in REG subjects. Estradiol, LH, and prolactin were significantly lower in AM athletes than in normal control subjects. These results support the idea that the incidence of secondary amenorrhea is higher in younger, nulliparous women and may be related to a later onset of menarche.

In one of the more recent and perhaps most comprehensive studies, Shangold and Levine distributed questionnaires to women who entered the 1979 New York City Marathon.[58] Of the 394 respondents, the incidence of oligo/amenorrhea was 24 percent during training and 19 percent prior to training. Of the women who had regular menses prior to training, 93 percent continued to have regular periods during training. Those subjects with amenorrhea were significantly lighter (p<0.005) and had lower weight/height ratios (p<0.005) than regularly menstruating women. Using these women as their own control group demonstrated that oligomenorrhea/amenorrhea during training is related to a similar pattern which occurred prior to training. Thus, it appears less likely that exercise alone is the causative factor in the development of such menstrual dysfunction. In agreement with the work of others, there did appear to be an association between amenorrhea and thinness. In contrast with other authors, they could find no relationship between weekly mileage and training pace. Table 3 summarizes these studies. A recent review of this subject is that of Gray and Dale.[50] These authors re-examined, through multiple correlation and regression analysis, those variables previously cited as being associated with menstrual dysfunction. Their analysis provided documentation of certain interrelationships and suggests possible causal linkages between variables. Significant correlations were shown between menstrual cycles/year and age, estimated oxygen uptake, training time/mile and percentage body fat. A path model (Fig. 1) is presented which indicates that training variables contribute significantly to body fat alterations, which is then related to menstrual cycle variation. The path coefficient reported therein indicated that a faster training time and increased frequency of running led to decreased percentage of body fat and this coupled with age (amenorrheic subjects were younger) was causal in menstrual alteration.[50] These observations contrast with a study by Wakat et al.[59] but are similar to those reported by Feicht.[48]

Table 3
Variables Related to the Onset of Oligo-Amenorrhea in Runners*

Factors	Reference (Sample Size)							
	Erdelyi (1976) (N = 552)	Feicht (1978) (N = 128)	Dale (1979) (N = 90)	Schwartz (1980) (N = 53)	Baker (1980) (N = 23)	Speroff (1980) (N = 885)	Lutter (1982) (N = 410)	Shangold (1982) (N = 394)
Previous menstrual irregularity	−					+		+
Nulliparity			+	+	−	+	+	+
Older age at menarche			−		+	−		−
Younger age at time of study					+	+	+	
Greater intensity of training	+	+	+		−	?		+
Increased weight loss/low % body fat		−		+	+	+	+	+
Increased life stress			?		?		?	?

+ = associated with oligomenorrhea or secondary amenorrhea.
− = not associated with oligomenorrhea or secondary amenorrhea.
? = Not measured but discussed.
Blank = not reported.
*Reprinted with permission from reference no. 62.

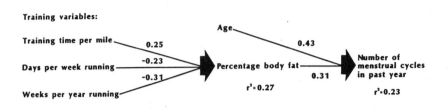

Figure 1: A path model relating training variables with number of menstrual cycles in past year. Used with permission.[50]

The studies summarized illustrate that menstrual alteration does occur in women who participate in vigorous exercise. This phenomenon is not limited to women runners but may also exist in swimmers and cyclists but is of lower prevalence.[60] Menstrual alteration also has been reported for skaters, gymnasts, and ballet dancers.[61] The general statement may be advanced that alteration of regular menstrual cyclicity may occur in women who exercise. The causal factor(s) or etiology of this dysfunction remains enigmatic. While the list of etiologies is legion, the most commonly stated ones include: (1) stress of running, (2) mileage per week, (3) intensity of training, (4) weight loss, (5) body fat loss, (6) hormone imbalance, (7) suppression of reproductive endocrine axis, (8) reduction of steroid hormone production, (9) reduction of gonadotropin stimulation, (10) short luteal phase, (11) hypothalamic dysfunction, (12) thermoregulatory dysfunction, (13) diet/nutrition changes, and (14) energy drain.[62] Some of these have been discussed briefly above; a detailed discussion appears below. Three recent reviews, each of excellent quality as well as thought-provoking, address these items in greater detail.[63-65] Presumably, because of these differences in survey design as well as populations studied and the lack of uniformity in clinical description of menstrual irregularity and the absence of endocrine data, the information obtained from these surveys has not clarified the incidence or even the existence of the phenomenon. Generally speaking, it can be stated that the incidence of secondary amenorrhea in the population of nonathletic women between the ages of 18−44 is low, approximately 1−5 percent. The incidence among runners, the most frequently studied group, is extremely variable at 1−43 percent, and the incidence among dancers, another highly studied group but usually much younger, is invariably higher at

18–45 percent but with an average age of less than 18 years. From the surveys reported above, it is probably safe to conclude that the patient presenting with menstrual dysfunction associated with high-intensity physical fitness orientation is more likely to be younger and more highly trained and possibly nulliparous. The recreational less-trained group will also be participants in fitness programs and will exhibit some degree of associated menstrual dysfunction. This group will be of lower incidence but still slightly more so than the general population. With these observations as an introduction, an examination of the mechanisms suspected of causing athletic-associated amenorrhea will follow.

Nonendocrine Etiology

In the following discussions, it is true that some endocrine mechanisms may be operative. Generally, however, it is felt that the described component, e.g., body composition, diet, etc., is a nonendocrine organ although not exclusively so.

Body Composition

Initially, the most widely accepted hypothesis for explaining the mechanisms for the development of secondary amenorrhea in women who exercised was the body fat or body composition data of Frisch and others.[66] More specifically, it was stated that amenorrheic athletes had a lower level of body fat, a lower total body weight, and had lost a greater percentage of body weight than had eumenorrheic athletes.[53] Furthermore, it was suggested that body fat served as a site for the certain biochemical steps in the aromatization of androgens to estrogens.[67] and the thought was extended that with less fat there was less estrogen produced leading to diminished stimulation of end-organs, e.g., the endometrium, leading to the absence of or a decreased menstrual flow. Additionally, the reduced production and secretion of steroid hormones may lead to inappropriate feedback at the hypothalamic-pituitary receptor sites thereby leading to altered GnRH and/or FSH/LH production.[51] Furthermore, it has been observed that women with anorexia nervosa, when challenged with estradiol, convert the substance more to 2-hydroestrone than to estriol as normally occurs in more obese women.[68] This latter observation suggests production of catecholestrogens as a possible stress-related endocrine adaptation. Its significance in normal endocrine economy is undetermined.

Despite the attractive endocrine possibilities described above, no clear association between body composition and menstrual function has been documented. The Frisch hypothesis has been critically attacked by several authors.[69,70] Furthermore, body measurements by various investigators have been conducted by differing methodologies and have sometimes employed inappropriate or incorrect equations applicable to young females.

Data from selected studies demonstrating inconsistencies in body weight as a determinant of amenorrhea is shown in the following examples.[63] In three studies, body weight was significantly lower in runners reporting amenorrhea when compared to runners reporting regular cycles. In two other studies with similar comparisons, there were no differences in body weight between the groups. In these five studies, the body weights of all amenorrheic runners were similar. The variability in body weight was found in those runners demonstrating regular cycles. In addition to attempts to establish body weight as a stable marker, the use of body fat measurements has also suffered from methodologic approaches. Examples from the literature are as follows. Studies by Frisch of amenorrheic dancers showed significantly lowered total water/body weight ratios.[63] Concurrently, Sanborn et al.[60] reported that the incidence of amenorrhea in athletes correlated with the estimated total water/body weight ratio. As body fat measurement may be estimated by a variety of techniques including Ponderal Index, sum of skinfold caliper measurements at defined anatomic sites followed by calculation from equations and hydrostatic underwater weighing, then it might be expected that different investigators would develop and publish differing results. This has been the case over the past decade and, to date, no satisfactory resolution of methodologic details has been agreed upon. Newer techniques of measurement by ultrasound, x-ray, or CT scan have been proposed. Measurement of lean body mass by isotope dilution of potassium related to creatinine excretion has also been employed. All have reached essentially the same endpoint and body fat measurements still tend to be estimated rather than determined by precise measurement. Also, the question of metabolic potential of adipose tissue from a "trained" person versus a sedentary person remains to be addressed. Laboratory model experiments are underway to attempt to provide answers to this question.[71]

Finally, the percentage of weight loss since onset of training has also been implicated as a causal factor. Runners reporting amenorrheic cycles also report having lost more weight or a greater percentage of their initial body weight since the onset of training.[54] Most of these reports were based on subject recall and, additionally, do give consideration to the changing distribution between body fat mass and lean tissue (muscle?) mass that may be occurring in response to training regimens. It may be that the rate at which weight loss occurs is more important than the percent or absolute amount lost.

There are other problems with the studies of the body composition hypothesis of exercise-associated amenorrhea as well as lack of consideration of other variables which may be interacting concurrently. These problems and variables include the observation that some thin (low fat) athletes are cyclic while some athletes with high-weight, high-fat composition are amenorrheic. Menstrual regularity may be regained (or lost) with no change in weight and some studies have compared body compositions to mixed groups of athletes. The variables of nutrition/dietary changes occurring with training, previous reproductive capabilities, stress of training, etc. have been omitted from the body composition mix. Each of these subjects will be addressed in the sections below. Suffice it to say that at this time, there appears to be no single critical body fat threshold for the maintenance of regular cyclic menses which applies to the majority of women of reproductive age whether or not they are athletically inclined. Additional studies on the role of body fat in the production and secretion of estrogens remain to be elucidated and then related to selected physical endeavors.

Diet and Energy Drain

An association between dietary/nutritional practices and athletic amenorrhea is only speculative at this time. The similarities between anorexia nervosa, stress of incarceration,[46] rapid and large weight losses, and their associated menstrual disruptions have been extended to that seen in the "exercise-induced" amenorrhea. Investigations of diet/nutrition patterns have not revealed any marked deficit of a single entity that might be considered etiologic. It is known that diets deficient in certain amino acids may alter neurotransmitter systhesis and this, in turn, may affect secretion of GnRH leading to the menstrual sequalae.[72] Diet diary histories may provide the basis for some speculation as is shown in the following examples.

A prospective 7-day dietary history of runners showed that daily protein intake of the amenorrheic athletes was significantly less than the regularly cycling ones and was further reduced when compared to nonrunner controls. The runners did not, however, consume fewer total calories than those who had regular cycles and thus calories consumed as protein may not have differed that much. The amenorrheic and cycling runners also differed in both body composition and training regimens and thus dietary protein intake alone may not have been the contributing variable.[55]

In a study by Dale and Goldberg,[73] it was shown through self-recorded 4-day diet diaries that runners (≥30 miles per week) consumed only 474 total calories per day more than did nonrunners. When consideration is given to the fact that these runners probably expended approximately 1,000 calories per day in their exercise program, they were probably calorically deficient compared to controls. The association between caloric deficiency and menstrual alteration, however, was not explored. In 1983, Gray compared diet histories between amenorrheic and cyclic runners, all of whom averaged over 40 miles per week, and did not find significant differences between the groups (unpublished data). Caloric deficits or deficiencies of specific nutrient items cannot be implicated, currently, as causal in the exercise-associated amenorrhea.

Recently, attention has focused on the incidence of secondary amenorrhea in high-mileage runners. These individuals, running greater than 35 miles per week, are believed to experience an exercise-induced state of undernutrition due to the large energy demands associated with their increased mileage. Several investigators have alluded to the concept of "energy drainage" to explain the incidence of amenorrhea resulting from physical training. Excessive energy expenditure, inadequate caloric intake, or a combination of the two can result in energy drainage or negative energy balance. In addition, alterations in normal body composition apparent in high-mileage runners have been proposed as being instrumental in the development of amenorrhea. Thus, energy drainage and body composition appear to work together to influence menstrual cycle alterations.[74] A negative energy balance would result in an alteration in body composition due to the increased reliance on adipose tissue stores for energy. Several investigators have examined the dietary habits of amenorrheic and eumenorrheic runners and have provided data which represent group mean calorie, protein, and fat intakes derived from 4- to 7-day food records. However, a well-controlled longitudinal study designed to determine individual energy balances in high-mileage runners with secondary amenorrhea has not been conducted; individual energy balance determinations should provide specific information concerning the presence of undernutrition.[75]

Reproductive History

Many authors have suggested gynecologic age, age at menarche, history of "irregular" cycles prior to onset of training, previous pregnancy, and oral steroid hormone contraceptive use as contributing to the etiology of athletic-associated amenorrhea.[50,52,54] Most authors agree and their data support the idea that the incidence of amenorrhea is higher in women of younger gynecologic age. Because the hypothalamic-gonadal endocrine axis may not be established in younger women, the axis may be amenable to disruption through exercise, stress, dietary or pscyhological changes occuring as a result of strenuous training. Studies involving women of low gynecologic age may be suspect because of this "immaturity."

It has been suggested that the athletes with a later menarchal age may be more susceptible to the athletic menstrual irregularity.[76] It has also been suggested that the "better" athletes are those with a later time of menarche. The endocrinology of puberty and its relation to achievement and athletic performance has not been studied to date. The endocrine changes that occur at this time need to be documented and the participants followed longitudinally in order to produce evidence showing causal relationship between hormones, menarche, and subsequent dysfunction. Much of the data concerning age of menarche is recall from subjects who may be anywhere from 1 to 20 years beyond menarche. This, quite obviously, suggests possible error. The same type of critical examination might be given to the "regular" or "irregular" designations used when obtaining information prior to onset of training. Again, we are faced with recall of situations that may not have even been important to the subject at her younger age. Data presented in 1979 by Dale and others[52] suggested that previous pregnancy was evidence of reproductive maturity, and in those women who had had a previous pregnancy, only 21 percent reported oligo or secondary amenorrhea compared to 51 percent who had never been pregnant and reported some type of menstrual alteration. The interpretation was given that endocrine maturity as evidenced by initiation of pregnancy conferred some type of "protective" effect or stabilization of the hypothalamic-gonal endocrine axis. This has not been accepted by all authors.

Finally, the widespread use of oral steroid hormonal contraceptives, and their discontinuance, should also be considered in relation to menstrual alteration. Very few studies have considered oral contraceptive usage. While pill use obviously induces artifically determined cycle length and flow, it may also be associated with absence of menses. Post-pill amenorrhea carries a reported incidence of 2.2 percent and may be contributory. The use of the intrauterine device (IUD) may be a confounding variable that has not been documented in many studies. During the late 1970's and early 1980's, many women discontinued pill and IUD usage because of health fears. These same women began to jog, exercise, participate in health food diets, and generally alter their own life-styles. These changes occurring concurrently may have contributed to the reported increased incidences of amenorrhea and may be a part of the nonendocrine etiology of the syndrome. The studies providing evidence in any direction have not been reported.

Sport Sepcificity

Is the reported exercise-associated amenorrhea specific to a particular endeavor, e.g., running, dancing, etc., or is it found in all areas of strenuous exercise? Current thinking suggests that the physiological alteration may, in fact, be sport-specific.[60] As stated above, runners and dancers do have a higher incidence of reported menstrual dysfunction whereas swimmers and cyclists have a lower incidence. It is interesting to speculate that swimmers may be "protected" by their ambient medium and body core temperature may not be elevated as it may be in runners. Because of the close anatomic proximity in the hypothalamus of the heat-regulating and reproductive centers, the suggestion has been made that this area may be involved in the etiology of menstrual dysfunction. There is, however, no evidence, to date to support this speculation.

Another area of current interest is that of weight (power)-

lifting. Some women may be employing anabolic steroids in order to promote the development of muscle bulk. These hormones could certainly influence not only menstrual characteristics but other secondary sexual characteristics, such as voice pitch or hair distribution.

Stress

As is well known clinically, the character of the menstrual cycle may be altered by many extraneous stresses.[46] Commonly, fear of pregnancy, death of a family member or friend, failure of achievement, incarceration, and entry into strenuous programs, e.g. West Point Military Academy, all have been considered as forms of stress that have led to menstrual alterations.[77] Usually when the stress situation has been resolved, "normal" menses return. Strenuous exercise has been proposed as a stress and is causal in the etiology of menstrual dysfunction. Some have commented that the everyday stresses of home, occupation, family, school, etc. are compounded by the scheduling of daily exercise activities and the sum of these stresses induces the physiological alteration.

Stress, as in the "fight or flight" reaction, brings about many rapid endocrine and metabolic changes in the organism. Stresses may increase dopamine release, or the release of endogenous opiates or other neurotransmitters and their increased production and secretion leads to alterations of reproductive function. Adrenal hormones, epinephrine and nonepinephrine, as well as cortisol may be elevated in response to exercise. Insulin, glucose, and the thyroid hormones may be altered simultaneously in response to chronic or acute stress. Perhaps the most convincing evidence of a stress-related change is the measurement of circulating catechol-estrogens. This mechanism leading to secondary amenorrhea will be discussed under endocrine mechanisms in a later section.

The usual approach to monitoring stress and relating it to the regularity of the menstrual cycle has been through the administration of a variety of psychological profile tests. Schwartz et al.[55] used four standardized tests, the Faschingbauer Abbreviated Multiphasic Personality Inventory, The Beck Depression Inventory, The Hopkins Symptom Checklist, and the Schedule of Recent Events in order to measure depression, hypochrondia, obsessive/compulsive patterns, and recent stressful events. They found no differences between cyclic and acyclic runners. Gray and Dale[50] used the Schedule of Recent Events and could find no differences between scores and number of menstrual cycles within the past year. Hendry (unpublished data) has suggested that runners are less depressed and more compulsive and introverted when compared to nonrunners. His data did not address reproductive function. Boyle (unpublished data) could not determine sexual preferences or frequency of sexual intercourse after administering a battery of profile tests to several hundred runners and controls. In summary, the results of test scores may show occasional differences between regular and acyclic runners but they are all within the range of normalcy.

Training Patterns

The time and intensity given to the training regime have been suggested by some as contributing to the induction of athletic-associated amenorrhea. In fact, one of the first studies attempted to correlate distance in miles run per week (mpw) as being related to increasing frequency of secondary amenorrhea.[48] Some studies, e.g. Lutter and Cushman,[56] suggest a high correlation with high mileage. In a study of recreational runners, Speroff and Redwine[54] could find no such relationship. Gray,[50] in her study of runners, showed no difference in miles per week between the amenorrheic group (n=9) and the eumenorrheic group (n=54), 42.2 mpw vs. 40.0 mpw. Also, the average number of days per week and weeks per year did not differ. The amenorrheic runners did train at a slightly faster pace (453 seconds/mile) than did the "regular" runners (499 seconds/mile). In other similar studies there do not appear to be marked differences in training regimens between women who become amenorrheic and those who retain regular menstrual cyclicity. Which parameters of training, distance, frequency, speed, duration, or level of performance may be causal in the etiology of menstrual disruption remains undetermined at this time.

The picture that emerges from examination of the variables described above which may be considered as etiologic in the onset of menstrual irregularity is that in which the female athlete at greatest risk for onset of athletic-associated amenorrhea is one who is of a younger age group, has a lower than average percent of body fat, trains at a relatively faster pace than her eumenorrheic counterpart, is a runner (≥30 miles/week) or a dancer, is nulliparous, is likely to be calorically or nutritionally deficient and spends a great deal of her daily dietary intake meeting her energy-draining exercise requirements. Additionally, she is psychologically stable and does not exhibit the extremes of anorexia or other stress-related phenomena. As stated above, there is probably no single factor which predisposes to or is pathognomonic of menstrual dysfunction in response to exercise. The associated nonendocrine factors discussed above may be acting singly or in concert, and all must be considered in evaluation of the patients with this concern. It is more likely that the causal underlying mechanisms leading to menstrual disruption are to be found through investigations of the endocrine systems. We now turn our attention to presentation of the currently proposed endocrine mechanisms.

Endocrine Mechanisms

In this section, major endocrine pathways presumably causal in the etiology of exercise-associated menstrual dysfunction will be considered, including discussions of studies that have looked at steroid hormones, pituitary hormones, neurotransmitters, and catecholestrogens. An attempt will be made to arrive at a unifying hypothesis. Three preliminary considerations, however, must be presented in order for the reader to better assess the endocrine studies described below.

Hormone measurements are made from body fluids obtained from volunteers. Plasma and serum are the most common sources. Occasionally urine samples have been utilized. Three important methodologic considerations must be remembered. (1) Concentrations of hormones measured will vary with plasma volume, the day of the cycle, the time of the day, and the inherent pulsatile nature of secretion of certain of these substances. (2) Because of the range of values encountered in measurements of hormones, a sufficiently large number of determinations must be made in order to give statistical validity to the differences of the results obtained between various subject groups. (3) The physiological importance of hormone concentration in trained vs. untrained and amenorrheic vs. eumenorrheic subjects must be appreciated. Not all studies have addressed these considerations. Studies to demonstrate these points as well as to pinpoint the site of endocrine defect(s) include the following.

In a study by Dale et al.,[78] serum hormone determinations of estradiol (E_2) progesterone (PRO) prolactin (PRL), FSH, and LH were made weekly for 5 weeks in groups of runners and control subjects. Menstrual histories were known for each of the subjects. Serum measurements of PRO documented ovulation in controls and cyclic runners, FSH, LH, and E_2 were lower in the amenorrheic groups as was PRL. While the measurements were descriptive, they gave little information to daily fluctuation, hormone clearance rates, or other aspects of metabolisms.

Bonen et al.[79] analyzed daily blood samples in four regularly menstruating teenage swimmers throughout a complete menstrual cycle. Their results were consistent with anovulation and corpus luteum defects. LH was elevated and FSH, PRO, E_2 and 17 hydroxy progesterone were all significantly lower in the swimmers when compared to gynecologically age-matched controls. The luteal phase length for the swimmers was also less than that of controls, viz. 4.5 ± 6.0 days vs. 6.7 ± 3.0 days near $\pm$ Standard Error.

Continuing the theme of shortened luteal phase, Prior et al.[80] examined Basal Body Temperature (BBT) and running and weight records of women attending a marathon clinic. Most of the patients would be considered as "normal and ovulatory by history." Of the 48 cycles examined, one-third were normal as determined by BBT, one-third were anovulatory (monophasic), and the remaining one-third exhibited a luteal phase length of less than 11 days. Thus, two-thirds of "normal" women showed a luteal phase defect and would not have been characterized as such by history alone.

In a third study, Shangold[81] and co-workers measured serum progesterone in a runner through a number of cycles (seven) and found that the length of the luteal phase was negatively correlated to the average weekly distance run and that the mean progesterone values 8.2 ± 0.85 ng/ml were significantly lower during training cycles than during control cycles when values were 23.7 ± 2.9 ng/ml. These three studies certainly document a subfertile profile if not an amenorrheic condition in the runners studied.

Baker et al.,[82] Cumming and Belcastro,[83] and Schwartz et al.[55] have all presented sophisticated studies of basal concentrations of hormones in amenorrheic athletes. While each of these studies suffers from certain of the methodologic considerations described above, these three studies do represent the largest set of values to date. Results of these studies are consistent for dehydroepiandrosterone (DHEA), sulfate (S), androstenedione (A), testosterone (T), and FSH in that amenorrheic and cyclic runners, amenorrheic runners and cyclic nonrunners, and cyclic runners and cyclic nonrunners are essentially similar. In these same group comparisons, results are inconsistent for estrone (E_1), E_2, cortisol, LH, PRL and TSH. Isolated data are presented for the three groups for DHEA, E_1, E_2, sex hormone binding globulin (SHBG) and growth hormone (hGH).[63]

These three studies, while varying slightly, do indicate that the amenorrheic athlete does have basal concentrations of androgens DHEA-S, DHEA, T and A within the normal range. Estrone and E_2 are within the low normal range. FHS is described as low normal and LH was elevated. These data are consistent with that of McArthur et al. and suggest the defect may be hypothalamic—wherein GnRH is not released appropriately, perhaps in response to inappropriate steroid hormone feedback. Many patients with delayed menarche, oligomenorrhea, or luteal phase inadequacy demonstrate an exaggerated response to GnRH therapy thus suggesting that the observations reported for menstrual dysfunction may also have a hypothalamic origin.

A synopsis of other studies including information obtained from measurements of gonadotropins, thyroid hormone, ovarian steroids, androgens, and prolactin, respectively, is now given. This will be followed by a description of studies involving catechol compounds and formulation of an endocrine hypothesis for menstrual dysfunction.

Dale et al.[52] found lowered FSH values in amenorrheic runners and cyclic values in ovulatory runners. Demers et al.[85] found similar results with decreased FSH after running. The only author finding increased levels of FSH was Jurkowski.[86] Schwartz et al.[55] and Shangold et al.[87] found no change in FSH values in runners. Reports of luteinizing hormone (LH) levels are also inconsistent. Schwartz et al.[55] found increased LH levels in the amenorrheic runners and cyclic values in runners with normal cycles. Demers et al.[85] and Dale et al.[52] both reported decreased LH values in amenorrheic women. Shangold et al.[87] and Jurkowski et al.[86] found no significant LH changes in the women runners studied. As the gonadotropins are normally variable throughout the menstrual cycle, a complete evaluation of pre-exercise, as well as daily variation, are needed to understand their change in relation to exercise.

Boyden et al.[88] reported thyroid changes in women who increased their training mileage from 13 to 30 miles per week. They also described a decrease in T_3 and reverse T_3, and an increase in

TSH response to TRH. Schwartz et al.[55] found lower TSH levels in amenorrheic runners.

Reported values for estrogen and progesterone levels in women studied are also conflicting except for those patients who participated in longitudinal evaluations. Dale et al.[52] showed cyclic values of estradiol and progesterone with low levels of both hormones in the women with amenorrhea. Bonen et al.[79] reported lower levels of progesterone, estradiol, and 17 OH progesterone in teenage swimmers. These values correlated with a short luteal phase in these subjects. Baker et al.[82] found lower estradiol levels in amenorrheic runners than in those with normal cycles. Boyden et al.[88] reported a significant decrease in estradiol concentrations in women participating in endurance training. Cumming et al.[89] showed changes in levels of estrone associated with exercise. Schwartz et al.[55] reported no change in either estradiol or estrone. Jurkowski et al.[86] demonstrated that progesterone levels are lower when evaluating runners over time. Shangold et al.[81] found a shorter luteal phase as well as lower progesterone levels in women running longer distances.

Androgen levels measured in exercising women have been found to be either increased or unchanged. No decreased levels have been noted. Dehydroepiandrosterone sulfate (DHEAS) levels were found to be increased in amenorrheic runners when compared to women with clinically diagnosed hypothalamic amenorrhea.[55] DHEA level elevations were found in exercising women by Cumming et al.[89] High normal plasma DHEA levels were noted in amenorrheic runners and in those runners less than 30 years of age by Baker et al.[57] Androstenedione levels were essentially the same in runners compared to controls. Dale et al.[52] and Demers et al.[85] reported an increased level of testosterone in runners. Boyden et al.[88] showed normal testosterone levels in their subjects. Shangold et al.[87] found that exercise increased the testosterone levels with the higher levels found during the follicular phase of the cycle. Post-exercise testosterone levels were noted to be higher than those prior to exercise.

Prolactin (PRL) levels have been shown to increase significantly immediately after exercise; however, levels return to normal if values are obtained at 1 hour post-exercise.[87] Boyden et al.[90] reported increases in prolactin responsiveness as subjects increased their running. Brisson et al.[91] found elevations in PRL responses to acute exercise. Bonen et al[79] reported lower prolactin levels in the luteal phase in teenage swimmers participating in endurance training. Whether these changes are due to stress or state of breast maturation is debatable.[92]

Additional investigations which address hypothalamic-pituitary interactions include those of McArthur,[84] Wakat,[59] Russell[93] and Carr.[94] A review of endorphin studies was given by McArthur in 1985. Each of these studies attempts to provide a mechanism whereby gonadotropin secretion changes may be related to altered hypothalamic function.

Increasing knowledge of the "catechol" compounds, specifically catecholamines and catecholestrogens, has advanced our awareness of the hypothalamic-pituitary regulation of hormones. Catecholamine levels have been determined and these data show increases of these entities to be greater in the follicular than in the luteal phase. Catecholestrogens are important in relating conversion of estrogens to a weaker metabolic level and thus diluting their effects on gonadotropin release. The catecholestrogens have hydroxyl groups at the 2- and 3- positions in their A-ring which is similar to the structures of dopamine (DA) and norepinephrine (NE). Catecholestrogens are potent inhibitors of the enzyme catechol-o-methyl transferase (COMT) which methylates, thus inactivating catecholamines. Catecholestrogens can also inhibit tyrosine hydroxylase, one of the major enzymes of catecholamine synthesis; they can occupy DA and NE receptor sites and therefore can stimulate or block synthesis. Adashi et al.[96] showed that with increased catecholestrogens, gonadotropins were decreased and prolactin levels did not change because of the catecholestrogen effect on dopamine receptors. Demers found dopamine, the inhibitor of prolactin, to have a fourfold increase immediately after a 42-kilometer run.[85] Physical activity also increases catecholamine output by a threefold increment. The catecholamines have been shown in animal studies to regulate gonadotropin release from the hypothalamic-pituitary axis. If one relates this information to the knowledge that adipose tissue is a site of estrogen metabolism and that anorexia nervosa patients have a low percent body fat with high levels of urinary catecholestrogens, an extrapolation may be made to the female athlete (Fig. 2).[97] Women participating in exercise programs that reduce body fat may have a shift of metabolism from estradiol to catecholestrogens which, in turn, has a positive effect on the cathecholamine regulation of gonadotropin release. However, other parameters besides body fat may have an influencing factor on anovulation, namely beta-endorphins. The C-terminal end of beta-lipotropin, beta-endor-

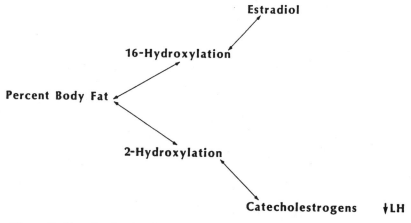

Figure 2: Hypothesized pathway of increased catecholestrogen production leading to decreased LH secretion and altered estradiol production. Used with permission.[97]

phin, has been reported to increase in response to exercise.[94,98,99] Beta-endorphin along with beta-lipotropins and ACTH, are synthesized in the pituitary from ACTH-lipotropin. Colt et al.[98] found endorphin levels to be related to intensity of exercise. After an initial run, only 45 percent of runners were found to have a rise in endorphins. However, after a strenuous run, 80 percent were found to have an increase in beta-endorphin levels. These data were confirmed by Carr who showed a rapid rise in beta-endorphins and beta-lipotrophins in competitively training athletes.[94] The upper limit of endorphin detection was exceeded in successive exercise sessions by these athletes, showing an additive effect. Coffery[100] reported that catecholamines are integrated in the breakdown of endorphins by blocking enkephalin amino peptidase, thus further potentiating endorphins.

The first correlation between gonadotropin release and beta-endorphins was shown by Barraclough and Sawyer.[101] They reported that ovulation in rats was blocked by an analog of beta-endorphin, morphine sulfate. Kalra[102] explained this finding by showing that beta-endorphin binds to hypothalamic cells that secrete LHRH, thus blocking stimulation by norepinephrine. In a recent study, a correlation of increased β-endorphin and catecholestrogens with a concomitant decrease in gonadotropins in women who were swimming competitively was found.[103]

These findings may be correlated with other data to explain

the hypothalamic control of amenorrhea in the female athlete. Increased levels of beta-endorphins, catecholestrogens, and dopamine, as a result of strenuous exercise and decreased body fat, interact to cause a suppression of the hypothalamic release of luteinizing hormone releasing hormone (LHRH). Elevated catecholestrogens compete with catecholamines for COMT. This elevation of catecholestrogens appears to potentiate the inhibitory effect of dopamine on LHRH. The stimulatory effect of LHRH by norepinephrine from exercise may be inhibited by the increased level of beta-endorphins. The beta-endorphins bind to norepinephrine receptors in the hypothalamus, resulting in suppression of LHRH (Fig. 3).[97] These metabolic changes result in a hypothalamic amenorrhea which appears to be reversible as hormone levels return to normal when the level of exercise is reduced. The percent body fat may be a modifying factor in the entire spectrum of endocrine events rather than a solitary cause of amenorrhea.

The total integration of neuroendocrine influences of exercise and subsequent menstrual dysfunction remains complex. However, with further research in these areas, information will be forthcoming and important in our understanding of the influence of exercise on the physiological and hormonal status of the female athlete.

From the data presented above, the practicing physician has at least two models from which to choose in order to explain secondary amenorrhea, viz. ovarian, i.e. luteal phase defect or hypothalamic, i.e. GnRH defect. The underlying basis for each defect may be the action of catecholestrogens altering steroid hormone and/or neurotransmitter synthesis and secretion. While the mechanism(s) require further elucidation, a tentative scheme may be presented at this time.

From the above studies, one may postulate that in response to

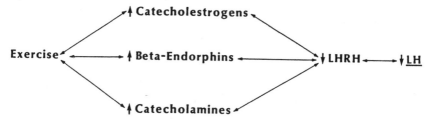

Figure 3: Hypothesized pathway of inhibition of LH synthesis and secretion by separate modalities acting synergistically. Used with permission.[97]

strenuous exercise the "stress" hormones increase leading to an inhibition of LH production and secretion. The decrease in LH may lead, in turn, to reduced progesterone production and secretion in the corpus luteum. The deficiency in progesterone contributes to diminished fertility and possibly altered menstrual intervals. The degree to which these changes occur cannot be quantitated at this time, that is, one cannot state that a certain increase in catecholamines or catecholestrogens results in a defined decrease in LH thus leading to a precise decline in progesterone which results in the observed menstrual alteration. The overall interaction of these hormones does give, at least, a hypothetical base for such a scheme.

In conclusion, it appears that the data currently available for explaining athletic menstrual irregularity on an endocrine base is in much the same state of confusion and controversy as those postulated on a nonendocrine basis. Several recent reviews cover similar information as given above and the reader is referred to them for the details of methodology as well as more comprehensive discussion than given above.[63,65]

Before discussing the management of secondary amenorrhea, which may or may not be related to exercise and/or athletic participation, two currently intriguing topics require address. These are (1) the association between exercise and lipoproteins and the currently popular method of contraception, birth control pills, and (2) the association between the hypoestrogenism accompanying menstrual dysfunction and the potential for the development of osteoporosis in the premenopausal woman. These two topics are perhaps the most novel since the previous edition of this book and require some elaboration.

Lipoproteins and Exercise (See Chapter 4 for more details)

Within the past decade, elevated serum levels of total cholesterol (TC), triglyceride (TG), and low-density lipoprotein cholesterol (LDL-C) have been associated with an increased risk of cardiovascular disease.[104] More recently, other studies have demonstrated a protective effect of increased levels of high-density lipoprotein cholesterol (HDL-C) on the incidence of coronary artery disease (CAD).[105] Because of the observed relationship between risk of CAD and abnormally elevated or depressed levels of the various lipid components, much research has been directed at identifying factors that alter serum lipid levels. Two factors that have been examined are oral contraceptive (OC) use and exercise. Because of the widespread use of OCs and the increasing number of women participating in athletics, either of these two practices could have a significant effect on female CAD morbidity and mortality. Studies of the effects of OC use on serum lipids have produced conflicting results.[106–109] In general, with the use of combined OCs, the estrogen component has been positively correlated with increased HDL-C, and the progestin component has been negatively correlated with decreased HDL-C. Elevations of TG, TC, and LDL-C have been reported in OC users when compared with control subjects not using OCs.[106–108] Lipid alterations have also been noted to occur as a result of consistent, strenuous exercise such as running. When compared with age-matched control subjects, women runners have lower TC, TG, and LDL-C levels and increased HDL-C levels.[110,111] These changes are regarded as protective against the development of CAD.[112]

A descriptive study by Gray, Harding, and Dale[113] was designed to examine differences between the serum cholesterol and lipoprotein levels in runners on the basis of their use of OCs. The data indicate that in a small sample of women runners, the use of OCs probably did not significantly alter serum lipid and lipoprotein levels. The non-OC-using controls were runners matched to the OC-using runners for percentage of body fat and cholesterol intake, two variables frequently associated with alterations in lipid levels. In addition, none of the participants were cigarette smokers, another variable believed to be inversely related to HDL-C levels. The cholesterol and lipoprotein levels in this group of women are similar to levels reported in other studies of women with increased levels of cardiovascular endurance as a result of regular strenuous aerobic exercise. OC users were expected to have elevated cholesterol, TG, and LDL-C levels with depressed HDL-C levels, as compared with non-OC-users. In this group of runners, no statistically significant differences were observed. Furthermore, the OC users had insignificant HDL-C and LDL-C changes in directions in contrast to what was expected. All runners had lipid profiles clearly indicative of low cardiovascular disease risk, without regard to OC use. It appears, therefore, that engaging in regular physical exercise may promote the development of a low-risk lipid profile in women without regard to OC usage.

The only significant differences observed between the two groups of women were in the testosterone (T) and estradiol (E_2) levels. The significantly lowered late follicular T and E_2 levels were expected, with the known effect of OC suppression of pituitary gonadotropin release. Again, the lower E_2 levels of the OC users, similar to levels in post-menopausal women, were not associated with adverse lipid profiles.

Much attention has been given to several large case-control studies, demonstrating excess mortality from diseases of the circulatory system among OC users.[114-116] It has been postulated that OC-induced lipid alterations have played some role in the pathogenesis of these deaths. Although this study consisted of a small sample of runners, the findings indicate that exercise may affect lipid alterations that have been shown to occur with OC use. Further investigation with a larger sample size, controlling for OC formulation and measuring lipid levels prior to both OC use and the initiation of a regular long-term, strenuous exercise program, is needed for definitive documentation of the combined effects of exercise and OC use.

Osteoporosis

In 1982,[117] it was reported that osteoporosis and subsequent bone loss might be an adverse side effect of nonmenstruating, hypoestrogenic women involved in sports. This observation was doubted by those supportive of the idea that exercise would actually prevent osteoporosis in the menopausal woman. Since that time several studies have appeared in the recent literature suggesting that exercise-associated amenorrhea and the consequent hypoestrogenism coupled with reduced dietary calcium intake may, in fact, lead to osteoposotic changes in the skeleton of very young women.

Drinkwater et al.[118] reported that 14 amenorrheic women had radial bone mineral content similar to that of 14 matched eumenorrheic controls but had lower vertebral mineral density. There were no major differences in diet, body fat, and frequency of training between the two groups except the amenorrheic subjects ran more miles per week. Additional data from this study show the amenorrheic subjects (A) with a vertebral mineral density of 1.12 g/cm^2 vs. 1.30 g/cm^2 for the eumenorrheic controls (E), serum estradiol concentrations were reported as (A) 35.58 pg/ml vs. 106.99 pg/ml (E), progesterone (A) 1.25 vs. 12.75 ng/ml (E), and miles per week was 41.8 (A) vs. 24.9 (E). Cann and colleagues, extending their earlier observations, also found a decrease in spinal trabecular bone in amenorrheic athletes.[117] It has been suggested that both the reduction in ovarian estrogen production and secretion and the excessive physical stress of running may contribute to bone deterioration.

A recent study by Linnell et al.[119] compared two groups of runners and could find no differences in body fat, average weekly running distance, or average daily intake of calcium and phosphorus. Also, there were no significant ($p < 0.05$) differences in bone mineral content at 3 cm distal radius and one-third distal radius. A significant difference, however, was noted between bone mineral content and body fat levels only within the amenorrheic group. Within the amenorrheic population, the five thinnest runners had significantly lower mean bone mineral content values at 3 cm (0.457 g. cm^{-2}) than the five runners with higher relative body fat levels (0.559 g. cm^{-2}). The conclusion was stated that amenorrhea was not related to reduced bone mineral content but the combination of excessive thinness coupled with amenorrhea may predispose to reduced bone mass.

Further research is needed relating the role of various dietary factors, exercise, and estrogens upon skeletal integrity of young women. It is necessary to determine whether exercise maintains that bone which is local to exercise in amenorrheic patients. On the basis of what has been reported recently, it appears there is no protection against systemic bone loss by exercise in women who are also hypoestrogenic. In fact, these recent results raise questions concerning the benefits of exercise in post-menopausal populations. The picture emerging from contemporary research suggests that in patients with chronically depressed levels of circulating estrogens, from whatever cause—exercise, surgical, or natural menopause—that there will be demineralization with a subsequent predisposition toward increased osteoporotic fractures. There is convincing evidence that replacement therapy in natural and surgically induced menopausal women is effective in preventing both cortical and trabecular bone loss. Such therapy must now be considered in the hypoestrogenic female athlete along with nutritional counseling and calcium supplementation.[120]

Management

For the physician dealing with patients presenting with what is generally considered to be an exercise-associated secondary amenorrhea, certain basic guidelines may be followed which, if the diagnosis is correct, will probably serve as a successful form of therapy. The therapy will, quite naturally, depend upon the end-point sought.

Initially, it must not be assumed that because a woman of reproductive age presents with amenorrhea and gives a history of exercise participation that the two are necessarily or causally related. The most common cause of amenorrhea in this age group is pregnancy. Furthermore, in the management of athletes, the same well-accepted guidelines that apply to nonathletes should be followed in the management protocol. Athletic participation is not novel or unusual and the life-style associated with it does not alter evaluation. It is not prudent to assume that low body weight, low body fat, poor diet, training regimen, etc. are the only causes of the amenorrhea. Underlying pathology should be evaluated for in the first stages following history and physical examination.

After a complete history, including athletic history, and physical, including pelvic examination, a series of serum hormone measurements should be performed. Complete blood count, electrolytes, and liver enzymes have not been proven to be cost-effective but may be included to complete the work-up. A pregnancy test is indicated if the patient has been sexually active. A serum prolactin measurement of less than 20 ng/ml infers a normal sella. Elevated prolactin suggests sella scan for pituitary microadenoma. Perhaps the next most important hormone measurement is that of serum estradiol, particularly if the physical examination shows evidence of hypoestrogenism. The serum estradiol level may suggest further testing, by appropriate technology, for osteoporotic changes and also serve as a basis for medical and dietary treatment. FSH and LH measurements will also document ovarian stimulation patterns. Individuals with elevated FSH and LH and under 35 years of age should be karyotyped for potential surgical management. Ovarian failure in women over 35 may be suggestive of premature menopause and appropriate therapy may be instituted for control of symptomatology. Thyrotropin, thyroxine, and tri-iodo thyronine resin uptake will serve to screen for primary or secondary hypothyroidism, a common cause of menstrual dysfunction.

For evaluation of ovarian function, a progesterone challenge, either I.M. or oral, is the simplest expedient. Withdrawal bleeding indicates adequate endogenous estrogen production. Absence of bleeding and serum estrogen levels of less than 50 pg/ml suggest treatment with conjugated estrogen replacement, 0.625 mg/day for 25 days. After day 19, an additional therapy of 10 mg/day of medroxyprogesterone acetate may be added to prevent unopposed estrogen effects. Depending on the end-point desired, this therapy, with supplemented calcium 1.5 gram/day, may be sufficient in absence of pathology. If prolactin levels are elevated and the sella does not show microademonatous changes, bromocriptine may be employed to reduce the hyperprolactinemia and lead to ovulation induction and subsequent menstruation.

For induction of ovulation in those patients desiring fertility, the medication clomiphene citrate, 50 mg/day, following reestablishment of body fat, or human menopausal gonadotropin or human chorionic gonadotropin preparations may be employed singly or in combination with clomiphene. The partner in the infertility work-up will also require evaluation. There is insufficient evidence to suggest that merely stopping or reducing exercise is sufficient to bring about resumption of ovulation, fertility, and menstruation. The physician must go beyond this in his evaluation.

FINAL COMMENTS

This chapter has addressed some of the major issues involved with exercise in the practice of obstetrics and gynecology. At the same time, it is only accurate to say that an equally large volume of literature pertaining to other equally important issues within the field has been omitted. Other issues include (1) the concerns of women in relation to exercise, (2) orthopedic injuries, (3) nutrition, (4) anemia, and (5) the performance of women in sports. Other specialists, such as orthopedists, nutritionists, and sports physiologists, will address some of the concerns, and yet some will remain overlooked because of time and space constraints. Let it suffice to say, at this time, that what has been addressed here are the current major reproductive or popular issues. These are the questions addressed in current research endeavors.[121] This is today's language; next year's words may be different. We can only look forward to learning more about the effects of exercise on our patients in our practices. We cannot guarantee that exercise will add years to our lives but we are aware that exercise does give life to our years, and, in that, we can be thankful that we can participate.

REFERENCES

1. Artal R, Wiswell RA (eds): *Exercise in Pregnancy*. Williams and Wilkins, Baltimore, MD. 1986, p. 221.
2. Cooper KH: *The New Aerobics*. New York, Bantam Books, 1970.
3. Cooper M, Cooper KH: *Aerobics for Women*. New York, Bantam Books, 1972.
4. *Medical World News* (Psychiatry Edition) 1984, p. 25.
5. *MMWR Weekly Report Annual Summary* 1982, 1983; 31:128.
6. Wirth V, Emmons P, Larson D: Running through pregnancy: Not only is it safe, it may save your life. *Runner's World* 1978; 13:55–59.
7. Wirth V, Larson D: Running after pregnancy: Positive steps to getting back on your feet fast. *Runner's World* 1978; 13:45–47.
8. Leaf D, Paul M: Giving birth to a new theory: Is running okay while pregnant? *Runner's World* 1983; 18:49–52.
9. Koro M: Pregnant jogger: What a record! *JAMA* 1981; 246:201.
10. Erdelyi GJ: Gynecological survey of female athletes. *J Sports Med Physical Fitness* 1962; 2:174–179.
11. Jokl E: Physical activity during menstruation and pregnancy. *Physical Fitness Res Dig* 1978; 8:1–25.
12. Zaharieva E: Olympic participation by women: Effects on pregnancy and childbirth. *JAMA* 1972; 221:992–995.
13. Zaharieva E: Survey of sports women at the Tokyo Olympics. *J Sports Med Physical Fitness* 1965; 5:215–219.
14. Jopke T: Pregnancy: A time to exercise judgement. *Physician Sports Med* 1983; 11:139–148.
15. De Swiet M: The cardiovascular system. In *Clinical Physiology in Obstetrics*. Hytten F, Chamberlain G (eds): Oxford, Blackwell Scientific Publications, 1980; pp. 3–42.
16. Edington DW, Edgerton VR: *The Biology of Physical Activity*. Boston, Houghton Mifflin Company, 1976.
17. Guzman CA, Caplan B: Cardiorespiratory response to exercise during pregnancy. *Am J Obstet Gynecol* 1970; 108:600–605.
18. Knuttgen HG, Emerson K: Physiological response to pregnancy at rest and during exercise. *J Appl Physiol* 1974; 36:549–553.
19. Artal R, et al: Maternal cardiovascular and metabolic responses in normal pregnancy. *Am J Obstet Gynecol* 1981; 140:123–127.
20. Orr J, et al: Effect of exercise stress on carotid, uterine and iliac blood flow in pregnant and non-pregnant ewes. *Am J Obstet Gynecol* 1972; 114:213–217.
21. Emmanouilides G, Hobel CJ, Yashira K, Klyman G: Fetal response to maternal exercise in the sheep. *Am J Obstet Gynecol* 1972; 112:130–137.
22. Clapp J, et al: Acute exercise stress in the pregnant ewe. *Am J Obstet Gynecol* 1980; 136:489–494.
23. Edwards M: The Effects of Hyperthermia on Pregnancy and Prenatal Development. In *Experimental Embryology and Teratology* Wodlam D, Morris G (eds): London, Elek Science, 1974.
24. Parker G: Central nervous system defects linked to maternal exercise, fevers. *Med Tribune 3 and 1B*, 1979.

25. Lotgering FK, Gilbert RD, Longo LD: Exercise responses in pregnant sheep: Oxygen consumption, uterine blood flow and blood volume. *J Appl Physiol* 1983; 55:842–850.
26. Lotgering FK, Gilbert RD, Longo LD: Exercise responses in pregnant sheep: Blood gases, temperatures and fetal cardiovascular system. *J Appl Physiol* 1983; 55:842–850.
27. Longo LD, Hardesty JS: Maternal blood volume: Measurement, hypothesis of control, and clinical considerations. *Rev Perinatal Med* 1984; 5:1–28.
28. Hon EH, Wohlegemuth R: The electronic evaluation of the fetal heart rate, IV. The effect of maternal exercise. *Am J Obstet Gynecol* 1961; 81:361–371.
29. Pomerance J, Gluck L, Lynch V: Maternal exercise as a screening test for uteroplacental insufficiency. *Obstet Gynecol* 1979; 44:383–387.
30. Hauth JC, Gilstrap LC, Widmer K: Fetal heart rate reactivity before and after maternal jogging during the third trimester. *Am J Obstet Gynecol* 1982; 142:545–547.
31. Dressendorfer RH: Fetal heart rate response to maternal exercise testing. *Physician Sports Med* 1980; 8:90–100.
32. Sibley L, et al: Swimming and physical fitness during pregnancy. *J Nurse-Midwife* 1981; 26:3–12.
33. Jarrett JC, Spellacy WN: Jogging during pregnancy: An improved outcome? *Obstet Gynecol* 1983; 61:705–709.
34. Dale E, Mullinax K, Bryan D: Exercise during pregnancy: Effects on the fetus. *Can J Appl Sports Sci* 1982; 7:98–103.
35. Clapp JF, Dickstein S: Endurance exercise and pregnancy outcome. *Med Sci Sports Exercise* 1984; 16:556–562.
36. Jones RL, et al: Thermoregulation during aerobic exercise in pregnancy. *Obstet Gynecol* 1985; 65:340–345.
37. Veille JC, et al: The effects of exercise on uterine activity in the last eight weeks of pregnancy. *Am J Obstet Gynecol* 1985; 151:727–730.
38. Collings C, Curet LB: Fetal heart rate response to maternal exercise. *Am J Obstet Gynecol* 1985; 151:498–501.
39. Paolone AM, Worthington S: Cautions and advice on exercise during pregnancy. *Contempory Ob/Gyn* Special Issue: *The Active Woman.* 1985; pp. 150–164.
40. Chamberlain G: Effect of work during pregnancy. *Obstet Gynecol* 1985; 65:747–750.
41. American College of Obstetricians and Gynecologists (ACOG) Technical Bulletins on Exercise in Pregnancy, 1985.
42. Gauthier MM: Guidelines for exercise during pregnancy: Too little or too much? *Phys Sports Medicine* 1986; 14:162–169.
43. Mullinax KM, Dale E: Some considerations of exercise during pregnancy. *Clin Sports Med* Freedson, PS, Katch FI (eds) 1986. (In press)
44. Kizer KW, Point B: Medical hazards of the water skiing douche. *Ann Emerg Med* 1980; 9:268–269.
45. Kizer KW: Women and diving. *Phys Sports Med* 1981; 9:84–92.
46. Drew FL: The epidemiology of secondary amenorrhea. *J Chron Dis* 1961; 14:396.
47. Erdelyi GJ: Effects of exercise on the menstrual cycle. *Phys Sports Med* 1976; 4:79–81.

48. Feicht CB, et al: Secondary amenorrhea in athletes. *Lancet* 1978; 2:1145–1146.
49. Foreman K: Seattle Pacific College, Seattle, WA. Unpublished Survey 1973, cited by Bloomberg R: Coach says running affects menstruation. *Phys Sports Med* 1977; 5:15.
50. Gray DP, Dale E: Variables associated with secondary amenorrhea in women runners. *J Sports Sci* 1983; 1:55–67.
51. Yen SSC: Chronic anovulation due to inappropriate feedback system. In *Reproductive Endocrinology.* Yen SSC, Jaffe RB (eds): Philadelphia, W.B. Saunders Co. 1978; pp. 297–323.
52. Dale E, Gerlach DH, Wilhite AL: Menstrual dysfunction in distance runners. *Obstet Gynecol* 1979; 54:47–53.
53. Dale E, Gerlach DH, Martin DE, Alexander CR: Physical fitness profiles and reproductive physiology of the female distance runner. *Phys Sports Med* 1979; 7(1):83–95.
54. Speroff L, Redwine DB: Exercise and menstrual function. *Phys Sports Med* 1980; 8(5):42–52.
55. Schwartz B, Cumming DC, Riordan E, Selye M, Yen SSC, Rebar RW: Exercise-associated amenorrhea: A distinct entity? *Am J Obstet Gynecol* 1981; 141:662–670.
56. Lutter JM, Cushman S: Menstrual patterns in female runners. *Phys Sports Med* 1982; 10(9):60–72.
57. Baker ER, Mathur RS, Kirk RF, Landgrebe SC, Moody LO, Williamson HO: Plasma gonadotropins, prolactin, and steroid hormone concentrations in female runners immediately after a long-distance run. *Fertil Steril* 1982; 38:38–41.
58. Shangold MM, Levine HS: The effect of marathon training upon menstrual function. *Am J Obstet Gynecol* 1982; 143:862–869.
59. Wakat DK, Sweeney KA, Rogol AD: Reproductive system function in women cross-country runners. *Med Sci Sports Exercise* 1982; 14:263–269.
60. Sanborn CF, Martin BJ, Wagner WW: Is athletic amenorrhea specific to runners? *Am J Obstet Gynecol* 1982; 143:859–861.
61. Erdelyi GJ: Gynecological survey of female athletes. *J Sport Med Phys Fitness* 1962; 2:174–179.
62. Dale E: Exercise and the menstrual cycle. *G O Dept Bulletin, EUSM.* 1984; 6:48–54.
63. Loucks AB, Horvath SM: Athletic amenorrhea: A review. *Med Sci Sports Exercise* 1985; 17:56–72.
64. Baker ER: Menstrual dysfunction and hormonal status in athletic women: A review. *Fertil Steril* 1981; 36:691–696.
65. Bonen A, Kizer HA: Athletic menstrual cycle irregularity: Endocrine response to exercise and training. *Phys Sports Med* 12:(8) 78–94.
66. Frisch RD, McArthur JW: Menstrual cycles: fatness as a determinant of minimum weight for height necessary for their maintenance or onset. *Science* 1974; 185:949–951.
67. Nimrod A, Ryan KJ: Aromatization of androgens by human abdominal and breast fat tissue. *J Clin Endocrinol Metab* 1975; 40:367–372.

68. Fishman J, Boyar RM, Hellman L: Influence of body weight on estradiol metabolism in young women. *J Clin Endocrinol Metab* 1975; 41:989–991.
69. Katch FI, Katch VL: Measurement and prediction errors in body composition assessment and the search for the perfect prediction equation. *Res Q* 1980; 51:249–260.
70. Trussel J: Menarche and fatness: Reexamination of the critical body composition hypothesis. *Science* 1978; 200:1506–1509.
71. Axelson JF: Personal communication, 1986.
72. Lytle LD, Messing RB, Fisher L, Phebus L: Effects of long-term corn consumption on brain serotonin and the response to electric shock. *Science* 1975; 190:629–694.
73. Dale E, Goldberg D: Implications of nutrition in athletes menstrual cycle irregularities. *Can J Appl Sports Sci* 1982; 7:74–78.
74. Warren MP: The effects of exercise on pubertal progression and reproductive function in girls. *J Clin Endocrinol Metab* 1980; 51:1150–1157.
75. Crognale DM: *Energy balance and menstrual cycle alterations in high mileage runners.* Master of Medical Science Thesis, Emory University School of Medicine. 1985, p. 62.
76. Malina RM, Spirduso WW, Tate C, et al: Age of menarche and selected menstrual characteristics in athletes of different competitive levels and in different sports. *Med Sci Sports* 1978; 10:218–222.
77. Anderson JL: Women's sports and fitness program at the US Military Academy. *Phys Sports Med* 1979; 7:72–80.
78. Dale E, Alexander CR, Gerlach DH, Martin DE: International Series on Sport Sciences, Vol. 11B. In *Biochemistry of Exercise* IV-B. Jacques Poortmans, Ph.D. and George Niset (eds): Baltimore, MD, University Park Press, 1981.
79. Bonen A, Belcstro AN, Ling WY, Simpson AA: Profiles of selected hormones during menstrual cycles of teenage athletes. *J Appl Physiol* 1981; 50:545–551.
80. Prior JC, Cameron K, Ho Yuen B, Thomas J: Menstrual cycle changes with marathon training: Anovulation and short luteal phase. *Can J Appl Sport Sci* 1982; 7:173–177.
81. Shangold M, Freeman R, Thysen B, Gatz M: The relationship between long-distance running, plasma progesterone and luteal phase length. *Fertil Steril* 1979; 31:130–133.
82. Baker ER, Mathur RS, Kirk RF, Williamson HO: Female runners and secondary amenorrhea: Correlation with age, parity, mileage, and plasma hormonal and sex-hormone-binding globulin concentrations. *Fertil Steril* 1981; 36:183–187.
83. Cumming DC, Belcastro AN: The reproductive effects of exertion. *Cur Prob Obstet Gynecol* 1982; 5(8):1–42.
84. McArthur JW, Bullen BA, Beitins IZ, Pagano M, Badger TM, Klibanski A: Hypothalamic amenorrhea in runners of normal body composition. *Endocrinol Res Commun* 1980; 7(1):13–25.
85. Demers LM, Harrison TS, Halbert DR, Santen RJ: Cited by Brunby P: Increasing numbers of physical changes found in nation's runners. *(Med News) JAMA* 1981; 245–547.

86. Jurkowski JE, Jones NL, Walker WC, Jounglai EV, Sutton JR: Ovarian hormonal responses to exercise. *J Appl Physiol* 1978; 44:109.
87. Shangold MM, Gatz ML, Thysen B: Acute effects of exercise on plasma concentrations of prolactin and testosterone in recreational women runners. *Fertil Steril* 1981; 35:699–702.
88. Boyden TW, Pamenter RW, Stanforth P, et al: Sex steroids and endurance running in women. *Fertil Steril* 1983; 39:629.
89. Cumming DE, Strich G, Brunsting L, Rebar RW, Greenberg L, Ries AL, Yen SSC: Acute exercise-related endocrine changes in women runners and non-runners. *Fertil Steril* 1981; 36:421–428 (abstract).
90. Boyden TW, Ramenter RW, Grosso D, et al: Prolactin responses, menstrual cycles, and body composition of women runners. *J Clin Endocrinol Metab* 1981; 54:911.
91. Brisson GR, Volle MA, DeCarutel D, et al: Exercise-induced dissociation of blood prolactin response in young women according to their sports habits. *Hormone Metab Res* 1980; 12:201.
92. Prior JC: Endocrine "conditioning" with endurance training: A preliminary review. *Can J Appl Sports Sci* 1982; 7:148.
93. Russell JB, Mitchell DE, Musey PI, Collins DC: The relationship of exercise to anovulatory cycles in female athletes. *Obstet Gynecol* 1984; 63:452–456.
94. Carr DB, et al: Physical conditioning facilitates the exercise-induced secretion of beta-endorphin and beta-lipotropin in women. *N Eng J Med* 1981; 305:560.
95. McArthur JW: Endorphins and exercise in females: possible connection with reproductive dysfunction. *Med Sci Sports* 1985; 17:82–88.
96. Adashi EY, Rakoff J, Divers W, Fishman J, Yen SSC: The effect of acutely administered 2-hydroxyestrone on the release of gonadotropins and prolactin before and after estrogen priming in hypogonadal women. *J Clin Endocrinol Metab* 1975; 41:989.
97. Mitchell DE, Russell JB: Endocrine aspects of exercise. *G O Dept. Bulletin, EUSM* 1984; 6:54–60.
98. Colt E, Wardlaw SL, Franta AG: The effect of running on plasma beta-endorphin. *Life Sci* 1981; 28:1637.
99. Fraioli F, Moretti C, Paolucci D, et al: Physical exercise stimulates marked concomitant release of beta-endorphin and adreno corticotropic hormone (ACTH) in peripheral blood in man. *Experientia* 1980; 36:987.
100. Coffrey JL, Hodges D: Inhibition of the enzymatic degradation of metenkephalin by catecholamines. *Endocrinology* 1982; 110:291.
101. Barraclough CA, Sawyer CH: Inhibition of the release of pituitary ovulatory hormone in the rat by morphine. *Endocrinology* 1955; 57:329.
102. Kalra PS, Kalra SP, Kunhich L, et al: Involvement of norepinephrine in transmissions of the stimulatory influence of progesterone on gonadotropin release. *Endocrinology*. 1972; 90(5): 1168.
103. Russell JB, Mitchell DE, Musey PI, Collins DC: The role of B endorphins and catecholestrogens on the hypothalamic-pituitary axis in female athletes. *Fertil Steril* 1984; 42:690–695.

104. Kannel WB, Castelli WP, Gordon T, Dawber TR: Serum cholesterol lipoprotein and risk of coronary heart diseases: The Framingham study. *Ann Intern Med* 1971; 24:1.

105. Gordon T, Castelli WP, Hjortlan MC, Kannel WB, Dawber TR: High density lipoprotein as a protective factor against coronary heart disease: The Framingham study. *Am J Med* 1977; 62:707.

106. Wynn Doar JMH, Mills GL, Stokes T: Fasting serum triglyceride, cholesterol and lipoprotein levels during oral-contraceptive therapy. *Lancet* 1975; 1:756.

107. Bradley DD, Wingerd J, Petitti DB, Krauss RM, Ramcharon S: Serum high-density lipoprotein cholesterol in women using oral contraceptives, estrogens and progestins. *N Engl J Med* 1978; 299:1.

108. Baggett B, Nash HA: Effects of contraceptive steroids on serum lipoproteins and cardiovascular disease scrutinized at workshop in Bethesda. *Contraception* 1981; 21:2.

109. Briggs M, Briggs N: A randomized study of metabolic effects of four low-estrogen oral contraceptives. 1. Results after 6 cycles. *Contraception* 1981; 23:5.

110. Wood PD, Haskell WL, Stern MP, Lewis S, Perry C: Plasma lipoprotein distribution in male and female runners. *Ann NY Acad Sci* 1977; 301:748.

111. Deshaies Y, Allard C: Serum high-density lipoprotein cholesterol in male and female Olympic athletes. *Med Sci Sports Exercise* 1982; 14:3.

112. Miller GJ, Miller NE: Plasma-high density-lipoprotein concentration and development of ischemic heart disease. *Lancet* 1965; 1:16.

113. Gray DP, Harding E, Dale E: Effects of oral contraceptives on serum lipid profiles of women runners. *Fertil Steril* 1983; 39:510−514.

114. Royal College of General Practitioners' Oral Contraception Study: Mortality among oral contraceptive users. *Lancet* 1977; 2:727.

115. Vessey MP, McPherson K, Johnson B: Mortality among women participating in the Oxford Family Planning Association Contraceptive Study. *Lancet* 1977; 2:731.

116. The Walnut Creek Contraceptive Drug Study: *A Prospective Study of the Side Effects of Oral Contraceptives*, Vol. 1. Ramcharon S (ed): Washington, DC, Department of Health, Education and Welfare Publication No. (NIH) 74−562, 1974, p. 1.

117. Gonzalez ER: Premature bone loss found in some nonmenstruating sportswomen. *Med World News* 1982; 248:513−514.

118. Drinkwater BL, Nilson K, Chestnut CH, Bremner WJ, Shainholtz MS, Southworth MB: Bone mineral content of amenorrheic and eumenorrheic athletes. *N Eng J Med* 1984; 311:277−281.

119. Linnell SL, Stager JM, Blue PW, Oyster N, Robertshaw D: Bone mineral content and menstrual regularity in female runners. *Med Sci Sports* 1984; 16:343−348.

120. Mitchell DE: Case presentation. *G O Dept Bulletin, EUSM* 1984; 6:74.

121. Puhl JL, Brown CH (eds): *The Menstrual Cycle and Physical Activity*. Champaign, IL, Human Kinetics Publishers. 1986, p. 166.

12

Exercise in Psychiatry

J. Brand Brickman, M.D.
Thomas A. Rodgers, M.D.

INTRODUCTION

A group of men, aged 40 to 55, meet six mornings a week to run. Professionals, executives, technicians, business people—these individuals deal continually with a variety of stresses: economic, familial, social, vocational, and "internal" (realized and unrealized ambitions, and personal expectations that may or may not be realistic). They also possess physiologies that are inevitably subject to the aging process.

They run each morning conscientiously, explicitly to improve their health. Over time, however, their activity has achieved a broader, more implicit objective. They talk as they run. They share feelings about their families, their finances, their multiple personal struggles. In doing so they derive many physiological, biopsychological, intrapsychic, and interpersonal benefits from their exercise.

It is our intention to explore how exercise, from a psychiatric perspective, has affected these men and is today more and more effective in the practice of medicine and to review a small portion of the current biosocial information that may account for the salutary effects of their daily running ritual.

From: Fletcher GF: *Exercise in the Practice of Medicine*, 2nd Revised Edition. Mount Kisco, NY, Futura Publishing Co., Inc., © 1988.

PHYSICAL ACTIVITY AND BIOPSYCHOLOGICAL RESPONSES

Although the literature which endorses the idea that exercise benefically affects both normal and pathological mental states continues to expand, few studies have shed light on the origins of these changes. The question continues to surface: Is the effect a direct one, or is it the result of changes in life-style, in interpersonal behavior, or in other aspects of everyday activity?[1]

Taylor et al.[2] list the results of physical activity in both clinical and nonclinical populations. They advance the notion that exercise decreases aggression, confusion, depression, phobias, tension, Type A behavior (if indeed that is a pathological phenomenon), and alcohol abuse. They also suggest that strenuous activity increases assertiveness, confidence, emotional stability, memory, mood, positive body image, work efficiency, sexual satisfaction, and the feeling of well-being.

An early and often-mentioned study[3] asserts that running is "at least as effective" a therapy for moderate depression as is psychotherapy, "time limited or time unlimited." Positive results are also mentioned for specific anxiety states, for example, simple phobias. Specifically related to alcoholism, one research group[4] found that alcoholics participating in a fitness program exhibited significantly higher abstinence rates 3 months after treatment than a nonexercise comparison population. As for tension states, other authors[5] examined the exercise effect via EMG studies, and concluded that "exercise has significantly greater effect upon the resting musculature, without any undesirable side effects, "compared to chemical relaxants" (mebrobamate). Social skill enhancement[6,7] and positive body image[8,9] were noted in mentally retarded populations.

Somewhat more random groups of observations on "normals" have also been reported in the literature. A study of the Irish Olympic cycling squad,[10] for instance, noted alterations after the competition racing season, including improved mood, less anxiety, heightened ambition. A report on a structured exercise program[11] recounts "improved psychological well-being" in normal adults. Similar studies have focused on effects of physical fitness on student volunteers[1] and also on aerobics and post-myocardial infarction depression.[12,13]

There are a variety of psychobiological theories about exercise and neurophysiology. Various research reviews[14,15] mention numerous mechanisms: changes in the biogenic amine metabolism of epinephrine, norepinephrine, serotonin, and corticosteroids. Endogenous opioid derivatives have been associated with enhancement of mood and anxiety reduction. More intuitively, one author[16] has remarked on the similarity between emotional changes brought about by strenuous exercise (particularly long-distance running) and in those individuals who have taken cocaine or other hallucinogens.

Clearly problematic, however, to many studies thus far is the varied methodology, as well as the lack of a standardized description of what constitutes "psychological well-being." For now, a troublesome portion of the available research publications has an often metaphorical and sometimes vaguely apocryphal quality.

PSYCHIATRIC CONCEPTS RELATED TO THE EXERCISE EXPERIENCE

In our introduction we alluded to certain clinically significant aspects of the exercise process which fall under the traditional constructs of psychiatry. The impact of the group setting was mentioned as a potential for psychotherapeutic interactions. Our clinical vignettes, to follow, will suggest other possibilities for psychological alterations as a result of physical activity.

Classical psychoanalytic theory has offered several notions about the relationship between body image (including body boundaries) and identity.[17] It has long been asserted that a major aspect of psychological well-being rests upon the developing individual's intrapsychic differentiation of the Self from its environment. This is in some part a physically mediated process, involving the development of motility. Throughout life, the human being's capacities for physical negotiation of the environment will represent a portion of the overall identity. Clearly, certain genetic givens are operant in this process. These include body build and potentials for strength, as well as intellectual and immunological factors.

Equally important, however, is the mental and physical education of the individual, including, for example, acquired skills. Insofar as the cardiovascular, muscular, and coordinative human function can be improved through exercise and games, overall "ego function" is also improved.

Beyond individuation through active, physical mastery of the environment, many exercise activities promote the complex results of socialization as well. If one views an exercise group as a potential therapy group, the available medical literature offers some enlightenment on the complex social events taking place. Yalom[18] has suggested the following: interpersonal input and output ("feedback"), catharsis (release of feelings through their expression), the sense of social cohesiveness, altruism, identification, guidance, and instillation of hope. Although the exercise-oriented group is at most a loose model for a psychotherapeutic experience, its unification and identity arises as a social grouping under the rubric of a common physical goal. Thus cohesiveness, which may well be one of the most powerful effects of groups,[19] is clearly present. Also clearly present in the "team" experience are altruism, identification, and hope.

Lest we ignore some of the literature concerning idiosyncratic responses to exercise, it should be noted that the activity may promote competition at the expense of feelings of cohesion and altruism. A recent publication on the "obligatory runner"[20] describes some of these individuals as inhibited, with very high expectations, and with an unusual tolerance for physical discomfort. Such individuals are often marathon and ultramarathon runners. Many tend toward the isolated exercise experience. A common thread of depression as well as introversion may characterize this population. Such people may not be able to utilize the group experience for psychological growth.

Overall, however, the majority of those who exercise (or play at physical games) in groups seem plainly to be on the road to substantial psychological benefits. Sociologists[21] have linked social support systems to "a kind of innate ego strength (which) accrues coincidental to an activity which may not begin as sociable." Group exercises may be initiated purely for "instrumental" purposes, that is, to improve physical fitness. But they have a way of evolving into "expressive" phenomena, with deep human significance.

USE OF EXERCISE FOR THE CLINICIAN

The literature has been equivocal about efficacy in certain psychiatric disorders (for example, schizophrenia), but it is consistent with the suggestion that routine exercise is helpful in treating depressive disorders.

The following four clinical case summaries represent typical referrals seen for mental health complaints.

Case #1

A 16-year-old male high school sophomore is referred because of a recent academic decline, increasing feelings of social isolation, insomnia, and a 25-pound weight loss. His physical examination is entirely unremarkable except for the weight loss. Metabolic screening is normal. The patient's father and paternal uncle had a history of psychiatric treatment for depression.

During the third interview, the patient admits that he is "upset" because a girl, whom he has secretly admired, turned down his invitation to a school dance. He is obsessed about the rejection and the prospects of "being alone forever." He also worries about patches of facial acne even though his dermatologist has reassured him that his is a mild transient case. In the past the patient has not been physically active or competitive except as demanded in school physical education classes.

Case #2

A 42-year-old mother of three teenagers describes a 2-month period of being "down in the dumps." In addition to her low mood, she describes the insidious onset of trouble getting to sleep, a 13-pound weight gain, restlessness, irritability, decreased libido, social withdrawal, a pervasive feeling of "emptiness," and anhedonia. She thinks her family would be better off without her but she denies specific suicidal plans.

The patient thinks she has completed menopause. Recently her family physician found her to be mildly hypertensive and prescribes hydrochlorothiazide 50 mg/day.

Background history shows no mental disorder although she did have a history of premenstrual "blues" and for a time after the birth of her second child was "depressed" but remained functional. Her family history is negative for mental or neurological disorders. She does not drink alcohol and has never abused drugs. In high school she was a member of the varsity volleyball team but for the past decade she has had "league bowling" as her only "vigorous" exercise.

Case #3

A 28-year-old carpenter suffered a low back "soft tissue" injury 1½ years ago. Prior to this he had been extremely physically and psychologically healthy. There is no family history of mental disorder. Since his injury he has been treated conservatively with bed rest, physical therapy, and muscle relaxants.

He is referred for psychiatric evaluation after an episode where he "lost control" in his Workers Compensation attorney's office. There he had threatened to kill the attorney.

Additional subjective complaints include "sciatic"-like pain daily, a 20-pound weight gain, decreased libido, constant fatigue, and 2:00 a.m. awakening with an inability to get back to sleep. His wife recently suggested a divorce and his vocational rehabilitation counselor just informed him that he is ineligible for further rehabilitative efforts. The patient admits to drinking two six-packs of beer per day and recently started smoking cigarettes again. He feels "lousy" because of physical inactivity. He had a pre-injury history of being very active in swimming, hunting, fishing, backpacking, and weight-lifting.

Case #4

A 33-year-old female loan officer is referred because of fatigability. She has been in excellent health and, in fact, 3 weeks prior to examination, completed her first 26-mile marathon. She has had a difficult time getting enthused about running since the race and for no apparent reason lost her appetite, quit taking vitamin pills, became sexually unresponsive, and has had trouble concentrating at work. She finds herself experiencing "packets of panic" during noontime business meetings. She no longer enjoys going to the beach with her children.

The patient's mother is described as a hard-driving, executive-type person who abused alcohol. The patient reports that she has not abused alcohol or drugs but that recently she took one of her husband's Valium pills and felt "terrible."

Although each clinical vignette represents a unique case, the initial data-gathering process, arriving at a differential diagnosis and enlisting the patient's cooperation, is basically the same. This also applies to the management of the sleep disorder, the use of psychoactive medication (antidepressants, anxiolytic agents, lithium), and initiating the process of supportive psychotherapy. What is unique in each of these cases, however, is the creation of a specifically tailored exercise program.

In Case #1, the clinician will have a difficult time convincing the 16-year-old that exercise is a must. The patient has a history of not being physically active except in PE classes. However, as treatment proceeds and as the teenager develops some understanding of his illness, he will begin to accept the fact that he can do something about altering the clinical course. He has better control over his sleeping patterns and feelings of rejection if he can "get his body moving." A specific plan was made to initiate a walking program 4 days a week. His progress was recorded and within 6 weeks he developed an interest in jogging. This led in 2 months to his first true success—a T-shirt as a prize for his first 10K run.

Examining the psychology of the adolescent yields further rationale for an exercise program. Identity is a major issue, and peer group approval rests on proof of accomplishment and mastery. Regressive considerations about "body image" are dealt with through weight redistribution and muscular development. Sublimation of aggressive drives leads to improved possibilities for socialization with peers.

In Case #2, rapport developed quickly and the patient accepts the fact that an exercise program may help alter her outlook on life and increase her mood and energy level. A referral is made to the newly opened YWCA near her home and she starts a beginner's swimming class. Although she "doesn't feel like going," her physician is insistent that she continue. In 3 months she pleasantly announces that she has lost 10 of the 13 pounds she had gained and that her clothes now fit her better. She develops a plan to take the summer aerobics class.

Early involutional concerns predominate in this instance. Not only does the patient gain reassurance about her control over the "aging process," but she also redirects her efforts toward socialization through membership in her "classes."

In Case #3, the disabled carpenter believes that his loss of physical activity has impaired his mood. Here, the treating physician works closely with the physical therapist and they develop a plan of regularly scheduled exercise that can be tolerated by the patient and that will not aggravate the underlying orthopedic condition. In this case, a program of swimming and "jogging" across the pool is helpful. This program gives the patient some structure and helps him understand that these are exercises he can control. This lifts his mood and his wife finds that he spends less time complaining about his pain.

The "laboring" individual has a natural avenue for aggression through strenuous daily physical activity. Deprived of that by a disability, he or she is automatically prone to depression. Additionally, the structured existence of a laborer has also provided external social controls. A new "program" that is physically demanding will counter the maladaptive aspects of social withdrawal and improve both marital and other interpersonal functions.

In Case #4, the patient is helped by learning that her condition is a rather common one for first-time marathoners. The approach in this case is to convince the patient that her condition will continue to deteriorate unless she remains physically active. She basically is in excellent physical shape and a refocusing of her physical activities to a "moderate" amount of bicycle riding each day is accepted. She reports that the depressed moods quickly dissipate as do the panic episodes. Three months later she terminates treatment and announces that she is training for her second marathon.

This patient's pattern is probably closest to that of the "obligatory runner" mentioned before. Perfectionistic, ambitious, pathologically identified with a "hard-driving" and addicted parent, she is vulnerable to irrational feelings of failure and consequent bouts of depression. Her "marathon" activities may well represent a defense against other, more destructive, addictions. Exercise is the immediate "treatment of choice" here, but concurrent psychotherapy remains essential.

SUMMARY

In summary, we have attempted to examine and discuss exercise in terms of its salutary effects upon mental health. It is presented not as a panacea but as an adjunct to a happier life and current data presented support that assertion. The biopsychological responses related to exercise are substantial and data will likely be more revealing in the future to enable a better understanding of the emotional, physiological, and metabolic changes that develop in persons who comply with long-term exercise training habits.

REFERENCES

1. Goldwater BC, Collis ML: Psychological effects of cardiovascular conditioning: A controlled experiment. *Psychosom Med* 1985; 47:174–181.
2. Taylor CB, Sallis JF, Needle R: The relation of physical activity and exercise to mental health. *Public Health Reports* 1985; 100:195–202.
3. Griest JH, Klein MH, Eischens RR, Faris JT, Gurman AS, Morgan W: Running as treatment for depression. *Comp Psychiatry* 1979; 20:41–54.
4. Sinyor D, Brown T, Rostant L, Seraganian P: The role of a physical fitness program in the treatment of alcoholism. *J Stud Alcohol* 1982; 43:380–386.
5. deVries HA, Adams, GM: Electromyographic comparison of single dose of exercise and mebroamate as to effects on muscular relaxation. *Am J Phys Med* 1972; 51:130–141.
6. Brown BJ: The effect of an isometric strength program on the intellectual and social development of trainable retarded males. *Am Correct Ther J* 1977; 31:44–48.
7. Nunley RL: A physical fitness program. *J Am Phys Ther Assoc* 1965; 45:946–954.
8. Maloney MP, Payne LF: Note on the stability of changes in body image due to sensory-motor training. *Am J Mental Def* 1970; 74:708.
9. Chasey WC, Swartz JD, Chasey CG: Effects of motor development on body image scores for institutionalized mentally retarded children. *Am J Mental Defic* 1974; 78:440–445.
10. Johnson A, Collins P, Higgins I, Harrington D, Connolly J, Dolphin C, McCreery M, Brady L, O'Brien M: Psychological, nutritional and physical status of olympic road cyclists. *Br J Sports Med* 1985; 19:11–14.
11. Blumenthal JA, Williams RA, Williams AG: Psychological changes accompanying physical exercise: A controlled study. *Med Sci Sports Exercise* 1981; 13:74 (abstract).
12. Doyne EJ, Chambless DL, Beutler LE: Aerobic exercise as a treatment for depression in women. *Behav Ther* 1983; 14:434–440.
13. Kavanagh T, Shephard RJ, Tuck JA, Qureshi S: Depression following myocardial infarction: The effect of distance running. *Ann NY Acad Sci* 1977; 301:1029–1038.
14. Dishman RK: Medical psychology in exercise and sport. *Med Clin North Am* 1985; 61:123–143.

15. Hughes JR: Psychological effects of habitual aerobic exercise: A critical review. *Prev Med* 1985; 13:66–78.
16. Mandell AJ: The second second wind. *Psych Ann* 1979; 9:153–160.
17. Fenichel O: *The Psychoanalytic Theory of Neurosis*. New York, WW Norton, 1945.
18. Yalom ID: *The Theory and Practice of Group Psychotherapy*. New York, Basic Books, 1975.
19. Orlinsky D, Howard K: Relationship of process to outcome in psychotherapy. In *Handbook of Psychotherapy and Behavior Change*. Garfield S, Bergin A (eds). New York, John Wiley and Sons, 1978.
20. Yates A, Leehey K, Shisslak C: Running: An analogue of anorexia? *New Engl J Med* 1983; 380:251–255.
21. Lin N, Dean A: Social support and depression. *Soc Psych* 1984; 19:83–91.

13

Exercise in Occupational Medicine

Robert T. Hyde, M.A.

Ralph S. Paffenbarger, Jr., M.D., Dr.PH.

EPIDEMIOLOGICAL BACKGROUNDS

Today's practical interest in leisure-time exercise is closely linked to occupational health. Opportunities for physical activity on the job now differ from those of a generation ago. Our work habits have been drastically altered by such developments as mechanization, automation, swift communication and transport, computers and display terminals. The resulting job patterns that tend to abolish vigorous occupational physical activity appear to be detrimental to the cardiovascular and other vital systems and hence even to life expectancy itself. Therefore we seek ways to adjust our work environment or alter other aspects of our life-style to compensate for the lack of healthful exercise at work. Physiologically and psychologically there are no real substitutes for adequate exercise, whether it is obtained on the job or at leisure.

Despite these observations, exercise has remained a controversial topic. Anecdotal testimonials and folk wisdom from antiquity are not sufficient grounds for acceptance of health programs without specific scientific evidence. Unfortunately, the medical

From: Fletcher GF: *Exercise in the Practice of Medicine*, 2nd Revised Edition. Mount Kisco, NY, Futura Publishing Co., Inc., © 1988.

aspects of physical activity are often too complex to permit experimental investigation with human subjects. Controlled clinical studies have made important findings and will continue to do so, but the broadest evidence that exercise has a key role in health maintenance has been coming from long-range, large-scale epidemiological investigations that are sometimes described as "natural experiments," i.e., based on the actual experience of specific subgroups in a total study population. The evidence so obtained may be deemed circumstantial, but also it appears to be very strong, as Thoreau said of finding a trout in the milk. The conclusions add up to a lot of common sense.

Coronary heart disease, first clinically defined by J.B. Herrick in 1912, became a 20th-century "epidemic," the risks of which were at first thought by many to be worsened by exercise. O.F. Hedley in 1939 found that white-collar workers in Philadelphia had higher rates of cardiovascular disease mortality than blue-collar laborers, but he did not attribute the difference to their activity patterns.[1] By the 1950's, however, J.N. Morris in England advanced a provisional hypothesis that physical activity could be protective against ischemic heart disease. He and his associates concluded that: "Men in physically active jobs have less ischaemic heart disease during middle age, what disease they have is less severe, and they tend to develop it later than similar men in physically inactive jobs." These views were supported by the findings from studies of two occupational groups. Among London transit workers on double-decked buses, the highly active conductors had significantly less heart disease than their relatively less active drivers. Also, among the thousands of British male civil servants whose desk jobs denied them much exercise while at work, those who habitually engaged in vigorous activity such as sports play during their leisure time had lower risk of ischemic heart disease than otherwise comparable fellow workers who did not include such exertion in their life-style.[2-4]

In the next 30 years many epidemiological studies in England and elsewhere supported the basic implications of Morris's findings, especially as refinements in data-gathering and analysis led to sharpening of observations in large populations. Only a few studies need be mentioned here to demonstrate that surveys of both occupational and leisure-time physical activity patterns have established the medical significance of exercise in the maintenance of good health. Physically active farmers in Puerto Rico and in Iowa had lower risk of coronary heart disease (CHD) than the more sedentary townspeople in those areas.[5,6] San Francisco cargo handlers whose work assignments required them to expend upward of 8,500 kilocalories per week on the job had less risk of CHD and of sudden death than dock workers with less demanding duties.[7] In Los Angeles County, the ergometer test performance of firemen predicted (inversely) their risk of myocardial infarction, especially if other predisposing influences (e.g., obesity, cigarette smoking, hypertension) were present.[8] That study resembled a clinical approach, as it used a specific measurement of "fitness" rather than physical activity levels. Epidemiological and clinical studies of exercise today routinely include attention to personal and life-style considerations such as age, weight, cigarette smoking, hereditary influences, and changes in duties, habits, or activities over time.

As physical work loads have been eased by technology, interest has shifted to the epidemiologic significance of leisure-time activity patterns. In the Framingham Heart Study and in a long-range survey among 50,000 alumni of Harvard University and the University of Pennsylvania, data from physical examinations, sports-play records, and follow-up questionnaires have been studied along with clinical and official death certificate information. Extensive series of reports have been published on life-styles, trends, physical activity, coronary heart disease, other chronic diseases, and all-cause mortality rates. The life experience of these large populations spans the 20th century to date and is still under scrutiny in these on-going studies. Many survivors are now entering the years of advanced old age, and there is much interest in learning more about their patterns of exercise, health, disease, and longevity. Findings on nearly 17,000 Harvard male alumni aged 35–85 have shown that regular habits of moderate but vigorous exercise are associated with delayed risk of all-cause mortality and hence with extended longevity.[9–15]

CHARACTERISTICS AND ASSESSMENT OF EXERCISE

With acceptance that exercise is important, attention has turned to its evaluation and characterization as to type, frequency, intensity, duration, constancy, and other aspects, especially in relation to their influences on health.[16–23] When interest has centered on resistance to CHD, the concept of *cardiovascular fitness* has been emphasized, the idea being to train and condition the cardiovascular-respiratory system by exercising it sufficiently to demand about three-quarters of its maximal aerobic capacity for a period of time considered to represent *endurance exercise*, variously defined as 20 to 45 minutes three or four days a week. The extant recommendations for such endurance exercise have been derived chiefly from clinical studies based on cycle or treadmill ergometer tests. The specialized fields of sports medicine also offer detailed observations that, whether anecdotal or broader in their physiological implications, should be useful in dealing with individual cases, particularly as to the benefits, hazards, requirements, and characteristics of various kinds of exercise, and reducing risks of injury or overstress.

In general, the level of aerobic or cardiovascular *fitness* is defined in terms of functional capacity or VO_2 max, which may be measured but is routinely assessed by the length of time of performance of exercise at a given rate or load established by the ergometer setting. Electronic motion sensors have been coming into use to record actual physical activity not restricted to a treadmill, exercycle, or exercise machine. Exercise level also may be monitored by the individual's pulse rate, respiration, sensations of fatigue, or other physiological responses. Much information has been published on these procedures as providing a useful standard, but further studies of exercise suggest that the concepts of cardiovascular fitness, however important, do not express the full value or total health implications of physical activity. Lately a more inclusive term, *health fitness*, has been coming into use, with or without a precise definition. It may be assessed (high or low) as a set of characteristics representing the state of one's health (good or bad), each being measurable and modifiable by exercise: (1) cardiovascular-respiratory endurance; (2) musculoskeletal strength, endurance, and flexibility; (3) body composition, or weight-for-height and percent body fat; (4) metabolic attributes; and (5) psychosocial attitude. In addition to these, a concept of *athletic fitness* would assess such refinements as skill, speed, strength, power, agility, balance, reaction-time, and coordination. A fit athlete must be in good health, but an individual may be fit and in good health without being an athlete.

Be that as it may, endurance fitness is often a central aspect of exercise assessment, and it should be viewed in individual terms involving age, general life-style pattern, health history, body mass index (weight-for-height), body composition, reasonable performance objectives, and so on. Since ergometers and exercise machines often are not readily available to the ordinary person, who is more likely to obtain his leisure-time workouts by walking, jogging, or some form of sports-play suited to his local opportunities and taste, it is fortunate that tables of exercise equivalents have been published widely in both professional and lay media, usually listing standard or average energy output requirements for specific physical activities.[16,21] These requirements have been variously expressed as kilocalories (Kcal) per unit of time (e.g., per minute), per distance (as, per mile), per pace of performance (MPH), or per activity (as, stairs climbed, chores performed, or sports played). Some scales have been refined to give Kcal per kilogram (of body weight) per time; others have been converted to estimates of METS or metabolic equivalents defined as multiples of the basal metabolic rate (approximately 3.5 ml O_2 per kilogram per minute, or 1 Kcal per kilogram per hour). Since metabolic rate is paralleled by heart rate, the METS system offers a means of estimating the probable load or level of exertion represented for an individual by a particular exercise regimen. Age and other limitations are considered to determine whether a proposed regimen would be appropriate or extreme in view of the individual's recommended maximum heart rate.[17,21,24,25]

For example, if his heart-rate range is estimated by 220—age in years—resting heart-rate, an exercise such as walking rated at 3.7 METS would demand of him a heart rate calculated by heart rate range $\times$ .60 + 3.7 + resting heart rate. Since walking at 1 mph = about 1 MET, the example given represents walking at a fairly brisk pace of 3.7 mph. In general, depending on terrain, efficiency, weight, etc., walking a mile expends about 100 Kcal, and our subject would expend about 370 Kcal during his hour of brisk walking. Application of such rules of thumb would appear useful on a day-to-day basis, especially since any individual may be instructed how to take his own pulse under resting and post-exercise conditions. Of course, estimates for exercise involving variations in level of activity or energy output must take its extremes and intervals into account.

Another convenient rule of thumb is the Borg scale of perceived exertion, by which the individual assesses his own perceptions of exertion as *weak, moderate, strong, very strong,* etc. Such approximations tend to parallel actual measured output.[21]

While the assessment of endurance fitness has a strong clinical basis, which in turn has been evaluated in many test subjects ranging from cardiac rehabilitants to world-class athletes, other aspects of exercise have been studied chiefly by epidemiological methods. In particular, the college alumni studies showed plainly that lower risk of CHD among middle-aged men was associated not with any athleticism they may have had in youth, not even varsity athlete status, but with their current and continuing habits of adequate physical activity and especially their leisure-time vigorous sports-play. The studies rated the physical activity levels of these men in terms of kilocalories per week expended in walking, stair climbing, and sports-play, compiled into a *physical activity index* intended to represent just that, an *index* of their physical activity level but *not* its actual total per week (which would be very difficult to determine in this study population). On this scale, the alumni were distributed as about 60 percent whose index was below 2,000 kilocalories per week and 40 percent who rated 2,000 or more. The latter men had significantly less risk of developing CHD at any age, and the index displayed a gradient effect reaching a maximum benefit at about 3,500 kilocalories per week.[14,15] Although certainly of value as indicators from broad experience, these ratings should not be construed as quantities for determining prescription. For each individual, many other considerations are essential.

Here an important caveat is that the relationships of exercise level to body weight are often ignored or misunderstood: a 200-pound man walking a mile does more work and expends more energy (Kcals) than a 150-pound man walking the same distance. But the difference is not simply linear and they may or may not be expending energy at the same rate in kilocalories per pound. Their weight difference is likely to involve differences in efficiency, diet, heredity, body composition, metabolism, heat transfer, energy utilization, and other complex variables.[28] Or again, the lighter person would have to walk more miles than the heavy person to expend 2,000 Kcal in a week, but it should not be assumed that both men will achieve equal benefit from walking a mile or expending 2,000 Kcal/week. Therefore the physical activity index breakpoint of 2,000 Kcal/week ought not to be regarded as a "magic number" applicable to everyone, but only as a general guide or reference.

Many studies of the interactions of exercise and adiposity are underway because much is unknown about them, even though obesity has long been a familiar topic.[28-30] A 1983 report on Harvard alumni found that a physical activity index of 2,000+ Kcal/week predicted a lowered risk of hypertension only among the more obese men, i.e., those at least 20 percent overweight by Quetelet's body mass index.[31,32] In this subgroup the finding might reflect an association between exercise and body composition, or between hypertension and body composition, perhaps one less critical in lighter-weight men. Relationships of exercise to cardiovascular health have been widely investigated, but any roles it may have in cancer, with or without obesity, have only begun to be sought.[29,30] The finding that adequate exercise appears to defer all-cause mortality should add a further impetus to those investigations.

Epidemiologic studies have also produced some hints toward comparative analysis of the influences of exercise. Despite marked differences in study population characteristics, the lowering of CHD risk by relatively moderate exercise among the college alumni tends to parallel the results noted among the San Francisco longshoremen whose high physical activity levels were assessed on the basis of specific job energy output requirements. This parallel suggests that (a) the physical activity index fairly reflected weekly total energy output by alumni, (b) their weekly total was at least relatively comparable to that of the longshoremen, or (c) that the amount of exercise necessary to reduce risk of CHD is apparently modest, at least in an otherwise sedentary population. But also the alumni exercise index data have confirmed, as might be expected, that levels of vigorous sports activity usually increased along with increase in physical activity index in kilocalories per week. Therefore the index relates to type or intensity of exercise as well as to total energy output.

ATHLETICISM AND OCCUPATIONAL MEDICINE

A facet of physical activity yet awaiting clarification is the role of athleticism, which has received increasing attention with the great popularity and commercial expansion of professional athletics into virtually all fields of sports play. As will be discussed later, epidemiological data have shown that former varsity athletes among the college alumni appeared to be at different and higher risks of CHD and earlier mortality than their classmates, even if they continued or resumed vigorous exercise.[14,15] Alumni whose physical activity index extended beyond the optimum level of 3,500 Kcal/week did not acquire further longevity, while those classified as extremely active seemed to lose ground. Since high index tended to signify more participation in vigorous sports activity, and also to associate with former varsity athlete status, these findings suggest that athleticism or its effects can reach a point where its hazards begin to outweigh its benefits. A number of hypotheses may be proposed to account for such patterns— heredity, early maturation, physiological stress limitations, pathological changes of recent or remote origin, social pressures, simple habits of risk, or specific characteristics of exercise already of great interest. In view of the social and financial prominence of professional athletics, and especially as most professional recruits are former college varsity luminaries, a detailed epidemiological study of athleticism and health would address an important field of occupational medicine.

Questions arise continually as to how much and what kind of exercise is beneficial, and how too much may be harmful. Recent studies have already shown that, for example, marathon running does not preclude the development of atherosclerosis, and this sport has begun to show a decline in favor of brisk walking or other moderate exertion, as runners are prone to musculoskeletal injuries and the promotion of mass marathons has been going out of fashion. Various misinterpretations have greeted reports that habitually vigorous athletes were seven or eight times more likely to suffer primary cardiac arrest *while exercising* than at other times. A further point was that these same athletes were far less likely to have a primary cardiac arrest at all than sedentary persons who habitually did not exercise enough to maintain their health.[33,34] Observations such as these show that much remains to be learned about how the various kinds and characteristics of exercise and "fitness" actually influence health and longevity. Since CHD accounts for nearly half of all deaths, the finding that risk of CHD appears to be reduced or at least delayed by adequate habitual endurance exercise is widely accepted as of central importance. But physical activity defers all-cause mortality as well, which implies that the benefits of exercise in general must extend beyond the cardiovascular system. If exertion also presents hazards to the unwary—as does any other human activity—surely the hazards may be studied and understood. Current informed opinion is that most hazards of appropriate exercise are usually avoidable and represent risks far outweighed by its demonstrable benefits if the physical activity is naturally suited to the individual and wisely undertaken. How well professional athleticism meets these requirements is a recurring topic in the field of occupational medicine.

BENEFITS AND HAZARDS OF EXERCISE

Table 1 presents a classification of various benefits and hazards of endurance exercise. Some may be equally applicable to other kinds of exercise as well. The lists are neither detailed nor exhaustive, but they do show that there are a number of ways in which exercise affects many systems of the body. The accepted interrelationships of these body systems amply suggest reasons why the adequacy or inadequacy of habitual physical activity is likely to have significant influence on health and longevity. The table does not specify whether the exercise is occupational or at leisure. Some studies have hinted that leisure-time exercise is more beneficial than occupational physical work, however vigorous, because the leisure-time exercise can more readily be chosen, tailored, and timed to suit the needs of the individual.[35] If so, the decline of manual labor and the rise of popular sports-play eventually may have far-reaching favorable health effects on the general population. Professional athletics has fostered development of vastly improved sports equipment and safety procedures, although its contributions of role models often have appeared debatable. Table 1 might be modified considerably if it were intended to present the benefits and hazards of *athleticism.*

While the focus of Table 1 is stated to be on *endurance* exercise, most forms of physical activity are likely to involve several other kinds of exercise. Some of them may be implied in Table 1. For example, *static* or *isometric* exercise calls for the application of energy or forces without motion, as in some stages of gymnastics or weight-lifting. Such exertion imposes stresses or strains especially on the musculoskeletal and cardiovascular/respiratory systems and their components. Almost everyone has to do some of this kind of work, such as in carrying a heavy object or maintaining bodily poise or balance in a given situation but it can be a source of physical hazard, depending on age, strength, skill, preparation, and other considerations. These sorts of activity are the opposite of *dynamic* exercise that includes bodily motion such as running, walking, rowing, swimming. The nature of endurance exercise as a form of dynamic exercise believed important to cardiovascular fitness has been described earlier. Dynamic exercise also may tend to improve reflexes, such as in juggling or other physical activity requiring manipulative skill or dexterity. Games such as tennis or badminton involving rapid adjustments of position and coordination of sight and motion represent dynamic exercise comprised of

Table 1
Benefits and Hazards of Endurance Exercise with Regard to
Various Body Systems and Chronic Diseases

Body Systems Involved	Beneficial Effects	Potential Hazards
Cardiovascular-respiratory	Enhances physical work capacity, hemodynamic function, hematologic action, and cardiovascular fitness Reduces risks of atherosclerotic-hypertensive disease Increases maximum breathing capacity	Increases risk of sudden death in overstress Initiates asthmatic attacks in susceptibles Contraindicated for patients with acute coronary occlusion, acute myocardial infarction, myocarditis, dissecting aneurysm, severe aortic stenosis, or uncontrolled hypertension
Endocrine-metabolic	Weight regulation Stimulates metabolic processes Influences hormone production Decreases fat body mass and increases lean body mass Improves plasma lipid and lipoprotein fraction profiles Enhances fibrinolytic activity Improves glucose and insulin metabolism	Induces temperature imbalance (effects of hypothermia or hyperthermia
Musculo-skeletal	Enlarges and strengthens muscle fibers Increases oxygen utilization Strengthens connective tissues Eases low back pain syndrome Retards osteoporosis Reduces rheumatoid- and osteo-arthritic trends (?)	Produces acute and chronic injuries of cartilage, muscle, and bone Falling injuries "Overuse syndrome" Induces traumatic arthritis (?)

Body Systems Involved	Beneficial Effects	Potential Hazards
Gastro-intestinal	Promotes peristaltic and mixing action of intestine Shortens enteric passage time Modifies appetite	Induces electrolyte imbalance
Neurologic	Influences neuromyocardial action Enhances mood, thought and psychological behavior	Initiates dysrhythmia Induces compulsive-reactive syndrome (?)

Table 1 (continued)

continual episodes of action and reaction, braking and acceleration, shifts of direction, and other irregularities that differentiate such games from the more regular, rhythmic, large-muscle endurance exercises found in running, cross-country skiing, bicycling, swimming, and rowing.

Walking is surely the most common form of deliberate exercise, and even in a single individual its pace may vary from a slow saunter to a hurried rush. With an adequate rhythm, pace, and duration, it qualifies as an endurance activity beneficial to the cardiovascular system. But also, as a weight-bearing activity, walking is helpful to the musculoskeletal structures and reduces risk of developing osteoporosis. For these and other reasons, it is considered a better exercise for the elderly than running or jogging.[26]

Bicycling and swimming are rhythmic and well qualified as endurance exercise, but they involve far less weight-bearing activity than walking, running, skating, or cross-country skiing.[21] Swimming indeed is often regarded as a weightless condition useful in some types of therapy and for training of astronauts. The various limitations of different kinds of exercise point to the desirability of engaging in several kinds instead of only one favorite sport or physical activity. This also can help avoid seasonal lapses of exercise.

All in all, it appears that the early development of a life-long habit of varied, vigorous, and generalized physical activity is part of the best prescription to maintain vitality and achieve longevity. The role of an appropriately balanced diet in conjunction with the exercise pattern is not to be minimized, but also the effects of nutrition on body composition are altered by levels and kinds of exercise or physical activity. Diet and exercise, these two life-elements of energy intake and energy output, are mutually inter-active components that must achieve a balance between them-selves and in harmony with the cardiorespiratory, metabolic, and other physiologic mechanisms.

EXERCISE AND LONGEVITY

Discussions of relationships of athleticism to health and life expectancy date from antiquity. A survey of the literature would reveal that opinions on strenuous exercise have swung back and forth like a pendulum for centuries. The Greeks, Romans, and most other ancient civilizations esteemed physical prowess and sports proficiency. A series of 19th- and 20th-century papers debated the risks and longevity of university oarsmen.[36-39] Subsequently, H.J. Montoye raised provocative questions on chronic disease occurrence and life expectancy in an analysis of the life-styles and experience of men who had been varsity athletes of Michigan State University prior to 1938. The categorical numbers available at that time were insufficient to draw firm statistical conclusions. Prospective observations continue.[40]

In 1984 and 1986, some apparent adverse effects of athleticism in a larger population of Harvard alumni were noted by Paffenbarger et al.[13-15] If further analyses support the finding that ex-varsity athletes among the Harvard alumni tended to risk having a shorter life expectancy than their nonvarsity but energetic classmates, the search may indeed begin to focus on identification of any particular hazards that may be associated with athleticism as distinguished from apparently more healthful yet also vigorous life-patterns of physical activity. Studies have not yet ascertained to what extent the quality, quantity, pace, time, duration, frequency, regularity, stress level, training level, energy transfer demands, or other characteristics of exercise influence its relationships to health, vitality, and longevity. If, as mentioned earlier, leisure-time exercise appears to be more beneficial than occupational exertion because it is more readily suited to the needs of the individual, the pressures on a varsity or professional athlete to give a peak performance on demand may represent a similarly adverse burden in an ironic contrast to an appropriate, self-determined, leisure-time physical activity pattern.

Since cardiovascular disease accounted for 45 percent of the deaths among the Harvard alumni, the question arises of whether death rates from cardiovascular disease paralleled those of all-cause mortality in being somewhat higher for former varsity athletes who expended 2,000+ Kcal/week than for their less athletic classmates who had a similar physical activity index. The answer is affirmative. The ex-varsity athletes who reported being physically active to an index level of 2,000+ Kcal/week had higher risks than similarly active nonvarsity alumni, of death from coronary heart disease, other cardiovascular disease, stroke, cancer, or any other cause, according to a recent further analysis of the data. Although all these men had less risk of death than fellow alumni who had a lower activity index, the high-index ex-varsity athletes appeared to encounter more health hazards than their equally active nonvarsity classmates, even though they did benefit most from vigorous sports play as alumni.[13-15]

The reverse curve of death risk among ex-varsity athletes with increasing physical activity index as alumni may be partly due to apparent differences in life-style as evidenced by data on their tendencies toward extra obesity, cigarette smoking, a generally "macho" or superman attitude, or other excesses likely to induce overstress. "Athletic burnout" is a commonly used term in the professional sports industry, which, if it is valid, might be applied here with reference to the cardiovascular, musculoskeletal, neurosensory, or other systems of the body, or all together. To cite one example, if it can be assumed that there is a finite or average number of heartbeats in a lifetime, it can be shown that since the pulse rate is slowed by habitual moderate exercise but is accelerated by sedentariness or extremes of effort, personal longevity should be increased by moderate physical activity but reduced by habitual lethargy or overexertion. In practice, the life of a professional athlete or anyone else is far too complex for the simple application of any such yardstick, but even as statistical folklore, it might serve to illustrate a point for an athletic patient. Perhaps the story arose because pulse rate is used routinely to monitor states of disease and levels of physical activity.

The issues of athletic risk may relate additionally to certain other findings among the alumni. For example, a high physical activity index (2,000+ Kcal/week) reduced risk of developing hypertension, especially among men 20 percent or more overweight for their height.[31] Also an index of 2,000+ or even 500+ Kcal/week markedly reduced the risk of death among hypertensives (alumni with physician-diagnosed hypertension), from coronary heart disease, cardiovascular disease, or all-cause mortality.[14,15] It is also true among the alumni that obese men, especially those with a low physical activity index, were at increased risk of death, particularly from coronary heart disease, and many sedentary ex-varsity athletes (or professional athletes) might be expected to fall into that category. On the other hand, men who gained the least weight since college and had a low physical index as alumni were at the greatest risk of all-cause mortality. Some ex-varsity athletes might as logically be found in that group, whether or not they were heavy-weights as students or as alumni. The association of low weight gain and low physical activity index with high risk of all-cause mortality might imply a tendency toward cancer or wasting disease in such men. Those data would not account for the increased risk for ex-varsity men with higher physical activity index of 2,000+ Kcal/week.[14,15] Whatever observations are considered, however, their implications may apply as well to professional athletes as to any of the ex-varsity college alumni.

Table 2 presents the relative and attributable risks of death from cardiovascular disease among the Harvard alumni, as derived from a multivariate analysis and computed for the presence versus the absence of each of several influential adverse characteristics, with adjustment for differences in age and each of the other characteristics listed. The relative risk of 1.31 associated with sedentary life-style signifies that men expending fewer than 2,000 Kcal/week were at 31 percent higher risk of death than men more active. Likewise, men with physician-diagnosed hypertension had 118 percent greater risk than normotensive alumni, and cigarette smokers 84 percent over nonsmokers. Men who were 20 percent or more overweight for their height were at 18 percent greater risk than men less obese. Alumni of whom either or both parents had a history of coronary heart disease were at 33 percent greater risk than classmates whose parents did not have such a diagnosis. Alumni who reported having any one or more of the listed adversities were at more than triple the risk of men who had none of them. Each of the five characteristics, or the basic mechanisms they represented, contributed independently to the risk of death from cardiovascular disease.

Clinical attributable risks provide the physician's perspective of anticipated effects through prescription of hygienic, medical, or

Table 2
Relative and Attributable Risks of Death from Cardiovascular
Disease among 16,936 Harvard Alumni, 1962 to 1978, According
to Selected Adverse Characteristics*

Characteristic	Prevalence, % of Man-Years	Relative Risk of Death	P Value	Clinical Attributable Risk, %	Community Attributable Risk, %
Sedentary life-style	62	1.31	0.0172	24	16
Hypertension	9	2.18	<0.0001	54	9
Cigarette smoking	38	1.84	<0.0001	46	25
Overweight for height	37	1.18	0.1081	16	6
Parental coronary heart disease	37	1.33	0.0062	25	11
One or more of the above**	90	3.03	0.0003	67	65

*Adjusted for age and each of the other characteristics listed. Sedentary life-style is defined as an energy expenditure of <2,000 Kcal/week in walking, climbing stairs, and sports-play. Hypertension was diagnosed by the patient's physician. "Cigarette smoking" refers to any amount of smoking. Overweight for height is defined as 20% or more above ideal weight for height by the 1959 Metropolitan Life Insurance Company standards (i.e., a body mass index of >36). Parental heart disease refers to heart disease in either or both parents.

**Adjusted for age only.

surgical intervention. They are estimates of the potential percentage reduction in risk of death for individuals who exchange an unfavorable characteristic for a more healthful one. Thus in Table 2 sedentary men becoming active might reduce their risk of dying from cardiovascular disease by 24 percent. Any hypertensives who could achieve normal blood pressure might have 54 percent lower risk. Alumni who quit smoking cigarettes might have 46 percent less risk; heavy-weights who reduced, 16 percent less. Sons of ailing parents might have been 25 percent less at risk if their parents had been free of coronary heart disease (a finding that might have practical value for subsequent generations).

Community attributable risks relate to the public health perspective of group interventions or broader "environmental" alterations, as they are estimates that take prevalence into account. They reveal what percentage of risk might be avoided in a community or population if the adverse characteristics were eliminated by substituting a more favorable life-style throughout the community. In Table 2, there might have been 16 percent fewer deaths from cardiovascular disease if all the alumni had attained a physical activity index of 2,000 or more kilocalories per week. If none were hypertensive, 9 percent of the cardiovascular deaths might not have occurred. Abolition of smoking might have saved 25 percent from fatal cardiovascular disease during the study interval. Avoidance of obesity might slim the death rate by 6 percent. Absence of coronary heart disease in their parents might have meant 11 percent fewer cardiovascular deaths among the sons. If none of the alumni had had any of the adverse characteristics, there might have been a 65 percent cut in their cardiovascular disease death toll during the 16-year follow-up period.

The continuing long-range studies in the university alumni population have shown that adequate habitual exercise, even though it might be considered only moderate, appears to delay all-cause mortality.[14,15] Physical activity index levels and all-cause death rates among 17,000 Harvard alumni during 1962–1978 are shown in Table 3. Death rates and relative risks are substantially lower for the more active men expending 2,000–3,500 Kcal/week by physical activity index than for their less active classmates.

Longevity data on the longshoremen have not been examined, but risk of sudden death was markedly lower among the most

Table 3
Rates and Risks of Death from All Causes among 17,000 Harvard Alumni, 1962–1978, by Leisure-Time Physical Activity

Index Kilocalories per Week in Walking, Stair-Climbing, and Sports-Play	Prevalence, % of Man-Years	Number of Deaths	Deaths per 10,000 Man-Years*		Relative Risk of Death	
<500	16	308	94		1.00	
500–999	21	322	74		.78	
1000–1499	15	202	68	75	.73	1.00
1500–1999	10	121	59		.63	
2000–2499	8	89	58		.62	
2500–2999	7	62	49		.52	
3000–3499	5	42	43	54	.46	.72
3500+	18	203	58		.62	

*Age-adjusted figures.

energetic cargo handlers. As machinery and containerization have abolished most of their manual labor, many longshoremen might need to take up some adequate leisure-time physical activity to compensate for their loss of occupational exercise. For several reasons, a further follow-up of this unique occupational study population would be of considerable interest.

A basic philosophical question naturally arises when the topic of exercise and longevity is brought up: Do these highly active groups or populations live longer than the rest of us? The answer is not that simple, because, for example, the life-styles of the longshoremen differ from those of the college alumni, and both differ somewhat from the general population. In fact, mortality rates for the longshoremen have not been different from the U.S. averages, while those of the college alumni were slightly lower—in keeping with the usual finding that levels of health and death rates tend to correlate with socioeconomic status and level of education. However, the results of each study are particular to the population studied: the more active longshoremen had less CHD risk than the less active longshoremen; similarly, the more active alumni had less CHD and better longevity estimates than their less active classmates. The same was true in subgroups within those populations, whether the subgroup was defined by age, blood pressure status, body mass index, weight gain category, or other characteristics of person or life-style. The logical conclusion is that each individual in any population is likely to fare better in health and longevity if he is habitually vigorous and active than if he is chronically sedentary, other things being equal. The findings add that he will fare still better if he is prudent also about other aspects of his life-style, such as by maintaining a suitable weight and not smoking cigarettes. Various studies have noted that habits of healthful exercise tend to promote weight management, dietary balance, favorable blood lipid profile, and other physiological benefits.[12] More have been listed in Table 1, discussed earlier. These findings offer clues to some of the mechanisms by which physical activity makes its essential contributions to vitality and longevity.

Table 4 is a modified life table showing estimates of added longevity gained by Harvard alumni up to age 80 if they had a physical activity index of 2,000+ Kcal/week versus classmates with a lower index, calculated from mortality among the alumni during the interval 1962–1978. Estimates are also given for those who reported vigorous sports-play versus those who did not.

Table 4
Added Life from an Active Life-Style in Men to Age 80, Estimated from Mortality among Harvard Alumni, 1962 to 1978*

Age of Entry	Years Gained with Physical Activity Index of 2000+ Kcal/Week** Vs. Less Physical Activity	Years Gained with Vigorous Sports-Play Vs. No Sports
35−39	1.50	1.55
40−44	1.39	1.45
45−49	1.10	1.23
50−54	1.20	1.32
55−59	1.13	1.21
60−64	0.93	0.95
65−69	0.67	0.55
70−74	0.44	−0.11
75−79	0.30	−0.09
35−79[#]	1.25[#]	1.28[#]

*Adjusted for differences in blood-pressure status, cigarette smoking, net gain in body mass index since college, and age of parental death.
**Kilocalories expended in walking, climbing stairs, and playing sports.
[#]Weighted averages.

IMPLICATIONS FOR THE PHYSICIAN

Whether in the practice of occupational or family medicine, in cardiology, or in community health, the physician has a key role in the promotion of favorable exercise habits for young and old, active and inactive, all with whom he has professional or more casual contact. Better facilities, better educational and evaluation programs, broader understanding and acceptance of the importance of appropriate exercise as an essential element of disease prevention and health promotion are some of the projects in which he may have continuing influence. Without the physician's support, indeed, they might be less likely to flourish, even though the urge to exercise is probably a basic drive that has been around since prehistoric times. Only in our day has natural physical activity become routinely withheld from entire societies of people, but now the solutions to this whole matter are being given a lot of thought and new impetus.[18,41,42] The field of occupational medicine has broadened with the recognition that the promotion of healthful exercise for employees is good business that reduces sick-leave absenteeism and enhances efficiency on the job. Costs of health insurance and work-related injuries should tend to be lowered. When considerations such as these and the quality of life are taken into account, prevention of disease is far less costly than cure.[43] The safety and welfare of employees is a constant responsibility both at work and at play, but even so, a baseball field, swimming pool, bicycle path, or exercise room is a better symbol of health care than an enlarged company clinic or hospital.[42,44,45]

One of the most encouraging developments of the modern "exercise revolution" has been the active participation of thousands of physicians everywhere, whose sincere advice and leadership have tended to keep the emphasis not so much on glamorous athleticism as on a wiser development of individual life-styles in which exercise is included both for health maintenance and personal enjoyment.[18,42,44,45] Physical activity has always been a requirement of good living, but never before have so many people needed to have it prescribed for them.[41,42]

Acknowledgment: Supported by research grant HL34174 from the National Heart, Lung, and Blood Institute of the U.S. Public Health Service, and by the Marathon Oil Foundation, Inc.

REFERENCES

1. Hedley OF: Analysis of 5,116 deaths reported as due to acute coronary occlusion in Philadelphia, 1933–1937. *US Weekly Public Health Report* 1939; 54:972.

2. Morris JN, Heady JA, Raffle PAB, Roberts CG, Parks JW: Coronary heart disease and physical activity of work. *Lancet* 1953; 2:1053–1057, 1111–1120.

3. Morris JN, Kagan A, Pattison DC, Gardner M, Raffle PAB: Incidence and prediction of ischaemic heart-disease in London busmen. *Lancet* 1966; 2:552–559.

4. Morris JN, Chave SPW, Adam C, Sirey C, Epstein L, Sheehan DJ: Vigorous exercise in leisure-time and the incidence of coronary heart disease. *Lancet* 1973; 1:333–339.

5. Garcia-Palmieri MR, Costas R Jr, Cruz-Vidal M, Sorlie PD, Havlik RS: Increased physical activity: A protective factor against heart attacks in Puerto Rico. *Am J Cardiol* 1982; 50:749–755.

6. Pomrehn PR, Wallace RB, Burmeister LF: Ischemic heart disease mortality in Iowa farmers: The influence of life-style. *JAMA* 1982; 248:1073–1076.

7. Paffenbarger RS Jr, Hale WE, Brand RJ, Hyde RT: Work-energy level, personal characteristics, and fatal heart attack: A birth-cohort effect. *Am J Epidemiol* 1977; 105:200–213.

8. Peters RK, Cady LD Jr, Bishoff DP, Bernstein L, Pike MC: Physical fitness and subsequent myocardial infarction in healthy workers. *JAMA* 1983; 249:3052–3056.
9. Dawber TR: The Framingham Study. *The Epidemiology of Atherosclerotic Disease.* Cambridge, Massachusetts, Harvard University Press. 1980; pp 151–171.
10. Kannel WM, Sorlie P: Some health benefits of physical activity: The Framingham Study. *Arch Intern Med* 1979; 139:857–861.
11. Paffenbarger RS Jr, Wing AL, Hyde RT: Chronic disease in former college students. XVI. Physical activity as an index of heart attack risk in college alumni. *Am J Epidemiol* 1978; 108:161–175.
12. Paffenbarger RS Jr, Hyde RT: Exercise as protection against heart attack. *New Engl J Med* 1980; 302:1026–1027.
13. Paffenbarger RS Jr, Hyde RT, Wing AL, Steinmetz CH: A natural history of athleticism and cardiovascular health. *JAMA* 1984; 252;4:491–495.
14. Paffenbarger RS Jr, Hyde RT, Wing AL, Hsieh C: Physical activity, all-cause mortality, and longevity of college alumni. *New Engl J Med* 1986; 314:605–613.
15. Letters to the Editor. *New Engl J Med* 1986; 315:399–401.
16. Passmore R, Durnin JVGA: Human energy expenditure. *Physiol Rev* 1955; 35:801–840.
17. Astrand P-O, Rodahl K: *Textbook of Work Physiology.* New York, McGraw-Hill, 1970 (3rd edition, 1986).
18. Powell KE, ed: Workshop on epidemiologic and public health aspects of physical activity and exercise. *Public Health Rep* 1985; 100:113–224.
19. Kannel WB, Wilson P, Blair SN: Epidemiological assessment of the role of physical activity and fitness in development of cardiovascular disease. *Amer Heart J* 1985; 109(4):876–885.
20. Morris JN: *Uses of Epidemiology.* London, Churchill Livingstone, 1975 (3rd edition).
21. Blair SN, Gibbons LW, Painter P, Pate RR, Taylor CB, Will J (eds): *Guidelines for Exercise Testing and Prescription. Amer Coll Sports Med.* Philadelphia, Lea & Febiger, 1986 (3rd edition).
22. LaPorte RE, Montoye HJ, Caspersen CJ: Assessment of physical activity in epidemiologic research: Problems and prospects. *Public Health Rep* 1985; 100(2):131–146.
23. Montoye HJ, Washburn R, Servas S, et al: Estimation of energy expenditure by a portable accelerometer. *Med Sci Sports Exercise* 1983; 15:403–407.
24. DeVries HA: Physiological effect of an exercise-training regimen on men aged 52–88. *J Gerontol* 1970; 23:325–336.
25. DeVries HA: Intensity thresholds for improvement of cardiovascular-respiratory function in older men. *Geriatrics* 1971; 26:94–101.
26. Shephard RJ: *Physical Activity and Aging.* London, Croom Helm Books, 1978.
27. Fries JF, Crapo LM: *Vitality and Aging.* San Francisco, W. Freeman & Co., 1981.
28. Buskirk ER, et al: Exercise in the treatment of obesity. Proceedings of a symposium. *Med Sc Sports Exercise* 1986; 18(1):1–30.

29. Paffenbarger RS Jr, Hyde RT, Wing AL: Physical activity and incidence of cancer in diverse populations: A preliminary report. *Am J Clin Nutri* 1987; (Suppl) 45;1:312–317.

30. Vena JE, Graham S, Zielezny M, Brasure J, Swanson MK: Occupational exercise and risk of cancer. *Am J Clin Nutrition* 1987; (Suppl) 45;1:318–327.

31. Paffenbarger RS Jr, Wing AL, Hyde RT, et al: Physical activity and incidence of hypertension in college alumni. *Am J Epidemiol* 1983; 117:245–257.

32. Wood PD, Haskell WL, Blair SN, et al: Increased exercise level and plasma lipoprotein concentration: A one-year randomized controlled study in sedentary middle-aged men. *Metabolism* 1983; 32:31–39.

33. Siscovick DS, Weiss NS, Fletcher RH, Lasky T: The incidence of primary cardiac arrest during vigorous exercise. *New Engl J Med* 1984; 311:874–877.

34. Thompson PD, Funk EJ, Carleton RA, Sturner QQ: Incidence of death during jogging in Rhode Island from 1975 through 1980. *JAMA* 1982; 247:253–255.

35. Morris JN, Everett MG, Pollard R, Chave SPW, Semmence AM: Vigorous exercise in leisure-time: Protection against coronary heart disease. *Lancet* 1980; 2:1207–1210.

36. Morgan JE: *University Oars*. London, MacMillan & Co., 1873.

37. Hartley PH-S, Llewellyn GF: The longevity of oarsmen: A study of those who rowed in the Oxford and Cambridge boat race from 1829 to 1929. *Br Med J* 1939; 1:657–662.

38. Rook A: An investigation into the longevity of Cambridge sportsmen. *Br Med J* 1954; 1:773–777.

39. Prout C: Life expectancy of college oarsmen. *JAMA* 1972; 220:1709–1711.

40. Montoye HJ: Health and longevity of former athletes. In Johnson WR, Buskirk ER (eds): *Science and Medicine of Exercise and Sport*, New York, Harper & Row, 1974. pp 366–376. (2nd ed)

41. Thomas GS, Lee PR, Franks P, Paffenbarger RS Jr: *Exercise and Health: The Evidence and the Implications*. Cambridge, Massachusetts, Oelgeschlager, Gunn & Hain, 1981.

42. Morris JN, et al: *Exercise, Health and Medicine*. Proceedings of a Symposium at Lilleshall Sports Centre, Shropshire, May 3–6, 1983. Health Education Council, Medical Research Society, National Sports Council, London, 1984.

43. Russell LB: *Is Prevention Better than Cure?* Brookings Institution, Washington DC, 1986.

44. Dishman RK, Sallis JF, Orenstein DR: The determinants of physical activity and exercise. *Pub Health Rep* 1985; 100(2):158–171.

45. Blair SN, Jacobs DR Jr, Powell KE: Relationships between exercise or physical activity and other health behaviors. *Public Health Rep* 1985; 100(2):172–195.

14

Influence of Environmental Factors on Exercise Activities in Patient Care

Barbara J. Fletcher, R.N., M.N.

Exercise activity for patient care has received nationwide attention in recent years. Since exercise activities and centers have been established in various geographic locations, the influence of temperature, humidity, altitude, air-pollutants, and terrain during exercise or activity must be considered.

HEAT AND HUMIDITY

The body produces heat through metabolism of carbohydrates, fats, and proteins and loses heat by convection, radiation, conduction, and evaporation. At rest in a comfortable environment, the body achieves a balance between heat produced and heat lost. Maintenance of thermal balance (approximate body temperature of 98.6°F) during physical work and constantly changing environmental conditions is accomplished primarily through vasoconstriction and dilation of skin arterioles.

Exercise in warm environments reveals initial cutaneous

From: Fletcher GF: *Exercise in the Practice of Medicine*, 2nd Revised Edition. Mount Kisco, NY, Futura Publishing Co., Inc., © 1988.

vasoconstriction but sufficient hyperthermia abolishes this response.[1] As body temperature increases, skin vessels dilate and there is a decrease in central blood volume resulting in an increase in circulation near the surface of the skin.[2] This decrease in central blood volume results in a reduction in stroke volume, triggering a compensatory increase in heart rate and physiologically maintaining cardiac output, thus allowing a continuation of the specific physical activity.[3,4]

Skin vasodilation is the body's physiological mechanism for dissipation of excess heat through physical forces such as radiation, convection, and evaporation.[2] With exercise, 75 percent of oxygen utilized in the production of energy is converted into heat. Therefore, the greater the metabolic demand of the activity, the greater the thermal load added to the body. When one exercises in a hot environment, the body is exposed to both internal and external sources of heat. A major function of the circulation at this time is to deliver necessary oxygen to the working muscles and to transport heat generated by these muscles to the skin's surface for dissipation.[5]

Evaporation of sweat is an important natural mechanism for heat dissipation. Sweat alone does not cool the body, but as sweat evaporates, the blood near the body's surface is cooled. This blood then flows more centrally to cool the body.[2] Individuals without sweat glands can participate in summer activities but they should periodically wet their skin so that evaporation can take place.[6] If air moisture content (humidity) is elevated, sweat cannot evaporate. Heat dissipation then becomes a significant problem when humidity is higher.[2]

The more highly trained individual expends less energy to dissipate heat for a specific activity and as a result has a lower central body temperature for a given task. Exercise in hot environments exposes the body to greater external heat, but this can be tolerated for short periods of time. As the activity continues in the hot environment, body temperature (internal heat) continues to increase until the activity ceases or the environment becomes cooler.[6]

In order to maintain the body's thermal balance, dehydration must be prevented. When an activity continues after 1−3 percent of body weight is lost due to sweating, central body temperature increases in a linear fashion with increasing fluid loss.[2] Studies have shown that fluid intake before, as well as during, the activity will prevent a marked elevation in body temperature.[7] Intake of

200–300 cc of fluid every 15–20 minutes is ideal and necessary in high level competition held in hot environments. The beverage should contain less than 25 grams/liter of glucose, 10 mEq sodium, and 5 mEq potassium/liter.[8]

Exercise in subjects with normovolemic, hypovolemic, and hypervolemic conditions produces various body fluid and sweating responses. Significantly greater decreases in blood volume occur in the hypervolemic subjects as compared to both normovolemic and hypovolemic individuals. In addition, the amount of sweating in the hypovolemic group is significantly less. Both the body fluid and sweating response are compensatory mechanisms to conserve circulating blood volume during exercise.[9]

Knochel and associates[10] reported significant potassium depletion in men undergoing intense physical training in hot climates with sweating as the major means of potassium loss. In contrast, subjects undergoing the same intense physical training in cooler environments did not develop potassium depletion. These data should make one aware of the need for close follow-up of serum electrolytes as well as fluid replacement in cardiac patients. This is especially true if their medication regimen includes potassium-depleting medications, such as diuretics, and if they reside or exercise in hot, humid climates.

Prophylactic salt (sodium) intake is not considered necessary when participating in moderate levels of activity in hot environments. More water than salt is lost through sweating. By ingesting salt, one may increase sodium concentration to a potentially harmful imbalance. Individuals obtain enough salt in a normal diet to compensate for the amount of salt lost in 6 pounds (6 pints) of water.[11]

Since cardiac patients are often limited in cardiovascular reserve capacity and hot, humid conditions increase cardiac work load, their activities should be modified when these conditions exist. When the exercise environment consists of temperature greater than 94°F and humidity in the range of 70–80 percent, exercise should be cancelled.[12] For additional safety during hot, humid months, all exercise prescriptions for cardiac patients should be decreased by 25 percent intensity or duration. The patients should be advised of early signs of hyperthermia such as throbbing cranial pressure, dizziness, nausea, and slight disorientation.[13] Patients should be advised to reduce activities at the first sign of hyperthermia.

Proper clothing in hot temperatures will aid in heat dissipation. The clothing should fit loosely and be made of cotton (rather than types of polyester or plastic) to allow for free convection flow of air. Light clothing (both in color and in weight) should be encouraged. Lighter colors reflect rays of heat while darker colors tend to absorb heat rays. Clothing wet with perspiration need not be replaced because wet clothing is more conducive to heat loss through evaporation. Obese patients desiring to lose weight rapidly often wear heavy clothing while exercising to increase fluid (weight) loss through sweating. This can lead to rapid depletion of electrolytes which may be potentially dangerous and should be discouraged.[2]

COLD

Cold temperatures precipitate peripheral vasoconstriction and decreased pulmonary ventilation. As one is exposed to cold, endogenous epinephrine and norepinephrine stores are released to enhance the production of internal heat. The epinephrine is also responsible for vasoconstriction, which is the body's effort to retain heat centrally. The resulting increase in peripheral resistance increases cardiac work or oxygen consumption in addition to causing a reduced stroke volume as venous return decreases.

As body temperature decreases, the delivery of oxygen at the tissue level is decreased. With less oxygen available, there is a tendency to develop metabolic or lactic acidosis which, in patients with coronary heart disease, may provoke ischemia and arrhythmias.[14] As one becomes colder, there is a tendency to shiver. Muscle tension and shivering can require energy of up to four times the resting metabolic rate.[15] Some cardiac patients are not capable of performing tasks requiring more energy than this and would expend the major portion of their energy through shivering.

Cardiac patients can safely exercise in cold environments if precautions are followed. However, extremely cold temperatures may precipitate angina pectoris[16–18] and should be avoided. A cold weather mask may be effective in these situations.[19,20] Environmental temperature changes are also known to affect one's diastolic blood pressure.[21,22] As temperature rises, diastolic pressure falls and conversely, diastolic pressure increases with colder temperatures. DeServi et al.,[23] as well as others,[24,25] demonstrated that exercise in a cold environment resulted in a significant increase in heart rate, blood pressure, and double product. Buonanno et al.[26] demonstrated significant changes in angiographic parameters in coronary artery disease (CAD) patients when exposed to cold. End-diastolic volume increased 11 percent, ejection fraction decreased 8 percent, and there was a significant reduction in segmental wall motion in the area of the diseased artery. Both CAD patients and non-CAD subjects demonstrated an increase in arterial pressure and double product when exposed to cold.

Cardiac patients require alterations in activity guidelines in winter as well as in summer. A wind-chill factor leads to colder perceived temperature; in addition, when one walks or runs against wind, the energy cost of the activity increases as the square of the wind velocity in meters per second increases.[27] Riggs et al.[28] demonstrated a 15-beat reduction in heart rate response in normal subjects exercising in cold wind (10°C). Cardiac patients exercising in cold, windy environments need to be aware of the possibility of a reduced heart rate to routine activity. As a general policy, cardiac patients should be advised to exercise indoors if the temperature is 40°F or less, and cancel exercise if environmental temperatures approach 4°F. Proper clothing is important in winter for conserving body heat. Clothing may be dark in color and should cover extremities. If the garment becomes damp with perspiration, it should be replaced, since dry clothing tends to conserve heat.[2] Layering of clothing is advised in both hot and cold temperatures. This provides a mechanism for the body to adjust to minute-to-minute changes in both internal and external temperature.

ALTITUDE

With increased altitude, there is a decrease in oxygen saturation of arterial blood due to a decrease in partial pressure of oxygen in the environment.[29] Until recently, it was thought that man needed supplemental oxygen when ascending to altitudes above 10,000 feet. Recently men have demonstrated their ability to climb Mount Everest (29,000 feet) without supplemental oxygen. Studies of cardiopulmonary parameters have currently been conducted on Mount Everest.[30] Karliner et al.[31] have demonstrated transient ECG changes consistent with increased pulmonary artery pressure in healthy subjects at extreme altitudes of Mount Everest. These changes had no adverse effect and returned to baseline after descent.

A series of altitude studies were performed by Inama and Halhuber[32] in the Austrian Alps on patients with cardiovascular disease. The majority of data was collected at an altitude of 6,000 to 8,000 feet above sea level (moderate altitude). These studies involved patients with high blood pressure, previous myocardial infarction, and angina pectoris and arrhythmias. In the high blood pressure study, 220 patients were treated with a carefully supervised activity program for 4 weeks at the above-stated altitude. They found that with training, both the resting and submaximal blood pressure showed a significant decrease and this lower blood pressure persisted as long as 8 months after returning to lower altitudes. Patients in the myocardial infarction study lived at similar altitudes of 6,000 to 8,000 feet above sea level and their training included daily hikes of 1,700 feet (one-third mile) to additional elevations. No serious complications occurred and an increase in functional capacity was demonstrated. A similar study was done with patients with angina pectoris and arrhythmias. Again, no complications were reported and most demonstrated an increase in functional capacity. Additional studies have noted maximal oxygen uptake to decrease and heart rate to increase in normal subjects at high altitudes.[33-35] Conversely, heart rates have been shown to decrease 14–23 percent in depths of 2–132 feet seawater gauge.[36]

Prolonged exposure of 20 days to a moderate altitude of 5,700 feet has been shown to decrease oxygen affinity after the first 9 days. A decrease in oxygen affinity facilitates oxygenation of tissues by allowing an increased oxygen release from red blood cells at a given partial pressure of oxygen. This decreased oxygen affinity reflects enhancement of tissue oxygenation. In addition, the increase in oxygen delivery to the tissues takes place without increase in cardiac output or other energy processes.[37]

Based on the above data, exercise at moderate altitudes should not be a contraindication in selected cardiovascular patients. Cardiac patients should be aware of the effects of altitude on alterations in heart rate. A period of time for acclimatization is ideal. Patients should be advised to be aware of signs of altitude sickness such as drowsiness, lassitude, mental fatigue (decreased mental proficiency), headache, nausea, or euphoria.[38] Proper clothing is most important, especially for skiing and should be light in weight, layered, and well-insulated since heavy weighted layers of clothing may impose added work during exercise.[2]

AIR-POLLUTANTS

Ozone (O_3) is one of the more common air-pollutants and primarily affects the pulmonary system. Since cardiac patients may have a problem with oxygen supply, the effect of ozone may be more pronounced. Ozone is a product of the interaction of light energy with automobile exhaust and is one of the chief constituents of photochemical smog. Ozone at near-ambient smog alert levels has been shown to cause decreases in pulmonary function and maximal oxygen consumption. Photochemical oxidants can result in eye irritation, chest tightness, dyspnea, cough, and gastrointestinal disturbances such as nausea and "dry heaves."[39-42]

Savin and Adams[43] in 1979 studied the effect of ozone on exercise test performance in healthy male subjects. Each subject performed three tests while breathing 0.00, 0.15, or 0.30 parts per million (ppm) of ozone. The order of the tests was randomly exposed. Maximal expired minute ventilation was decreased ($P <$ 0.05) in a dose-dependent fashion. However, there was no significant effect on maximal work rate, aerobic threshold, or other pulmonary function indices. They concluded that exposure of healthy young men up to 0.30 ppm O_3 for no more than 30 minutes of high-level exercise is insufficient to cause a significant decrease in work capacity or maximal oxygen consumption. It is noteworthy that some industrialized areas have reported a monthly maximum level of 0.54 ppm O_3. The higher the humidity and temperature, the greater the detrimental effect of O_3.[44]

Illing and co-workers[45] reported data supporting a decrease in resistance to infection in exercising mice after exposure to pollutants (O_3 and NO_2). The mice were divided into two groups. Both groups were exposed to pollutants but only one group was exercised. Both groups of mice were then exposed to *Streptococcus pyogenes*. The exercised mice had a significantly higher mortality rate from the streptococcus than those not exercised. Humans are often engaged in physical activities involving exposure to air-containing pollutants. If exercise and pollutants do indeed decrease resistance to infection in man, as has been demonstrated in mice with exercise, further studies are needed to establish acceptable exposure levels of pollutants.

Little is known about the pollutant effect of sulfur oxides on maximal working capacity. However, when sulfur oxides reach the level of 1 ppm, subjects may be "significantly uncomfortable" and cardiac patients should limit activity. Sulfur oxides at these levels occur more frequently in highly industrialized areas.[46]

Carbon monoxide (CO) is an air-pollutant prevalent in most geographical areas. Cigarette smoke, industrial waste products, and automobile exhaust produce CO.[47] Several animal studies have supported harmful effects of CO. Astrup and colleagues[48] have shown that rabbits with carboxyhemoglobin (COHb) levels of 13 percent developed marked degenerative changes in their major arteries and myocardium over a 3-month period. Debias[49] reported monkeys exposed to CO were more susceptible to ventricular fibrillation after 6 hours exposure to 100 ppm of CO than monkeys not exposed to CO.

An additional study[42] evaluated ten subjects with angina pectoris and tested each twice on a treadmill. The first test was conducted after each subject drove 90 minutes on an "industrialized" freeway with open windows which enabled them to inhale typical air-pollutants (mainly CO) from car exhaust. The second test was conducted after each subject was placed in an environment for a period of time breathing purified air. The data demonstrated a decrease in treadmill test time and an earlier development of angina pectoris in the test after driving on the freeway.

CO may be harmful within the body when levels exceed minimal values. Normal COHb levels seldom exceed 1 percent. The average city commuter may increase his/her COHb by 2–3 percent and smokers are reported to have COHb levels in excess concentrations of 4–10 percent per day.[50,51] Recent evidence indicates that maximal oxygen consumption of healthy males is reduced linearly relative to increased levels of COHb ranging from 5–35 percent.[52] In accord with this and the recent Surgeon General's report, nonsmoking individuals should request a smoke-free environment.

In summary, air-pollutants decrease oxygen availability and increase heart rate response to submaximal work loads. This is very similar to the effect of heat exposure. Oxygen debt with various activities is also increased which could possibly precipitate arrhythmias. One needs to advise cardiac patients very carefully regarding activity in environments with an abundance of air-pollutants. This problem is compounded in hot, humid environments and especially if the patient is a smoker.

TERRAIN

Terrain hiking along mountain trails was used by Oertel[53] in the late 1800's as one of the first efforts in cardiac rehabilitation. Since many of today's cardiac patients have musculoskeletal problems, specific terrain factors should be considered when discussing activities. Weak ankles, back problems, and general loss of flexibility may quickly lead to greater problems if activity such as running or brisk walking is done in areas with unlevel surfaces or surfaces that are "cluttered" with obstacles. Calisthenics to increase strength and flexibility should be strongly encouraged for those planning outdoor exercise regimes. One should also consider positive features of being outdoors in natural terrain. Pleasant surroundings of mountains, foliage, or seashore can provide a "relaxing effect" on the cardiovascular system.

GENERAL RECOMMENDATIONS

Advice is frequently requested regarding environmental factors and specific activities for cardiac patients. This advice should be individualized and based on the length of time since the particular cardiovascular event, as well as the stability of the current condition. Data are available quantitating various activities and energy requirements.[54] It is important for the patient to recognize his or her end-point. These vary from generalized fatigue, increase or decrease in heart rate, elevated blood pressure, cardiac arrhythmias, to angina pectoris. One must always use terminology the patient understands such as "skipped beats" instead of "premature ventricular contractions," and "chest discomfort" rather than "chest pain." Advice for the patient needs to be based on scientific research, personal experience, and objective evaluation such as exercise testing and ambulatory ECG monitoring when necessary. Each patient should have had a minimum of at least one exercise test to establish individual end-points for activity.

Cardiac patients are generally concerned about *specifics*. They desire to know exactly when, what, and how much of a certain activity they can do outside a medically supervised exercise program. Patients should be aware that their end-points on the exercise test should always surpass end-points with all activities they choose. They should also be aware that the time of end-points with specific activities will vary with the environment.

Running is probably the most common activity that cardiac patients desire to do alone. Cardiac patients engaging in running may develop hemodynamic compromising situations. With this in mind, cardiacs are generally discouraged from running when they are not supervised. Exceptions to this policy are those with total myocardial revascularization, normal high-level exercise test, and patients with documented one-vessel disease, good ventricular function, and a normal exercise test and ambulatory ECG recording study. *Brisk walking* is an excellent substitute for running.

Swimming is another popular activity. Water activity can be more strenuous on one's cardiovascular system as compared to other activities. This is most likely related to the higher cardiac output and stroke volume that occurs with water exercise as compared to land exercise.[55] Studies have been done on the amount of energy involved in *walk/jogging, exercise dancing,* and *swimming* in post-infarction patients.[56] Swimming was found to have almost twice the energy requirement than either exercise dancing or walk/jogging. In addition, Magder and associates noted that cardiac patients are more often unaware of their routine symptoms when swimming as compared to awareness of symptoms at the same work level on the bicycle ergometer.[57] Based on these data, it is advisable to give cardiac patients a 5 percent lower target heart rate for water activity than for running or dancing. It has been demonstrated that cardiac subjects can safely achieve similar training effects with water and land exercise.[58] With swimming, walk/jogging, or dancing, environment plays a major role. One should consider the temperature, humidity, and air-pollution level when making specific recommendations. For example, suggest a temperature-controlled pool for water activity, a well-ventilated room for dancing, or a walk/jog course away from heavily traveled highways and apart from industrialized areas.

When one advises patients on *tennis*, it is wise to consider that "doubles" is most likely less strenuous than "singles." One should caution patients not to play in extreme temperatures. In summer it is preferable to play either early or late in the day, while in winter it would be more appropriate to play during midday.

Isometric activity is involved in *water skiing*. There have been two anecdotal cases of possible ventricular fibrillation associated with water skiing. For this reason, cautious advice is given to cardiacs with regard to water skiing and it is not advised if the patient has confirmed high-grade ventricular ectopy or moderate to severe hypertension. In addition to the physical activity parameters of water skiing, one should be aware of the cardiovascular effects of temperature; for example at a similar time and locale, river water is generally colder than lake or ocean water.

Snow skiing is permitted for stable selected cardiac patients. They are cautioned to remain at moderate altitudes, dress appropriately, utilize rest periods for fatigue and warmth, and be aware of wind factors present.[27] Cardiac patients receiving beta-adrenergic blocking agents may have peripheral vascular side effects. "Cardiac skiers" should be warned that these side effects can be more pronounced in cold environments. Patients with coronary spasm should be extremely cautious since severe cold may precipitate spasm. It would be wise to test these patients with the cold pressor test prior to making a recommendation.

A *stationary bicycle* is an excellent mechanism for activity apart from a medically supervised program. It can be done in a controlled environment and involve a specific exercise prescription based on previous testing. Safety for cardiac patients with arrhythmias can be enhanced by use of a telephone monitoring system.[59] With the monitoring system, patients may transmit electrocardiographic recordings at a given time before, during, and after each bicycle session.

Bicycling outdoors for pleasure or, more specifically, as a mode of transportation is becoming increasingly popular. As with other outdoor activity, one should consider temperature, humidity, air-pollution, terrain, and the patient's fatigue factor. Be aware of the patient's activity level and his need or lack of need for supervision.

With any activity, alcoholic beverages or large meals should be avoided prior to the activity. Timing of medication is important specifically in patients on antiarrhythmic agents since serum levels need to be maintained for effectiveness. Many patients who have angina take nitrates before, during, or after certain activities. This is individualized and should be encouraged with proper medical advice. Patients may be more appropriately advised if prophylactic use of nitroglycerin is initially evaluated by exercise testing. Patients should be aware of potential avenues of emergency care should signs and symptoms of cardiac compromise arise while exercising alone.

In conclusion, when advising patients to exercise, one should consider the individual's clinical data along with various environmental factors and the energy cost of the specific activity. In today's automated, mechanized, industrialized society located in environments of varied pollutants, temperature, humidity, and altitude, patients would likely perform activities more safely and effectively in controlled indoor or pollutant-free environments.[60]

REFERENCES

1. Johnson JM, Park MK: Effect of heat stress on cutaneous vascular responses to the initiation of exercise. *J Appl Physiol* 1982; 53(3):744–749.
2. Guyton AC: Body temperature, temperature regulation and fever. In *Textbook of Medical Physiology*. Philadelphia, WB Sanders Company, 1981; 886–898.
3. Rowell LB: Human cardiovascular adjustments to exercise and thermal stress. *Physiol Rev* 1974; 54:75–159.
4. Rowell LB, Marx HJ, Bruce RA, et al: Reduction in cardiac output, central blood volume, and stroke volume with thermal stress in normal men during exercise. *J Clin Invest* 1966; 45:1801–1816.
5. Raven PB: Heat and air pollution: The cardiac patient. In Pollock MC, Schmidt DH (eds). *Heart Disease and Rehabilitation*. Boston, Houghton Mifflin Professional Publishers, Medical Division, 1979; 563–586.
6. Gisolfi C: Thermal effects of prolonged treadmill exercise in the heart. *Med Sci Sports* 1974; 6:108–113.
7. Blyth CS, Burt JJ: Effect of water balance on ability to perform at high ambient temperatures. *Res Quart* 1961; 32:301–307.
8. American College of Sports Medicine. Position statement on prevention of heat injuries during distance running. *Med Sci Sports* 1975; 7(1):vii–ix.
9. Fortney SM, Nadel ER, Wenger CB, Bove JR: Effect of blood volume on sweating rate and body fluids in exercising humans. *J Appl Physiol* 1981; 51(6):1594–1600.
10. Knochel JP, Dotin LN, Hamburger RJ: Pathophysiology of intense physical conditioning in a hot climate. *J Clin Invest* 1972; 51:242–255.
11. Mathews DK, Fox EL: *The Physiological Basis of Physical Education and Athletics* (2nd ed). Philadelphia, WB Sanders Company, 1976; 379–380.
12. Fletcher BJ, Cantwell JD, Fletcher GF: *Exercise For Heart and Health*. Atlanta, Georgia, Pritchett and Hull Associates, Inc., 1985; pp 36–38.
13. Rowell LB: Human cardiovascular adjustments to exercise and thermal stress. *Physiol Rev* 1974; 54:75–159.
14. Blake B: Altitude and cold. In Pollock MC, Schmidt DH, (eds). *The Cardiac Patient: Heart Disease and Rehabilitation*. Boston, Houghton Mifflin, Professional Publishers, Medical Division, 1979; 551–562.
15. Pugh LGC: Accidental hypothermia in walkers, climbers and campers. *Br Med J* 1966; 1:123.
16. Franklin BA, Hellerstein HK, Gordon S, Timmis GC: Exercise pre-

scription for the myocardial infarction patient. *J Cardiopulmonary Rehabil* 1986; 6:62–79.

17. Hattenhauer M, Neill WA: The effect of cold air inhalation on angina pectoris and myocardial oxygen supply. *Circulation* 1975; 51:1053–1058.

18. Leon DF, Amidi M, Leonard JJ: Left heart work and temperature responses to cold exposure in man. *Am J Cardiol* 1970; 26:38–45.

19. Kavanagh T: A cold weather "jogging mask" for angina patients. *Can Med Assoc J* 1970; 103:1290–1291.

20. Franklin BA, Parker S, Mitchell M, Rubenfire M: Hazards of shoveling snow. *Physician Sports Med* 1980; 8:40–48.

21. Adams CE, Leverland MB: Environmental and behavioral factors that can affect blood pressure. *Nurse Practitioner* 1985; 10:39–50.

22. Thauer R: Circulatory adjustments to climatic requirements. In *Handbook of Physiology III*. Washington, DC, American Physiological Society, 1979.

23. DeServi S, Mussini A, Angoli L, Ferrario M, Bramucci E, Gavazzi A, Ghio S, Ardissino D, Specchia G: Effects of cold stimulation on coronary haemodynamics during exercise in patients with coronary artery disease. *Eur Heart J* 1986; 6:239–246.

24. Epstein S, Stampfer M, Beiser GD, Goldstein RE, Braunwald E: Effects of a reduction in environmental temperature on the circulatory response to exercise in man: Implications concerning angina pectoris. *N Engl J Med* 1969; 280:7–11.

25. Lassik CT, Areskog NH: Angina in cold environment: Reactions to exercise. *Br Heart J* 1979; 42:396–401.

26. Buonanno C, Vassanelli C, Arbustini E, Dander B, Paris B: Effects of the cold pressor test on the left ventricular function of patients with coronary artery disease. *Int J Cardiol* 1983; 3:295–306.

27. Menier DR, Pugh LGCE: The relation of oxygen intake and velocity of walking and running, in: competition walkers. *J Physiol* (London) 1968; 197:717–721.

28. Riggs CE Jr., Johnson DJ, Konopka BJ, Kilgour RD: Exercise heart rate response to facial cooling. *Eur J Appl Physiol* 1981; 47:323–330.

29. Riley RL, Otis AB, Houston CS: Respiratory features of acclimatization to altitude. In Boothby W (ed). *Respiratory Physiology in Aviation*. USAF School of Aviation Medicine, Report No. 21 2301–0003, 1954:153.

30. Sutton JR, Jones NL, Pugh LGCE: Exercise at altitude. *Ann Rev Physiol* 1983; 45:427–437.

31. Karliner JS, Sarnquist FF, Graber DJ, Peters RM, West JB: The electrocardiogram at extreme altitude: Experience on Mt. Everest. *Am Heart J* 1985; 109:505–513.

32. Inama K, Halhuber MJ: Der Herz-Kreislaufkranke in Hochgebirgs klima. Deutsche Zentrale fur Volksgesundheitspflege, Frankfurt, 1975.

33. Miles DS, Wagner JA, Horvath SM, Reyburn JA: Absolute and relative work capacity in women at 758, 586 and 523 torr barometric pressure. *Aviat Space Environ Med* 1980; 51 (5):439–444.

34. Drinkwater BL, Kramar PO, Bedi JF, Folinsbee LF: Women at

altitude: cardiovascular responses to hypoxia. *Aviat Space Environ Med* 1982; 53(5):472−477.

35. Aigner A, Berghold F, et al: Investigations on the cardiovascular system at altitudes up to a height of 7,800 meters. *Z Kardiol* 1980; 69(9):310−316.

36. Eckenhoff RG, Knight DR: Cardiac arrhythmias and heart rate changes in prolonged hyperbaric air exposures. *Undersea Biomed Res* 1984; 11:355−367.

37. Humpler E, Inama K, Deetjen P: Improvement of tissue oxygenation during a 20-day stay at moderate altitudes in connection with mild exercise. *Klin Wochenschr* 1979; 57:267−272.

38. Guyton AC: Aviation, high altitude and space physiology. In *Textbook of Medical Physiology*. Philadelphia, WB Sanders Company, 1981; 542−551.

39. Stokinger HE: Evaluation of the hazards of ozone and oxides of nitrogen. *AMA Arch Industrial Health* 1957; 15:181−190.

40. Scheel LD, Dobrogorski OJ, Mountain JT, et al: Physiologic, biochemical, immunologic and pathologic changes following ozone exposure. *J Appl Physiol* 1959; 14:67−80.

41. Folinsbee LJ, Silverman F, Shephard RJ: Exercise responses following ozone exposure. *J Appl Physiol* 1975; 38:996−1001.

42. Aronow WS, Harris CN, Isabell MW, et al: Effect of freeway travel on angina pectoris. *Ann Intern Med* 1972; 77:669−676.

43. Savin WM, Adams WC: Effect of ozone inhalation on work performance and Vo_2 max. *J Appl Physiol* 1979; 46:309−314.

44. Folinsbee LJ, Horvath SM, Raven PB, et al: Influence of exercise and heat stress on pulmonary function during ozone exposure. *J Appl Physiol* 1977; 43:409−413.

45. Illing JW, Miller FJ, Gardner DE: Decreased resistance to infection in exercised mice exposed to NO_2 and O_3. *J Toxicol Environ Health* 1980; 6:843−851.

46. Hazucha M, Bates DV: Combined effect of ozone and sulfur dioxide on human pulmonary function. *Nature* 1974; 257:50−51.

47. Stewart RD, Petersen JE, Baretta ED, et al: Experimental human exposure to carbon monoxide. *Arch Environ Health* 1970; 21(2):154−164.

48. Astrup P, Kjelsden K, Wanstrup J: Effect of carbon monoxide exposure on the arterial walls. *Ann NY Acad Sci* 1970; 174:294−300.

49. Debias DA, Banerjee CM, Burkhead NC, et al: Carbon monoxide inhalation effects following myocardial infarction in monkeys. *Arch Environ Health* 1973; 27(2):161−167.

50. Raven PB, Drinkwater BL, Horvath SM, et al: Age, smoking habits, heat stress and their interactive effects with carbon monoxide and peroxyacetylnitrate on man's aerobic power. *Int J Biometeorol* 1974; 18:222−232.

51. Lindquist VAY: Carbon monoxide: Its relationship to air pollution and cigarette smoking. *Public Health* (London) 1971; 86:20−26.

52. Vogel JA, Gleser MA, Wheeler RC, et al: Carbon monoxide and physical work capacity. *Arch Environ Health* 1972; 24:198−203.

53. Oertel MJ: *Therapie der Kreislaufstorungen*. Handbuch des allg.

Therapie Siemmsen Bd IV. Leipzig, Germany, Verlag FCW Vog. 1884.

54. Fox SM, Haughton JP, Gorman PA: Physical activity and cardiovascular health. III. The exercise prescription: Frequency and type of activity. *Mod Concepts Cardiovasc Dis* June 1972; 41:25−30.

55. Nielsen B, Rowell LB, Petersen FB: Cardiovascular responses to heat stress and blood volume displacements during exercise in man. *Eur J Appl Physiol* 1984; 52:370−374.

56. Fletcher GF, Cantwell JD, Watt EW: Oxygen consumption and hemodynamic response of exercise used in training of patients with recent myocardial infarction. *Circulation* 1979; 60(1):140−144.

57. Magder S, Linnarsson D, Gullstrand L: The effect of swimming on patients with ischemic heart disease. *Circulation* 1981; 63(5):979−986.

58. Lloyd A, Theil J, Holloman P, Fletcher BJ, Fletcher GF: Water exercise versus land exercise in cardiac patients. *J Cardiopulmonary Rehab* 1986; 6:434 (Abstract).

59. Fletcher GF, LeMay MR, Thiel JE: Telephonically monitored home exercise early after coronary artery bypass surgery. *Chest* 1984; 86:198−202.

60. Johnston BL: Infuence of environmental factors on exercise activities of cardiac patients. *Cardiovascular Nursing* 1982; 18:7−12.

15

The Dangers of Unwise Exercise

Gerald F. Fletcher, M.D.

INTRODUCTION

The popularity of exercise continues to increase in the United States both in the allegedly healthy individual as well as in those with known cardiovascular disease. The popularity of exercise is evident by the prevalence of runners, joggers, walkers, bicyclers, racquet ball players, tennis players, and swimmers seen in parks, gymnasiums, recreation areas, school facilities, and neighborhoods. In the past several years there have been efforts to acquire significant data with reference to this popularity. This has been done largely by means of surveys and polls.

Available data[1-3] reveal that adult runners grew in number from a handful in 1960 to approximately 6 million in 1972. In 1975 there were approximately 11 million and in 1978 there were 17 million runners. Tennis enthusiasm has increased to involve more than 10 million players and racquet ball has grown from a relatively unknown sport with only 50,000 participants in 1972 to a popular activity in 1978 with about 3.1 million participants. This trend continues in the 1980's.

Over and above this, the intensity of exercise has increased

From: Fletcher GF: *Exercise in the Practice of Medicine,* 2nd Revised Edition. Mount Kisco, NY, Futura Publishing Co., Inc., © 1988.

along with the greater number of individuals involved in exercise. It has been estimated that about one of every six adult Americans invest an average of 300 minutes a week in vigorous activity and an equal number spend about 200 minutes a week in the same way. There are now about 200 or more marathon races (26-plus miles) in the United States every year and more than 50,000 Americans have successfully completed at least one marathon. Probably more than 4,000 have run the marathon distance in less than 3 hours.

Exercise participation is higher in younger age groups; however, nearly 38 percent of all Americans (age 50 years or older) say they exercise regularly. In several activities, namely bicycling, tennis, and swimming, the number of female participants actually exceeds the number of males. There appear to be several reasons for this increase in participation in recent years. The reasons most frequently cited are increases in leisure time, increased affluence, growing concern about health and health care costs, and intensive efforts by both public and private agencies to promote exercise and sports.

In accord with the aforementioned data, physicians and others in the health field are becoming more involved with patients who have questions about exercise—its *benefits, consequences,* and potential *dangers.* Many studies are available on the probable benefits of exercise from the standpoint of the effect on the hemodynamics of the cardiovascular system (improved oxygen consumption and decrease in resting and exercise heart rate).[4] There are also other reported effects on various aspects of health maintenance, i.e., prevention of coronary artery disease, control of high blood pressure, body weight, certain blood lipid abnormalities, and psychiatric implications.[5] An "infrequently mentioned" aspect of exercise, however, is the potential danger that one may incur with moderate and reasonable exercise levels but even more with extremely high levels. For any clinical intervention into medical practice, it is important for physicians and other health personnel to be aware of the possibility of side effects, dangers, misuses, and abuses of the intervention. This is certainly true with regard to exercise.

It is not the purpose of this chapter to minimize the usefulness of exercise when properly prescribed and utilized in the practice of medicine. The purpose is to emphasize, from the "preventive" standpoint, the possible dangers that may be encountered when exercise is used improperly.

BACKGROUND AND EXPERIMENTAL DATA

In discussing dangers of exercise, it is important to include certain experimental data supporting the possibility of myocardial damage from exercise. One of the most remarkable studies reflecting the dangers of exercise is that of Arcos et al.[6] who analyzed mitochondrial changes in young female rats by electron microscopy after repeated exercise by swimming. With moderate exercise, there was an increase in the size and number of mitochondria and a few scattered foci of degenerative changes. With advanced stages of exercise (361 to 490 hours of swimming), the animals showed evidence of physical exhaustion and were unable to maintain the same rate of exercise. The distribution and extent of focal degenerative myocardial changes were much more pronounced. These findings suggest that increase in myocardial mass is a compensatory response to exercise and this increase brings about focal regions of hypoxia during overexercise which are responsible for the degenerative changes (Fig. 1 A,B,C).

Vatner[7] has studied the effects of exercise in experimentally induced heart failure in dogs and found that the failing heart responded differently to the stress of exercise in that inotropic responses were markedly attenuated. Dowell et al.[8] studied rats and noted that in response to sustained pressure overload, stress-trained rats maintained pre-stress levels of contractility, whereas contractility was depressed in the control rats. In addition, studies by Grimm et al.[9] and Williams et al.[10] have shown that rats and cats trained by running demonstrate an unchanged or slightly depressed state of contractility of the myocardium, whereas rats trained by swimming manifest enhanced contractility.[11]

In addition to such animal studies, there have been studies in humans to support some of the aforementioned findings. One study by Holmgren et al.[12] showed that exercise training of at least moderate intensity and duration produced cardiac enlargement involving both hypertrophy and dilatation. This training effect seemed to persist after detraining regression occurred in other variables, i.e., bradycardia.

In addition, other studies[13-16] of cardiac chamber size and mass in highly trained individuals measured by echocardiography compared with measurements in sedentary control subjects have shown mild to moderate degrees of right and left ventricular dila-

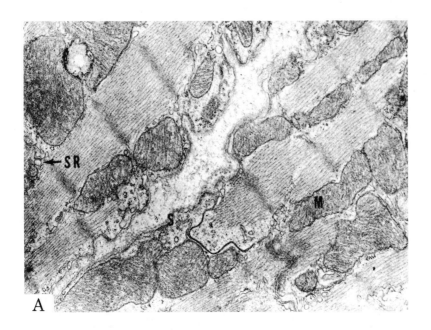

Figure 1: A. Longitudinal section of normal rat ventricular myocardium. The myofibers are bounded by a sarcolemma (S). The myofibrils present the usual bands. Mitochondria (M) and sarcoplasmic reticulum (SR) lie between the myofibrils; × 24,000. (From Aros JC, et al: Changes in ultrastructure and respiratory control in mitochondria of rat heart hypertrophied by exercise. *Exp Mol Pathol* 1968; 8:49. Used with permission.)

tation with hypertrophy. In addition, the study by Morganroth et al.[13] compared endurance training with strength or isometric training. These authors found that athletes trained with isometrics had normal ventricular volumes but increased ventricular wall thickness and significant degree of concentric hypertrophy.

Other indices of cardiac dynamics have been studied, specifically with reference to "cardiac fatigue." This has been addressed in the studies of Saltin et al.[17] and Ekelund et al.[18] These discussions reflect that, since the heart is a muscle that performs heavy levels of work for long periods of time during exercise, it is attractive to hypothesize that a gradual decrease in cardiac pumping ability occurs during prolonged exercise. As exercise continues, the heart becomes increasingly unable to respond to the demands placed upon it by exercise. However, available data do not substantiate a decrease in cardiac function in such states in normal people.

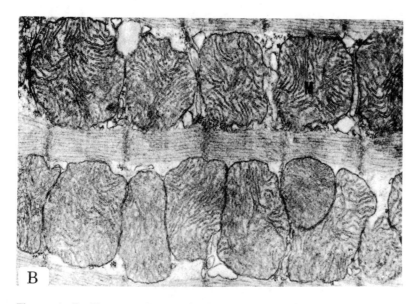

Figure 1: B. Electron micrograph of left ventricular myocardium from an exercised rat of group C (140–180 hours of swimming) indicating an increase in mitochondrial (M) size as compared to control rats; × 24,000. (From Aros JC, et al: Changes in ultrastructure and respiratory control in mitochondria of rat heart hypertrophied by exercise. *Exp Mol Pathol* 1968; 8:49. Used with permission.)

Therefore, the aforementioned work (both in animals and in humans) indicates the presence of residual cardiac chamber dilatation or hypertrophy after exercise at extreme levels. One might further hypothesize the development of potential secondary problems with this state of dilatation or enlargement. As heart disease (such as coronary artery disease) develops in our population, the effect of a previously hypertrophied ventricle may evoke more rapid deterioration in certain subsets of these disease states. For example, the availability of myocardial oxygen supply in the state of hypertrophy may be compromised with the development of occlusive coronary artery disease. In addition, dilatation of cardiac chambers might enhance the development of certain conduction disturbances or arrhythmias related to alterations of cardiac structure. Such implications are speculative, although experimental data are certainly suggestive.

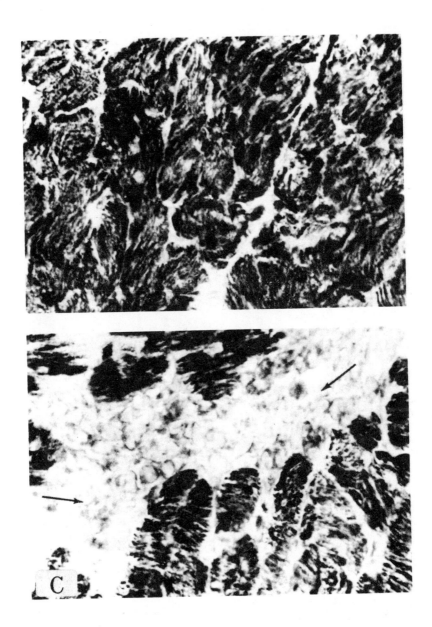

Figure 1: C. Normal rat myocardium (top). Myocardium of a rat that swam for 361−490 hours (bottom). Arrows indicate an area of extensive myocytolysis and the complete loss of mitochondrial enzyme activity in the degenerating muscle fibers. Original magnification × 480. (From Aros JC, et al: Changes in ultrastructure and respiratory control in mitochondria of rat heart hypertrophied by exercise. *Exp Mol Pathol* 1968; 8:49. Used with permission.)

POPULATIONS INVOLVED

There are several categories of subjects or patients involved in exercise today who are often subject to its dangers. These are specifically the *allegedly healthy group* who are involved in races, marathons, etc., the *post-myocardial-infarction group* who are frequently in supervised exercise programs (but often in their own individual program), *post-myocardial-revascularization patients, post-angioplasty patients,* and *subjects with documented coronary artery disease with stable angina pectoris.*

Another group of great importance and magnitude are the *coronary-prone* subjects. These are subjects with risk factors such as the cigarette smoking habit, high blood pressure, and abnormal blood lipids, who have undertaken health programs for the purpose of primary prevention. This particular group frequently has underlying coronary artery disease.

Allegedly Healthy Group

Early in our experience, we reported two cardiac complications that occurred in allegedly healthy people while jogging.[19] One of these subjects experienced an acute myocardial infarction and the other a cardiac arrest. Both were resuscitated effectively. These complications occurred while jogging the subjects were in an organized exercise program and alerted us at that time to these potential complications in allegedly healthy people.

Other data are available in a report in 1978[20] of two physicians who died suddenly while jogging. Autopsy studies were performed on both. One, a 52-year-old champion tennis player (anethesiologist) had severe atherosclerotic disease of all coronary arteries and evidence of multiple old myocardial scars. The other, a 28-year-old veteran jogger (orthopedic resident physician in training), had normal coronary arteries. Retrospective screening for coronary risk factors revealed multiple factors in the first and few in the second. It was felt that exercise testing may be useful in screening such individuals for effort-related myocardial ischemia and ventricular rhythm disturbances.

More recent studies of normal people have cited radionuclide angiographic evaluations of left ventricular function during strenuous exercise. One study reported by Foster et al.[21] revealed that during strenuous exercise, the left ventricular ejection fraction decreased in six of nine patients. Other signs of left ventricular dysfunction, such as exercise-induced regional wall motion abnormalities or dilatation, were not evident. The results of this study of maximal upright and graded bicycle exercise without warm-up support the concept of relative global subendocardial ischemia during sudden strenuous exercise in normal people.

Other studies of arterial hypoxemia during maximal exercise testing at high altitudes have been reported by Sutton et al.[22] In this study, progressive exercise tests by cycle ergometry were performed on 30 healthy subjects at sea level and after exposure to 5,300 meters. The study demonstrated profound arterial desaturation during exercise at high altitude. Desaturation persisted even with climatization. This implies that perhaps athletes as well as cardiac patients who are trained and climatized at high altitudes may suffer problems with hypoxemia when they exercise to extremes. This, of course, may impose deterimental effects on the cardiovascular system.

More interesting of late have been reports by Welton et al.[23] regarding the relationship of "vagal-related" arrhythmias to aerobic capacity in middle-aged joggers and marathoners. In this study the authors evaluated 10 marathoners, eight joggers, and eight control patients. They found a maximal oxygen consumption (VO_2max) of 60.8 ml/kg/minute for the marathoners, 53.3 for the joggers, and 36.4 for the control patients. Holter monitor evaluation during usual activities for the subsequent 24 hours (nonexercise) revealed that in the marathoners, eight of 10 had ventricular premature beats, and two of 10 had sinus exit block (2 to 1) with associated Mobitz I and first-degree atrioventricular block. Of the joggers, six of eight had ventricular premature beats and two had sinus exit block. Of the control patients, only two of eight had ventricular premature beats, none had sinus exit block, and only one had Mobitz I phenomenon. All subjects had similar double products with exercise testing and all exercise tests were negative for ischemia. Sinus exit block was seen in four of 13 or 31 percent of those with VO_2's greater than 55 ml/kg/minute. The significance of these types of arrhythmias remains to be seen; however, one might infer that the bradycardia of the training effect, perhaps with associated arrhythmias and conduction problems, might be instrumental in syncope or sudden death episodes in this population. This may be in the presence of perfectly normal coronary arteries.

To determine the incidence of arrhythmias and conduction

disturbances in trained athletes and the level of physical training at which they occur, 24-hour ambulatory electrocardiographic recordings were obtained in 80 healthy runners during both exercise and free activity. Subjects were grouped according to the number of miles per week (mpw) they had regularly run during the previous 3 months: Group I—0 to ≤5 mpw (≤8 km); Group II—>5 to ≤15 mpw (>8 to ≤24 km); Group III—>15 to ≤30 mpw (>24 to ≤48 km); and Group IV—>30 mpw (>48 km). Ectopic ventricular complexes occurred in 41 of 80 subjects (50 percent) and ectopic supraventricular complexes occurred in 33 (41 percent). There were two episodes of paired ventricular ectopic activity and a five-beat run of ventricular tachycardia with exercise. The study revealed no significant differences in the occurrence of arrhythmias or conduction disturbances in the different groups, although the two episodes of paired ventricular ectopic activity and five-beat run of ventricular tachycardia are of concern.[24]

Other data in marathon runners by Paulsen et al.[25] have been reported. In order to determine cardiac adaptations to prolonged endurance training, these authors performed left ventricular echocardiograms in eight active marathoners (mean age 27 years) and compared the results to 10 sedentary controls. When peak velocity of circumferential fiber shortening was corrected for changes in rate-pressure product, there was no significant difference between the runners and controls either at rest or during exercise. There was, however, an increased left ventricular chamber size and wall thickness in the runners. The implications of these latter changes are unknown. However, as mentioned previously, hypertrophy and dilatation of myocardial structure may be factors in future development of myocardial ischemia, arrhythmias, and conduction disturbances in certain individuals.

Nishimura et al.[26] reported an echocardiographic evaluation of 60 professional bicyclists and control subjects. They found evidence of enlargement of left ventricular end-diastolic dimensions in all of the bicyclists compared to controls. In the older subgroup, there was also significant depression of left ventricular function. In 14 percent of this subgroup, there was also enlargement of left atrial dimension and T-wave inversion in the left precordial leads of the electrocardiogram. Therefore, echocardiographic and electrocardiographic studies in middle-aged athletes suggest more susceptibility to electrocardiographic abnormalities and slight depression of left ventricular function which renders concern for this level of physical activity in this group of subjects.

In healthy females, Schoene et al.[27] have described menstrual fluctuation of respiratory drives in exercising women athletes. They found that menstruating females have augmentation of resting ventilatory drives and exercise ventilation and demonstrated decrease of VO_2max and exercise duration during mid-luteal phase. Although maximal exercise time is not decreased significantly, the combined decrease of VO_2 max and exercise time may affect women in highly competitive athletic situations.

A most interesting single case[28] we have seen is that of a 37-year-old orthopedic surgeon who ran 50 miles per week for many years. He began to have symptoms of fatigue and requested an exercise test (no previous test). The test revealed ischemic electrocardiographic ST segment displacement at a heart rate of 160 beats per minute. One ectopic ventricular beat was recorded after exercise. Further investigation revealed that for several months the subject had been on a vegetarian diet (no meat) and that he was anemic with a hematocrit of 27 percent. Further tests for evaluation of the anemia were normal. Resumption of a more normal diet including some meat and decrease in exercise resulted in resolution of the anemia. This case is an example of the use of high-level exercise with extreme dietary modification which may be related to and causative of the abnormal clinical state.

More recent data with regard to risks of exercise in healthy persons have evolved through community studies and case reports. Siscovick et al.[29] reported on vigorous exercise and primary cardiac arrest as affected by other factors. They investigated 133 males without prior heart disease and 133 controls. Spouses were interviewed to quantify leisure time activity and persons who did not engage in high intensity activity($\geqslant$6 kcal per minute) for more than 20 minutes per week were grouped as nonvigorous. The risk of primary cardiac arrest was found to be more than doubled for nonvigorous males, both in the presence and absence of other coronary risk factors taken indvidually, i.e. age >60, hypertension, cigarette smoking, obesity, and family history. The authors therefore conclude that (in spite of anecdotal data to suggest that extremely vigorous exercise may be dangerous) males at increased coronary risk may benefit the most from vigorous exercise. To the contrary, however, case reports continue to appear, such as that by Chan et al.,[30] who reported a case of coronary thrombosis and acute anterior myocardial infarction after a marathon. The case was of particular interest in that the thrombosis (seen on initial angiography) had completely resolved 10 days later on repeat angiography. The authors mention possible increases in both coagulability and fibrinolysis with marathon running and emphasize that marathoning certainly does not confer immunity against coronary disease.

Niemela et al.[31] reported a provocative study of 13 experienced male ultramarathon runners who took part in a 24-hour competitive run completing distances of 114 to 227 km. Echocardiograms were done at various times—near the end of the race and as long as 25 minutes after the race. Stroke volume and fractional shortening declined by 24 percent and 16 percent, respectively, and the mean velocity of circumferential fiber shortening also decreased by an average of 9 percent (all changes were statistically significant but returned to normal within 2–3 days after the race). Therefore, it seems that prolonged strenuous exercise results in notable left ventricular dysfunction in part because of a reversible depression in contractile state of the myocardium. The implications of these changes may be quite significant if, for instance, a subject had a compromised coronary circulation. Of particular interest of late is a report by Northcote et al.[32] on deaths associated with playing squash. There were 60 sudden deaths (59 male, 1 female) with mean age of the subjects being 46 years. The deaths were associated with documented coronary disease in 51 cases. Forty-five of those dying had reported prodromal symptoms, most commonly chest pain, and 14 had a history of high blood pressure.

Therefore, increasing evidence is available in the "allegedly" healthy population supporting the potential dangers of exercise in this group. Certainly if this group has clinically inapparent coronary artery disease, the implications are obvious. However, even in the group that is completely healthy, studies and reports support a concern for the dangers and potential hazards of exercise because of the frequent presence of subclinical coronary disease.

Subjects With Known Cardiac Disease

Exercise has been incorporated for many years in rehabilitation programs for post-infarction patients as well as other subsets of patients with coronary disease.[33] Haskell[34] reported on the associated mobidity and mortality in post-infarction exercise programs and found that morbidity and mortality were no greater, and probably less than usually expected with such patients not involved in such programs. Mead et al.,[35] however, reported 15 cases of exercise-associated ventricular fibrillation occurring in the Seattle program since 1968. All were successfully resuscitated. They felt that, relative to this, treating patients exhibiting exercise-induced premature ventricular contractions with antiarrhythmic drugs, prompt attention to serum potassium levels, and strict adherence to training heart rates and warm-up will likely prevent similar events.

We have reported ventricular fibrillation in a medically supervised program in Atlanta.[36] In a group of five patients with ischemic heart disese, all were resuscitated after experiencing ventricular fibrillation under medical supervision. Four subsequently had successful myocardial revascularization (three prior to hospital discharge) and three returned to an exercise prescription of reduced intensity. Catheterization revealed that multivessel operative coronary disease is common in patients experiencing ventricular fibrillation and that ventricular fibrillation may occur unpredictably from 2 to 48 months in the duration of the exercise. It is emphasized that exercise programs for such patients should be medically supervised and equipped with a defibrillator and appropriate drugs.

Other studies[37] have measured oxygen consumption and hemodynamic responses to individualized exercise activities before and after exercise training in 22 male post-infarction patients. It was found that oxygen consumption obtained for post-infarction patients, when compared to available data on normal subjects, is significantly variable, suggesting the need for caution when prescribing exercises in this group of subjects. This was particularly relevant because of the significantly high oxygen consumption that occurred during swimming activities compared to calisthenic and walk/jog activities. The reason for the increased oxygen consumption with swimming activities is unclear. However, there may be effects of immersion, alterations in peripheral vascular resistance, or other unknown factors with patients in the "water environment."

Thompson et al.[38] have evaluated 18 cases of patients in the California area who died during or immediately after jogging. The group included 13 men who died of coronary artery disease and four men and one woman who died of other causes. Six of the coronary heart disease patients had medical histories relevant to the cardiovascular system but only one had diagnosed coronary disease. Six coronary subjects experienced prodromal symptoms but continued the vigorous exercise program. Two subjects had exercised less than 1 month but most had trained regularly for 2 years. The coronary risk factors did not differ from those for other age-matched physically active men. It was felt that superior physical fitness does not guarantee protection against exercise deaths. These data from Thompson et al.[38] emphasize the presence of extensive coronary disease in people who are in exercise programs and otherwise seem healthy. It also demonstrates that often the presence of disease is known both by physician and subject and the subject has been warned against exercise. However, because of intense interest in exercise, the subjects do not adhere to proper advice and continue to exercise. This provokes the question of a behavioral modification problem.

Viitasalo et al.[39] have described ventricular arrhythmias during exercise testing, jogging, and sedentary life summarized from the most current data available in a series of studies. These authors found that healthy, physically active men had fewer ventricular arrhythmias in all of the tested situations. They found that the greatest number and highest grades of ventricular arrhythmias during exercise were found in healthy sedentary men, whereas men with previous myocardial infarction had ventricular arrhythmias more during sedentary activity.

Probably one of the most publicized examples of the danger of exercise was the death of Representative Goodloe E. Byron. Byron died while jogging on the C & O canal towpath along the Potomac River. An aide running with Byron stated he had run 12½ miles before collapsing. Interesting data[40] revealed that Byron's younger brother had died of a heart attack at age 32 and an uncle died of the same at age 42. His older brother had one heart attack and two coronary bypass operations. Byron had been advised of "severe irregularities of his heart beat" and a cardiologist described his exercise test as abnormal. Byron had been advised to have an exercise thallium radionuclide test for further evaluation but this had been delayed on the part of the patient and was not done before his death. This example of exercise-induced death in a patient with known myocardial ischemia is likely not an uncommon occurrence for others in our society.

Swimming studies in patients with ischemic heart disease have been reported by Magder et al.[41] In this study, eight males (8 to 14 months post infarction) exercised to exhaustion or angina on a cycle ergometer as well as in a swimming flume. The authors summarized that the subjective comfort and the enlarged muscle groups involved make swimming a good exercise, but the high relative energy costs and failure to identify ischemic symptoms indicate caution in cardiac patients especially if swimming skills are poor. This supports previous data[37] acquired in other studies.

In addition to myocardial ischemia with known coronary artery disease, other cardiac conditions are thought to precipitate catastrophic events in patients. One example is that of a 20-year-old female college student who collapsed while jogging near the Medical University of South Carolina.[42] Luckily, paramedics were in the area and were summoned rapidly. Electrocardiographic rhythm strips revealed ventricular fibrillation prior to electrical shock, which resulted in normal sinus rhythm and successful resuscitation. This patient had cardiac catheterization which revealed normal coronary arteries and a normal functioning left ventricular cavity. One abnormality, however, found on catheterization was a very high left ventricular end-diastolic pressure (55 mmHg) after exercise. Interpretation was that the patient likely had severe left ventricular dysfunction with exercise compatible with a cardiomyopathy of unknown etiology. She was placed on digoxin and urged to participate in only mild to moderate exercise.

Therefore, the presence of heart disease may be more common than expected in our exercising population. The incidence of coronary artery disease is most likely the prevalent problem; however, cardiomyopathy (including obstructive), residual changes from previous myocarditis, and occult valvular disease are all possible mechanisms and documentation of these is becoming more frequent.

CATEGORIES OF EXERCISE DANGERS

The dangers of exercise can be categorized into two specific subgroups: *cardiac* and *noncardiac*.

Cardiac dangers include myocardial infarction and other levels of myocardial oxygen deprivation, sudden death, and catastrophic ventricular arrhythmias. The latter two (sudden death and arrhythmias) are probably interrelated and one in the same in most instances.

A recent review, Goldschlager et al.[43] discussed exercise-related ventricular arrhythmias. Table 1, abstracted in part from this review, lists conditions associated with exercise-related arrhythmias. Of particular note in this group is the normal cardio-

Table 1
Clinical Settings That May Be Associated With
Exercise-Related Arrhythmias

Normal cardiopulmonary status at various levels of exercise
Coronary artery disease including post-infarction and post-bypass patients
Mitral valve prolapse and variants of click-murmur syndrome
Cardiomyopathy—obstructive, hypertrophic, congestive
Aortic valve stenosis
Long QT interval syndrome
Electrolyte abnormalities
Cardiac drugs such as digitalis and quinidine
"Psychotrophic" agents

pulmonary status which heads the list of conditions (especially in our experience). Most likely this group includes occult coronary artery disease, but in many instances it appears that obstructive cardiomyopathy is becoming more prevalent. Of particular note is the commentary on therapy in this review in that no antiarrhythmic medication was found uniformly effective in reducing or abolishing exercise-induced ventricular extrasystoles. Seemingly, the most benefit accrued from the use of quinidine sulfate or propranolol alone or in combination with procainamide and/or long-acting nitrate preparations. The latter medication group (that is, the nitrates) increase the threshold of ventricular fibrillation in patients with known coronary artery disease.

These authors[43] further relate that exercise-related ventricular ectopic activity is a very common occurrence in the asymptomatic population as well as in populations with known heart disease. The predicted likelihood for sudden death in asymptomatic individuals, however, is considered small. In subjects with coronary disease, with or without prior myocardial infarction, exercise-related ventricular ectopic activity is often complex (R-on-T, multiform, salvos, or sustained runs of ventricular tachycardia), tends to occur at lower heart rates, and may coexist with electrocardiographic abnormalities indicative of myocardial ischemia. The prognostic significance of exercise-related ventricular ectopic activity appears to lie not in its occurrence *per se* but in its coexistence with extensive coronary artery disease with ischemia or with left ventricular dysfunction.

A specific cardiac disease entity of particular danger in exercise is aortic stenosis. This problem has been addressed by Mark et al.[44] The authors found that forearm vasoconstrictor responses to leg exercise are inhibited or reversed in patients with aortic stenosis, possibly related to activation of left ventricular baroreceptors. Their observations suggest that reflex vasodilatation resulting from activation of left ventricular baroreceptors may contribute to exertional syncope in patients with aortic stenosis. Another example of "aortic valve sensitivity" to exercise is described by Sainani and Szatkowski,[45] who describe a patient with rupture of a normal aortic valve causing aortic regurgitation. The event was precipitated by shoveling snow.

Data by Joplin[46] relate cardiovascular deaths while running from the standpoint of the epidemiologist. The author summarized that when a person dies of cardiovascular causes during recreation or running, the public frequently assumes that exercise caused the death. For a statistical perspective, the number of cardiovascular deaths while running that occur by chance alone was estimated. If white male runners resemble marathoners, being nonsmokers and at lowest lean weight, four deaths from cardiovascular disease would occur per year while running 20 minutes three times per week and 30 deaths per year if the 2 hours after running are considered as running-associated. However, if runners resembled the white male population, then 15 deaths would occur from cardiovascular disease per year while running and 104 during the associated period. Thus four to 104 cardiovascular deaths per year are predicted on a purely temporal basis in white males while running. This latter information infers that cardiovascular deaths are common and occur whether or not people are exercising at high or low levels or exercising at all.

Noncardiac dangers of exercise tend to debilitate the exercise enthusiast and cause drop-outs from exercise programs or interrupt exercises in an individual program. (Table 2 itemizes specific complications.)

Exercise-induced asthma is a well-documented phenomenon[47] occurring only with exercise in subjects who are normal between episodes both by clinical and functional criteria. Other allergic-type reactions to exercise (at times exhibiting a pulmonary component) include post-exercise hyperhistaminemia, dermographia, and wheezing,[48] and exercise-induced anaphylaxis to shellfish[49] and other foods such as celery and peaches.[50]

More recent studies have addressed other types of exercise-induced "allergic type" syndromes. Lee et al.[51] described exercise-induced *late asthmatic reactions* with neutrophil chemotactic activity. Two adults and 13 children with exercise-induced asthma

Table 2
Noncardiac Dangers of Exercise

Heat-induced illness (stroke-exhaustion)
Sprains, fractures, and tendon rupture
March fractures (stress)
Soft tissue bleeding (often with anticoagulants)
Penile or nipple frostbite
Exacerbation of arthritis
Encounter with objects and animals
"Runner's trots" (diarrhea)
Exercise asthma
Elevated plasma MB creatine kinase
Hyperammonemia
Hemo- and myoglobinuria and proteinurea
Myopathy and palsy of local neuromuscular groups
Petechiae
Gout
Syncope (reported in weight-lifters)
Anaphylaxis
Alterations of serum sodium
Gastrointestinal blood loss

had both immediate and late (4–10 hours) reduction in forced expiratory volume in 1 second (FEV_1) after treadmill exercise. Late reaction was associated with wheezing or chest tightness or both. Increases in neutrophil chemotactic activity (expressed as the absolute number of neutrophils per 10 random high-power fields or as a percentage change from values before challenge) measured in 13 subjects accompanied the reduction in FEV_1. The agent responsible was identical for both the immediate and late neutrophil reaction. Their observations suggest that some subjects with exercise-induced asthma have late reactions that, as with antigen-induced bronchoconstriction, are associated with the release of neutrophil chemotactic activity. Casale et al.[52] have elucidated features of exercise-induced anaphylaxis and developed challenges to differentiate exercise-induced anaphylaxis from cholinergic urticaria/anaphylaxis. In a study of two patients after passive heat challenge, inducing increases in core body temperature more that 0.7°C, only the subject with cholinergic urticaria developed anaphylaxic symptoms and had a rise in plasma histamine. Thus these authors felt that passive heat challenges are valuable in differentiating these two syndromes and that thermoregulatory mechanisms seem to be an intricate part of the pathophysiology of cholinergic urticaria/anaphylaxis.

Heat-induced illness related to exercise is a well-known entity. In addition to the exercise-associated morbidity of this problem, it remains the second leading cause of death among athletes in this country.[53] To avoid the "heat-stroke" problem from running, education in heat acclimatization, prehydration, hydration during running, and proper treatment of heat injuries with rapid cooling onsite has been effective in many areas.[54] Knochel et al.[55] have studied the specific pathophysiology of intense conditioning in a hot climate. They found significant potassium depletion in their subjects—probably a renal loss from increased production of aldosterone during the intense physical work in the heat. This electrolyte abnormality may, of course, be associated with muscular weakness as well as possible cardiac electrical instability.

*Hyper*natremia[56] as well as *hypo*natremia[57] have been more recently reported with exercise. In a study of *short burst intensive* swimming, Felig et al.[56] found that 30−60 percent of 16 subjects involved in a 100 m swim lasting 1 minute had frank hypernatremia (>150mEq/L). This was in contrast to no change in serum sodium with less intensive swimming, i.e. 800 m lasting 10 minutes. They felt that the hypernatremia is likely due to a shift of hypotonic fluid from the extracellular to the intracellular compartment. To the contrary, Frizzell et al.[57] in *ultramarathoners* (after the run) reported *hyponatremic* (123 and 118 mEq/L) encephalopathy. They felt the hyponatremia was likely caused by increased consumption of dilute fluids and by excessive sweat sodium loss. Therefore, alteration of serum sodium should be considered as possible consequences of exercise, i.e. hypernatremia with acute exercise and hyponatremia after endurance exercise.

Gastrointestinal problems with exercise are infrequently noted. However, Fogoros[58] has reported "runner's trots." He relates that the diarrhea in the two cases reported was likely "gut" ischemia based on published data showing that during maximal exercise in both trained and untrained subjects, blood flow to the gastrointestinal tract is reduced by as much as 80 percent.[59] Two more recent reports.[60,61] have focused on the possible role of gastrointestinal blood loss in explaining the anemia in long distance runners.

Renal problems of both hemoglobinuria[62] and myoglobinuria[63] and proteinuria[64] have been reported as well as specific neuromuscular problems including exercise myopathy of the extensor carpi ulnaris muscle[65] and radial palsy after muscular effect.[66] Other problems, usually involving the musculoskeletal system, are frequently seen. Harris et al.[67] reported seven subjects who developed acute gout in a group of 265 subjects who were involved in an exercise program. Other reported complications include development of petechiae,[68] jogger's heel,[69] exacerbation of osteoarthritis,[70] and severe persistent muscular soreness which accounted for 34 of the 98 drop-outs reported by Harris et al.[67]

Of particular interest in our program has been the possible role of vigorous exercise in aggravating or provoking arthritis and/or other musculoskeletal problems, particularly in the more elderly patients. Lane et al.[71] addressed this issue in 41 long distance runners (50–72 years in age) compared with 41 controls to examine for osteoarthritis and osteoporosis. They found that male and female runners have about 40 percent more bone mineral than controls and that female runners (not male) appeared to have somewhat more sclerosis and spur formation in spine and weight-bearing knee x-ray films, but not in hand films. There were, however, no differences between groups in joint space narrowing, stability, or symptomatic osteoarthritis. The authors concluded that, although running is associated with increased bone mineral, there is no increase in clinical osteoarthritis. Panush et al.[72] further confirmed these findings in 17 male runners stating that long-duration, high-mileage running need not be associated with premature degenerative joint disease. Therefore, some evidence suggests little consequence to high-level exercise with regard to the musculoskeletal system; however, we continue to be concerned about such consequences and therefore favor more moderate intensity and frequency of exercise which seems to enhance long-term compliance in most subjects.

Of particular interest to weight-lifters should be the syndrome of "weight-lifter's blackout."[73] This type of syncope is likely attributed to reduced cardiac output and cerebral blood flow associated with the Valsalva maneuver. With vascular dilatation having already been produced by hyperventilation and squatting, the cardiac output falls acutely during refilling of central vessels when the very high thoracic pressures are released at the end of the weight-lifting maneuvers. It is felt that limiting the degree of hyperventilation and duration of squatting, and lifting the weight as rapidly as possible will avoid this problem and potential danger.

In our experience with post-infarction exercise, a number of minor but notable problems have occurred. These include ecchymoses, sprained fingers secondary to volleyball, muscular strains, aggravation of pseudo-gout, aggravation of previous knee injuries (cartilage or ligament), and an occasional minor laceration. The most debilitating noncardiac complication occurred in the early years of the program in a 61-year-old man who fell in a seated position while playing volleyball. He suffered a compression fracture of the lumbar spine. X-ray changes are seen in Figure 2. He was treated conservatively and subsequently returned to the program.

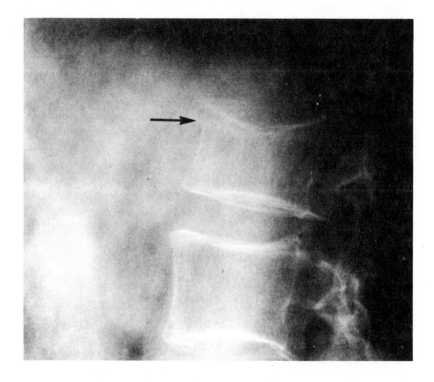

Figure 2: X-ray film of the lumbosacral spine showing compression fracture (arrow). (From Fletcher GF, Cantwell JD: *Exercise and Coronary Heart Disease.* 2nd ed. Springfield, Ill., Charles C. Thomas, 1979. Used with permission.)

It is therefore important that exercise programs be such that they are not interrupted by noncardiac complications which tend to impair compliance and enjoyability of such programs. These complications may delay the patient's progress in training but do not necessarily cause termination of participation.

The long-term effect of transient musculoskeletal injuries is not well known. It is felt that the musculoskeletal system can only tolerate a certain amount of "trauma" associated with exercise over a period of years. There are no data at this point to confirm the latter but as the high-level exerciser tends to progress with such activities, the effect on the musculoskeletal system will likely become apparent.

Another potential area of concern in exercise is that of the *psychological "addiction."* This seems to impose a very "beneficial effect" in most subjects. However, as we evaluate these people over the long term, it seems that their addiction to exercise causes them to increase their intensity and frequency of exercise to levels that are not practical and may be potentially harmful. Actually, some subjects seem to develop an "evangelical" approach to exercise. In many instances, this is associated with an obsession and often a compulsion to exercise over and above the level of benefit— probably to extremes that may be detrimental to both the musculo-skeletal and cardiopulmonary systems. As there are no data in this area of exercise, one can only "speculate"; however, it is an area of concern for medical and allied health professions.

POTENTIAL DANGERS OF THE EXERCISE TEST

In discussing the dangers of exercise, it is appropriate to consider exercising testing. The data available on the complications of exercise testing are somewhat limited and are not very impressive in "labeling" the test as a dangerous procedure. Rochmis and Blackman reported a survey in 1971[74] of exercise testing from 73 medical centers. They had results of 170,000 exercise tests and found a mortality rate of four per 10,000 tests. The combined mortality/morbidity rate was four per 10,000. In the experience of Detry et al.[75] in 10,000 exercise tests, there was only one episode of ventricular fibrillation. All subjects were successfully defibrillated. A more dramatic single occurrence has been reported of a 56-year-old man who died after a near-normal maximal treadmill test.[76] Autopsy showed hemorrhage in an intimal atherosclerotic plaque which produced total occlusion of the left anterior descending coronary artery.

A survey on exercise testing by Atterhog et al.[77] involved a prospective study of complication rates. This was done in Sweden through questionnaires sent to hospital departments of clinical physiology where the majority of exercise testing is done in that country. Twenty of 24 departments replied. These 20 departments then took part in an 18-month study of complications related to exercise testing. During the period of study, approximately 50,000 exercise tests were accomplished. Complications were defined as reactions occurring during or within 24 hours after the tests, constituting a risk or leading to mobidity or mortality. The study revealed a complication rate of 18.4, a morbidity rate of 5.2, and a mortality rate of 0.4 per 10,000 tests. The morbidity rate was higher but the mortality rate lower than that found retrospectively by Rochmis et al.[74] However, the difference may be due to the prospective technique in the study which probably resulted in higher reported rates of minor complications leading to morbidity. Another explanation for the higher incidence might be the nonrestrictive policy found in this study regarding criteria for exclusion from an interruption of tests in patients with severe heart disease. However, the reported rates of severe morbidity (that is infarction, cerebrovascular lesions, and persistent arrhythmias) were low.

The findings that 89 percent of the patients with complications suffered from suspected or proven heart disease and that 82 percent were at least 50 years old indicate that elderly patients with heart disease constitute a high-risk group for complications during testing. The Swedish data are in accord with results reported by McNiece.[78] The incidence of arrhythmias, supraventricular and ventricular, during exercise testing increased with age and for all age groups, it increased with the evidence of cardiovascular disease.

In the majority of cases reported in the Swedish group, complications occurred at a heart rate of 150 beats per minute or less, a systolic blood pressure of 200 mmHg or less, and at a respiratory frequency of 30 breaths per minute or less. In addition, it was felt that patients with aortic valve stenosis obviously perform exercise testing with a high risk of complications.

More recently, in an overall national survey of exercise testing facilities in the United States, Stuart and Ellestad[79] reported complications of 518,448 tests in 1,375 centers. Complications were 3.58 infarctions, 4.78 serious arrhythmias (those requiring cardioversion or intravenous medication), and 0.5 deaths per 10,000 tests. The total of all complications were 8.86 per 10,000 tests. Table 3 displays a conglomerate of exercise test complications from reported data.

With the constant increase in the use of exercise testing in both primary and secondary prevention, physicians interested in these areas often detect unexpected rhythm disturbances as endpoints in testing. Figure 3[28] is the exercise test result of a 28-year-old runner who had been resuscitated after experiencing ventricular fibrillation while running. He had been hospitalized for the latter and had a benign hospital course with normal coronary arteriography and ventriculography. Exercise testing on disopyramide revealed no arrhythmia. The exercise test was repeated later to assess the effect of discontinuing therapy and revealed paired ventricular ectopic beats and ventricular tachycardia with exercise. This was followed by atrial fibrillation after exercise with subsequent resumption of sinus rhythm with ventricular bigeminy. Therapy with disopyramide was reinstituted by the subject's private physician and he has done well with continued lower intensity exercise.

Standards for adult exercise testing laboratories have been published by the American Heart Association.[80] This report emphasizes the need for a proper physical environment, laboratory staffing, and laboratory equipment as well as emergency equipment and drugs. It further emphasizes that one physician should be in charge of the exercise testing laboratory. A physician must also be immediately available for exercise testing but may delegate the actual conduct of the test to personnel that are deemed

Table 3
Complications of Exercise Testing

Authors	Number of Tests	Morbidity	Mortality
Rochmis et al.[74]	170,000	4/10,000	4.0/10,000
Detry et al.[75]	10,000	10/10,000 (VF)	
Atterhog et al.[77]	50,000	5.2/10,000	0.4/10,000
Stuart and Ellestad[79]	518,448	3.58 MI and 4.78 serious arrhythmias per 10,000	0.5/10,000

Abbreviations: VF = ventricular fibrillation; MI = myocardial infarction.

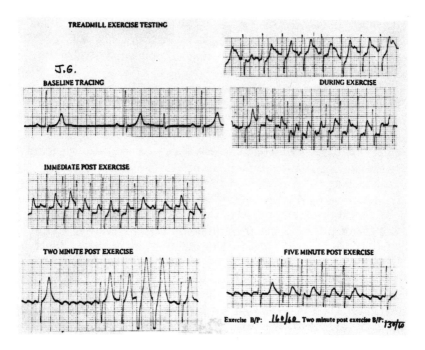

Figure 3: Exercise electrocardiogram of a 28-year-old runner (done after resuscitation for ventricular fibrillation while running) to assess need for antiarrhythmic treatment. The test reveals paired ectopic ventricular beats and ventricular tachycardia with exercise. After exercise, atrial fibrillation developed (immediate) with some sinus beats followed by sinus rhythm with ventricular bigeminy at 5 minutes after exercise. The test shown was done while on no treatment. Further testing on treatment revealed no arrhythmias. See text for more details.

capable. Each laboratory should have a written plan for handling cardiopulmonary complications that might occur during testing. The plan should provide for procedures to follow for myocardial infarction, ventricular dysrhythmias, and pulmonary edema. The laboratory itself should be designed to permit rapid evacuation of emergency cases and the plan should specify in detail the route for transfer to the hospital. The written plan should also contain specific provisions for care of the patient during transport to the hospital if the laboratory facility is not within the hospital setting.

In cardiac emergencies, the patient should be stabilized and then moved to a hospital as quickly as possible. In the instance of cardiac arrest, basic and advanced life support should be initiated immediately according to the standards of the American Heart Association.

The guidelines state specifically that the patient should be evaluated prior to exercise testing and outlines specific contraindications to testing:

> These contraindications are acute myocardial infarction, myocarditis or pericarditis, rapid atrial or ventricular dysrhythmias, second or third degree heart block, heart failure, known high grade left main coronary artery disease, aortic stenosis, uncontrolled hypertension and unstable progressive angina.

It is felt that if the aforementioned guidelines are followed, exercise testing is a safe mechanism as part of our armamentarium in the evaluation of patients. The section herein discussed is only to warn against the possible dangers of such testing and to emphasize the precautions that must be utilized to prevent such dangers.

RECAPITULATION

The data herein discussed with reference to the dangers of exercise are not intended to suppress interest or enthusiasm for exercise. The purpose is to emphasize some of the "cons" as well as the "pros" of exercise as we evolve this area of activity in our system of health and medical care. The popularity of exercise has been made clear in the data presented and the reasons are outlined as a basis for concern of the health profession in this area.

Prevention of exercise dangers is an important topic that physicians must address. This is often overlooked because in prescribing exercise we are not always aware of the intense enthusiasm with which a subject may accept and implement our advice. Cardiac complications are certainly clear. Over and above this, noncardiac complications that may detract from or alter compliance may be even more of a problem. Proper clothing and footwear are important and consideration must be addressed to proper running and exercising surfaces.

Exercise should be prescribed in moderate intensity with appropriate frequency. The type of exercise should be tailored for the individual subject. It seems that low- to moderate-intensity activities engender compliance and that persons who do not "overexercise" tend to be compliant for longer periods of time. The variety of exercise is also important in preventing specific dangers as well as avoiding the danger of noncompliance.

Finally, the definition of exercise is most important. Exercise does not necessarily imply only running or jogging. Effective dynamic exercise may be done with stationary bicycle, conventional bicycling, racquet ball, swimming, and in some instances with tennis, basketball, or other sports that are done by subjects in which the attained oxygen consumption is of the proper magnitude. It is suggested that oxygen consumption be measured in selected individuals when there is question of the effectiveness of a type of exercise. An example might be that of a regular tennis player who feels that he is exercising properly but, when actually tested by oxygen consumption studies, his level of exercise training or conditioning is found to be surprisingly low.

In summary, it is intended that this chapter will stimulate physicians and others in the health field to be aware of the growing arena of health care that we must address with regard to proper exercise. This is not just for patients with occult or manifest coronary or other cardiovascular disease. It applies to patients with pulmonary, gastrointestinal, psychiatric, and other disease problems as well as to the healthy population. Exercise must be precisely prescribed and its potential dangers clarified in all of these areas. If done more in a "preventive" manner, it is felt that the dangers of exercise will often be avoided or diminished as this area of interest evolves as a major factor in our health care system.

REFERENCES

1. The President's Council on Physical Fitness and Sports. *Adult Physical Fitness Survey.* Opinion Research Corporation, 1972, 1975.
2. The Gallup Poll. *American Exercise Survey, 1978.*
3. Louis Harris and Associate, Inc.: *Perrier Survey of Fitness in America.* August 1979.
4. Fletcher GF, Cantwell JD: *Exercise and Coronary Heart Disease.* (2nd ed.) Springfield, Ill, Charles C. Thomas Publisher. 1979; p. 11.
5. *Ibid:* 63.
6. Arcos JC, Sohal RS, Sun SC, et al: Changes in ultrastructure and

respiratory control in mitochondria of rat heart hypertrophied by exercise. *Exp Mol Pathol* 1968; 8:49−65.

7. Vatner SF: Response of the failing heart to severe exercise. *Clin Res* 1976; 24:422A (Abstract).

8. Dowell RT, Cutilletta AF, Ruduik MA, et al: Heart functional responses to pressure overload in exercised and sedentary rats. *Am J Physiol* 1976; 230:199−204.

9. Crimm AF, Kubota R, Whitehorn WV: Properties of myocardium in cardiomegaly. *Circ Res* 1963; 12:118.

10. Williams JF, Potter RD: Effect of exercise conditioning on the instrinsic contractile state of cat myocardium. *Circ Res* 1976; 39:425−428.

11. Mole PA: Increased contractile potential of papillary muscles from exercise-trained rat hearts. *Am J Physiol* 1978; 234:H421−H425.

12. Holmgren A, Strandell T: The relationship between heart volume, total hemoglobin and physical working capacity in former athletes. *Acta Med Scand* 1959; 163:149−160.

13. Morganroth J, Maron BJ, Henry WL, et al: Comparative left ventricular dimensions in trained athletes. *Ann Intern Med* 1975; 82:521−524.

14. Roeske WR, O'Rourke RA, Klein A, et al: Noninvasive evaluation of ventricular hypertrophy in professional athletes. *Circulation* 1976; 53:286−291.

15. Gilbert CA, Nutter DO, Felner JM, et al: Echocardiographic study of cardiac dimensions and function in the endurance-trained athlete. *Am J Cardiol* 1977; 40:528−533.

16. Underwood RH, Schwade JL: Noninvasive analysis of cardiac funtion of elite distance runners: Echocardiography, vectorcardiography and cardiac intervals. *Ann NY Acad Sci* 1977; 301:297−309.

17. Saltin B, Steinberg J: Circulatory response to prolonged severe exercise. *J Appl Physiol* 1964; 19:833−838.

18. Ekelund LG, Holmgren A, Ovenfors CO: Heart volume during prolonged exercise in the supine and sitting positions. *Acta Physiol Scand* 1967; 70:88−98.

19. Cantwell JD, Fletcher GF: Cardiac complications while jogging. *JAMA* 1969; 210:130−131.

20. Cantwell JD, Fletcher GF: Sudden death and jogging. *Physician and Sports Med* 1978; 6:94.

21. Foster C, Anholm J, Hellman C, et al: Left ventricular function during sudden strenuous exercise. *Circulation* 1979; 60II−21 (Abstract).

22. Sutton JR, Powles ACP, Gray GW, et al: Arterial hypoxemia during maximum exercise at altitude. *Clin Res* 1977; 25:673A (Abstract).

23. Welton DE, Mokotoff DM, Squires WG, et al: Relationship of vagal-related arrhythmias to aerobic capacity in middle aged joggers and marathoners. *Circulation* 1979; 60:II−15 (Abstract).

24. Pilcher GF, Cook AJ, Johnston BL, Fletcher GF: Twenty-four-hour continuous electrocardiography during exercise and free activity in 80 apparently healthy runners. *Am J Cardiol* 1983; 52:859−861.

25. Paulsen WJ, Boughner DR, Cunningham DA, et al: Left ventricular

function at rest and during exercise in marathon runners. *Am J Cardiol* 1980; 45:431.

26. Nishimura T, Yoshihisa Y, Chuichi K: Echocardiographic evaluation of long-term effects of exercise on left ventricular hypertrophy and function in professional bicyclists. *Circulation* 1980; 61:832–840.

27. Schoene RB, Pierson OJ, Robertson HT, et al: Menstrual fluctuation of respiratory drives and exercise in women athletes. *Clin Res* 1980; 28:60A (Abstract).

28. Unpublished data, courtesy JD Cantwell: Preventive Cardiology Clinic, 1980.

29. Siscovick DS, Weiss NS, Fletcher RH: Vigorous exercise and primary cardiac arrest: effect of other factors on the relationship. *Clin Res* 1983; 31:238A (Abstract).

30. Chan KL, Davies RA, Chambers RJ: Coronary thrombosis and subsequent lysis after a marathon. *JACC* 1984; 4:1322–1325.

31. Niemela KO, Palatsi IJ, Ikaheimo MJ, Taakkunen JT, Vuori JJ: Evidence of impaired left ventricular performance after an uninterrupted competitive 24-hour run. *Circulation* 1984; 70:350–356.

32. Northcote RJ, Flannigan C, Ballantine D: Sudden death and vigorous exercise: A study of 60 deaths associated with squash. *Br Heart F* 1986; 55:198–203.

33. Fletcher GF, Cantwell JD: *Exercise and Coronary Heart Disease.* Springfield, Ill., Charles C. Thomas Publisher, 1979; p. 168.

34. Haskell W: Cardiovascular complications during medically supervised exercise training of cardiacs. *Circulation* 1975; 51:II–118 (Abstract).

35. Mead WF, Pyfer HR, Trombold JC, et al: Successful resuscitation of two near simultaneous cases of cardiac arrest with a review of 15 cases occurring during supervised exercise. *Circulation* 1976; 53:187–189.

36. Fletcher GF, Cantwell JD: Ventricular fibrillation in a medically supervised cardiac exercise program. *JAMA* 1977; 238:2627–2629.

37. Fletcher GF, Cantwell JD, Watt EW: Oxygen consumption and hemodynamic response of exercises used in training of patients with recent myocardial infarction. *Circulation* 1979; 60:140.

38. Thompson PD, Stern MP, Williams P, et al: Death during jogging or running. *JAMA* 1979; 242:1265–1267.

39. Viitasalo MT, Kala R, Eisalo A, et al: Ventricular arrhythmias during exercise testing, jogging and sedentary life. *Chest* 1979; 76:21–26.

40. Bulletin of President's Council on Physical Fitness and Sports. *Death of Rep. Byron was loss to Physical Fitness Movement.* 1979; p. 11.

41. Magder SA, Linnarsson D, Gullstrand L, et al: Physiological work load of swimming in ischemic heart disease. *Circulation* 59, 60 1979:II–76 (Abstract).

42. Personal communication: Grady Hendrix, M.D., Department of Medicine (Cardiology), Med Univ SC, 1979.

43. Goldschlager N, Cohn K, Goldschlager A: Exercise-related ventricular arrhythmias. *Mod Con Cardiovasc Dis* 1979; 48:67–72.

44. Mark AL, Kioschos JM, Abboud FM, et al: Abnormal vascular re-

sponses to exercise in patients with aortic stenosis. *J Clin Invest* 1973; 52:1138.

45. Sainani GS, Szatkowski J: Rupture of normal aortic valve after physical strain. *Br Heart J* 1969; 31:653–655.
46. Koplan JP: Cardiovascular deaths while running. *JAMA* 1979; 242:2578–2579.
47. Rebuck AS, Read J: Exercise-induced asthma. *Lancet* 1968; 429–431.
48. Mathews KP, Pan PM: Postexercise hyperhistaminemia, dermographia, and wheezing. *Ann Int Med* 1970; 72:241–249.
49. Maulitz RM, Pratt DS, Schocket AL: Exercise-induced anaphylactic reaction to shellfish. *J Allergy Clin Immunnol* 1979; 63:433–434.
50. Buchbinder EM, Bloch KJ, Moss J, Guiney JM: Food-dependent, exercise-induced anaphylaxis. *JAMA* 1983; 250:2973–2974.
51. Lee TH, Nagakura T, Papageorge N, Iikura Y, Kay AB: Exercise-induced late asthmatic reactions with neutrophil chemotactic activity. *N Engl J Med* 1983; 308:1502–1505.
52. Casale TB, Keahey TM, Kaliner M: Exercise-induced anaphylactic syndromes. *JAMA* 1986; 255:2049–2053.
53. Sprung CL: Heat stroke: A modern approach to an ancient disease. *Chest* 1980; 77:461–462.
54. Sutton JR: Heatstroke from running. *JAMA* 1980; 243:1896.
55. Knochel JP, Dotin LN, Hamburger JR: Pathophysiology of intense physical conditioning in a hot climate. I. Mechanisms of potassium depletion. *J Clin Invest* 1972; 51:242–255.
56. Felig P, Johnson C, Levitt M, Cunningham J, Keefe F, Bboglioli B: Hypernatremia induced by maximal exercise. *JAMA* 1982; 248: 1209–1211.
57. Frizzell RT, Lang GF, Lowance DC, Lathan SR: Hyponatremia and ultramarathon running. *JAMA* 1986; 255:772–774.
58. Fogoros RN: Runner's trots. Gastrointestinal disturbances in runners. *JAMA* 1980; 243:1743–1744.
59. Clausen JP: Effect of physical training on cardiovascular adjustments to exercise in man. *Physiol Rev* 1977; 57:779–815.
60. Stewart JG, Ahlquist DA, McGill DB, Ilstrup DM, Schwartz S, Owen RA: Gastrointestinal blood loss and anemia in runners. *Ann Intern Med* 1984; 100:843–845.
61. McMahon LF Jr, Ryan MJ, Larson D, Fisher RL: Occult gastrointestinal blood loss in marathon runners. *Ann Intern Med* 1984; 100:846–847.
62. Blum SF, Sullivan JM, Gardner FH: The exacerbation of hemolysis in paroxysmal nocturnal hemoglobinuria by strenuous exercise. *Blood* 1967; 30:513–517.
63. Fletcher GF, Humphrey WT: Myoglobinuria and strenuous exercise. *JAMA* 1965; 193:77.
64. Poortmans JR: Postexercise proteinuria in humans. *JAMA* 1985; 253:236–240.
65. Tompkins DG: Exercise myopathy of the extensor carpi ulnaris muscle. *J Bone Joint Surg (Am)* 1977; 59:407–408.
66. Lotem M, Fried A, Levy M., et al: Radial palsy following muscular effort. *J Bone Joint Surg (Brit)* 1971; 53:500–506.

67. Harris WF, Bowerman W, McFadden RB, et al: Jogging: An adult exercise program. *JAMA* 1967; 201:759–761.
68. Cohen HL: Jogger's petechiae. *N Engl J Med* 1968; 279:109.
69. Siegel IM: Jogger's heel. *JAMA* 1968; 206:2899.
70. Hunder GG: Harmful effect of jogging. *Ann Intern Med* 1969; 71:664.
71. Lane NE, Bloch DA, Jones HH, Marshall WH, Wood PD, Fries JF: Long-distance running, bone density, and osteoarthritis. *JAMA* 1986; 255:1147–1151.
72. Panush RS, Schmidt C, Caldwell JR, Edwards NL, Longley S, Yonker R, Webster E, Nauman J, Stork J, Pettersson H: Is running associated with degenerative joint disease? *JAMA* 1986; 255:1152–1154.
73. Compton D, Hill PM, Sinclair JD: Weight-lifters' blackout. *Lancet* 1972 (2): 1234–1237.
74. Rochmis P, Blackburn H: Exercise test. *JAMA* 1971; 217:1061–1066.
75. Detry JMR, Mengeot P, Rousseau MF: Maximal exercise testing in variant angina. *Br Heart J* 1976; 38:655–656 (letter).
76. Lintgren AB: Death from myocardial infarction after exercise test with normal result. *JAMA* 1976; 235:837–839.
77. Atterhog JH, Jonsson B, Samuelsson R: Exercise testing: a prospective study of complication rates. *Am Heart J* 1979; 98:572–579.
78. McNiece HF: Legal aspects of exercise testing. *NY State J Med* 1972; 72(2):1822–1824.
79. Stuart RJ, Ellestad MH: National survey of exercise stress testing facilities. *Chest* 1980; 77:94–97.
80. Ellestad MH, Blomqvist CG, Naughton JP: Standards for exercise testing laboratories. *Circulation* 1979; 59:421A.

Recapitulation and Future Implications

The second edition of this book has considered and covered exercise in many specialties and subspecialties of the practice of medicine. Considerable emphasis has been placed on the field of cardiovascular disease and cardiovascular health as this is obviously the subset of medicine in which there is currently more interest and from which most data have been derived.

In addition to the information covered in this book, in the future efforts will be made to address the issues of the elderly with regard to exercise, high- versus low-level exercise (particularly in cardiovascular disease rehabilitation), and more attempts at earlier exercise after cardiac events.

Addressing the elderly is of vast importance in today's society. Life expectancy is greater year by year and, according to many speculations, at or about the year 2000+, 30 percent of our population will be 65 years of age or older. In this population (with regard to exercise), there are often more musculoskeletal problems, more connective tissue problems, and care must be given to address these appropriately. Of course, as one becomes older, the heart rate deceases and maximal oxygen consumption decreases. These changes must be addressed with regard to the exercise prescription and the proper type of training. Research is now being addressed towards this population and will be available in the future.

From: Fletcher GF: *Exercise in the Practice of Medicine,* 2nd Revised Edition. Mount Kisco, NY, Futura Publishing Co., Inc., © 1988.

The particular issue of low- versus high-level exercise after cardiac events has been addressed only in a limited fashion. Some data suggest that perhaps higher levels of exercise impose a better protective effect from the cardiovascular standpoint. However, such studies are not supported by randomized trials and this is most important to consider in the future. Many of these currently mentioned topics will be forthcoming in studies in the literature and will be addressed more in the future.

As this book goes to press, there are many areas of exercise and medicine that have not been covered in detail. It is our hope, however, that this second edition has addressed more in detail the areas that were covered previously and that forthcoming work will be supplementary to this book for the reader audience.

Index